XANDRIA

WILLIAMS

CANCER CONCERNS

A Practical 10-Step Programme

Described and Explained

Xtra Health Publications

Cancer Concerns

by

Xandria Williams

ISBN: 978-0-9568552-0-6

This book is published by Xtra Health Publications in conjunction with Writersworld Limited and is available to order from Internet book retailers, most book shops throughout the United Kingdom, and from the author at xandria@xandriawilliams.co.uk or Tel: 44 (0)20-7824-8153.

Copy edited by Ian Large

Cover design by Simon Potter

Printed and bound by www.printondemand-worldwide.com

www.writersworld.co.uk

WRITERSWORLD
2 Bear Close
Woodstock
Oxfordshire
OX20 1JX
England

The text pages of this book are produced via an independent certification process than ensures the trees from which the paper is produced come from well managed sources that exclude the risk of using illegally logged timber while leaving options to use post-consumer recycled paper as well.

DISCLAIMER

This book is for educational purposes only and is not intended to be prescriptive or to replace appropriate professional diagnosis, guidance and help. The information given in the following pages is for information only and is not intended to replace appropriate medical, naturopathic or other health care advice. In no way should anyone infer that the author claims to treat cancer. The reader is strongly advised, throughout the text, to obtain appropriate professional help for any problems that they may have.

The author and publisher have made every endeavour to ensure the accuracy of the information provided in this book. However, they assume no responsibility for unwitting errors, omissions or inaccuracies. They assume no responsibility for any inaccuracies in the source materials, nor in how that material is used. The text is not intended to be comprehensive, but rather to provide general protocols that the author considers to be of value in the maintenance of homoeostasis.

More research results and evidence become available daily and many new developments may have been reported by the time this book is in print. Feel free to consult the author for further information.

ABOUT THE AUTHOR

Xandria Williams, MSc, DIC, BSc, ARCS, MRSC, ND, DBM, MRN, studied chemistry at Imperial College, London and began her career as a field geochemist involved in mineral and oil exploration, working in a variety of countries in the southern hemisphere. Xandria Williams was in Sydney, Australia when she changed the focus of her career and turned to biochemistry and the study of human metabolism, nutrition, naturopathy and herbal medicine. Later, Xandria Williams studied psychotherapy and related mental and emotional therapies such as neurolinguistic programming (NLP) and the Emotional Freedom Technique (EFT). Xandria Williams has explored and used these and other methods ever since to help people with both physical health problems and emotional issues.

Xandria Williams has been head of the Nutrition and Biochemistry Departments in, and lectured extensively at, several naturopathic, chiropractic and osteopathic colleges in both Australia and London. Xandria Williams has been a guest lecturer at colleges and events in these and other countries, and she continues to give lectures at conferences and seminars to public interest groups and to post-graduate students. Xandria Williams has a lucid and readily comprehensible style of lecturing and writing, even when covering complex topics. Her published works include over 400 articles and 20 books, published in several different languages, on physical and mental health care, and Xandria Williams has appeared frequently on radio and television.

Xandria Williams has evolved her unique and highly effective approach to tackling life's physical and emotional problems over more than three decades of research, writing, teaching and helping patients.

Xandria Williams has been in private practice for thirty years, initially in Sydney, Australia and now in Central London and County Kildare in Ireland. Xandria Williams has always helped people with a wide range of physical and emotional problems, but in recent years she has specialised in cancer and has focused progressively on researching the cancer process, the problems leading to it and how these can be corrected.

This book is the result of her many years as a lecturer, writer and practitioner and, specifically, of her own work with people wanting to prevent, or needing to recover from, cancer.

Xandria Williams sees clients at her clinics in both Central London and County Kildare, Ireland at her **CanSurvive Resource Centres.**

She also works long distance with clients by phone or by Skype.

She can be contacted:

By phone on   (44) 020-7824-8153 (UK) or
              (353) 046-973-1191 (Ireland)

By mobile   (44) 07509-121-303 (voice) or
              (44) 07940-83-66-73 (texts)

By email: xandria@xandriawilliams.co.uk.

Skype address: xandriaw

For more details see her website: www.xandriawilliams.co.uk

XANDRIA'S OTHER BOOKS INCLUDE:

Vital Signs for Cancer   Protect yourself from the onset and recurrence of cancer.

The Herbal Detox Plan   The revolutionary way to cleanse and revive your body.

Liver Detox Plan   The revolutionary way to cleanse and revive your body.

Overcoming Candida   The ultimate cookery guide.

Fatigue   The secrets of getting your energy back.

Living with Allergies   Food intolerances explained with recipes and food alternatives.

You're not Alone   A guide to understanding and overcoming feelings of isolation.

The Four Temperaments   How to achieve love, health and happiness.

From Stress to Success   10 steps to a relaxed and happy life.

Beating the Blues   A guide to avoiding and lifting depression.

Choosing Weight Intentionally   How to lose weight without dieting.

What's in my food?   The nutrient content of foods in relation to their calorie content.

Choosing Health Intentionally   Unlocking your subconscious for a better physical and emotional future.

How to Prevent Osteoporosis Building Stronger Bones Naturally   The osteoporosis diet and exercise plan.

Ideal Weight Ideal Shape

Nutritional Supplements formulated by Xandria Williams:

Liver Support

Adrenomax

Books and supplements are available from Xandria Williams:

By phone on: (44) 020-7824-8153 (UK) or (353) 046-973-1191

By email: xandria@xandriawilliams.co.uk.

The supplements are also available from Nutri Imports on 0-800-212-742 or 44 (0)-1663-718-804.

ACKNOWLEDGEMENTS

All research and development is based and built on the work and research of countless people. It is impossible to list all those who have added immensely to our knowledge of the development of cancer, as outlined in this text, and who have explored, developed and provide the many avenues of support that are now available to people suffering from cancer and who do not want to rely partially, or wholly, on the medical model.

Clearly an immense debt is owed to the specific researchers whose work is discussed in this book, Dr. Otto Warburg, Dr. Waltraut Fryda, Dr. Toru Abo, Dr. John Beard, Dr. Mario Biava, William Kelley and Dr. Johanna Budwig, and to the many others who worked with them.

Huge and heartfelt thanks go to Chris Burley, Naturopathic Physician, for her support both intellectually and practically, her professional suggestions and input, her excellent contributions to the detailed editing of the book, even more so for her warm and deeply valued friendship and finally for her very thoughtful Foreword .

Thanks to Susan Taylor who read and commented on the manuscript from the perspective of the general reader. Thanks to Stuart Gregory for his many hours of help with all matters relating to computers and the Internet.

Thanks are due to Graham Cook of Writersworld for the smooth way in which his company has published this book, at great speed and with great care and efficiency, keeping me informed of every step along the way, and to Ian Large for his meticulous copy editing.

As always, I owe heartfelt thanks to my agent, Sara Menguc, for her ongoing support and her commitment.

This book could not have been written without the indirect contributions of all the wonderful patients with whom it has been my privilege to work over the years, and without a variety of colleagues and patients who have provided sounding boards for my ideas and much valuable feedback.

DEDICATION

From the original Hippocratic Oath:

"I will prescribe regimens for the good of my patients according to my ability and my judgment and ***never do harm*** *to anyone."*

This is commonly translated by many as
"first do no harm".

This book is dedicated to people who are aware of and concerned about the escalating increase in the incidence of cancer over recent years, the limited success that results from drugs, radiation and surgery, and conscious of the significant harm that can be done by these treatments. It is dedicated to those who are keen to explore other options and rational methods of cancer prevention and treatment that are in harmony with their bodies, and who also require a strong evidence base for the benefits of the suggestions made to them.

It is dedicated to all those who recognise the wisdom of their body as a potentially self-maintaining and self-healing entity, provided its nutrient and other needs are met and it is spared the onslaught of avoidable toxins and other damaging agents.

It is dedicated to all people who are working hard to prevent cancer, in themselves and others, by rational and natural means, to people who care for those with cancer and to people who have cancer and are looking to take some personal responsibility for their care and their future, and who have the commitment and discipline to follow through on the many lifestyle changes that are required for the harmonious recovery of optimum health without adverse and toxic side effects.

FOREWORD
by Chris Burley, Naturopathic Physician

Cancer remains a scary word but it has also become 'Big Business'. In fact, the amount of money pumped annually into cancer research – the so-called 'War on Cancer' optimistically championed by successive US presidents – now exceeds six billion dollars a year. Yet, the number of people diagnosed, and tragically dying from cancer, continues to climb ever upwards. Indeed, the World Cancer Report for the World Health Organisation (WHO) suggests an increase by 50%, to 15 million, new cases by the year 2020, up from 10 million in 2002. Thankfully, there have been improvements in the treatment of certain cancers, but these have hardly impacted on the spiralling mortality figures. WHO also informs us that, *"...the most advanced forms of treatment may produce a 5-year survival rate of 75% or more for certain types of cancer, e.g. cancers of the endometrial, breast, testis, and melanoma."* This isn't good. How can it be so low, and why with such few cancers?

Why, with an industry employing two million people involved exclusively in cancer research all over the world, especially in the West, has so little progress been made? Why do we keep hearing about these 'magic bullet' drugs, invariably due out in only three, five or seven years time, which, this time, will definitely be the cure for this or that cancer – even all cancers – and then nothing materialises? The latest wonder drug disappears off the radar and, with it, our hopes as further human trials fail, sometimes at great personal cost to the previously healthy young people who took part. Why does this model of pharmacological medicine continue to let us down?

Could it be, is it just possible, that there is another way of dealing with cancer? Perhaps an even better way, which does not involve smashing the immune system and destroying the very mechanisms within the body designed to defend us from cancer whilst, at the same time, causing painful, exhausting and often life-threatening side effects. Sadly, it is not uncommon for patients to die not from the cancer itself, but from the effects of the very therapy prescribed to cure them – including radiation burns to internal organs, lymphoedema (damaging the immune-helping lymphatic system) plus a range of other destructive consequences. and all this aside from the so-called 'minor' side effects such as constant nausea and vomiting, loss of appetite and inability to eat, hair loss, skin damage, insomnia – even severe depression leading to suicide – to name but some. A sad catalogue indeed, for anyone involved in healing the sick.

Is it not right that we would, and should, spend the earth if it saves the life of a beloved child, partner, relative or friend? It does cost the earth, and yet, for all this costly research and medication, there is a proven overall treatment effectiveness of just 11%[1]. This is an appalling and shocking statistic which takes no account of the enormous cost in non-monetary terms, of the pain, worry and despair suffered by patient and family – often for it all to be repeated if, and often when, the cancer returns. Surely, surely – it must be time to look for another solution?

The time has come to take other options more seriously. Other approaches and treatments that, although not heralded in the press, perhaps surprisingly to some have already helped people recover from cancers, even terminal cancers. These are treatments and protocols that work, even if they're not designed to make people richer, and they work without negative or harmful side effects. Amazingly, such treatments, which do not rely on chemotherapy, radiation and surgery, are effective against cancers of all types, even really tricky ones like pancreatic and brain cancers. They've been found to be effective because they work with the body, not against it, working alongside nature and not with man-made synthetic substances or machines. Quietly, motivated neither by financial gain nor job security, this return to natural, non-harmful medicine has been pioneered by hard-working, 21st-century biochemists, doctors, professors and researchers dedicated to their task.

Nor is any of this new. This 'Other Way', which is similar to and based on 'The Way' of Hippocrates, has stood the test of time throughout the world for thousands of years, unlike the inappropriately named 'conventional', drug-based medicine of the last century or so. Instead, we have natural, metabolic and functional medicines, harnessing the best that nature offers us, and leading to the development of new, highly effective, scientifically-based protocols. Indeed, we frequently hear and read about people's 'miraculous' cures often at the hands of courageous, yet sometimes perceived as maverick, medical scientists and non-mainstream qualified doctors. Thinking outside the box, often whilst being ostracised by their own profession because they've dared to consider another way, these people have found answers as to how to heal the body, using nature's way. But, precisely for this reason, there is little or no money to be made and no commercial incentive to market these therapies because natural substances cannot be patented.

This is what you will read about in this pioneering and exciting book – about methods that have worked for hundreds and thousands of people, many of whom had been declared hopeless cases with terminal cancer, and they work with nature, with the body, gently, yet effectively, supporting its own ability to heal. Even from the brink. To the amazement of their oncologists, these people are still alive, decades later.

Xandria Williams presents us with a foundation protocol on which you can build. She offers past and current research, generally 'gold standard', and explains, in straightforward terms, what underpins the protocols she has suggested, and what makes these therapies work, what biological mechanisms are at play, and suddenly it all makes perfect sense. We can avoid cancer in the first place, but even if we are unlucky, we can still get rid of it. For good.

She doesn't claim it is easy. Although pain-free and practically entirely without adverse side effects, the naturopathic approach is more difficult in many ways. Because, instead of being passive and relying on others, the patient determined to get well needs to be profoundly pro-active. Again, thinking outside the box. It's not enough to keep to one's old lifestyle, indeed, that may well be what caused the problem in the first place. Think about it. One's whole life must be examined and changes made to restore the harmony and balance (homeostasis) the body likes best. In this way, it can work optimally to help the gastrointestinal system absorb what is required to provide the building blocks and enzymes for all forms of renewal and healing. Blood will be at its correct pH, with normal glucose and other values, the endocrine and other systems will be working harmoniously with the immune system, and all body functions will be normalised.

This book shows how you can help with all this, providing insight and information to help the reader understand what needs to be done, whether patient or therapist, and should this book be read when the body seems to have passed the point of recovery, these therapies will still help, easing suffering and ensuring the best possible quality of life even in decline.

Many streams make a river and many natural ways unclog a messed-up body. There is no magic bullet cure for cancer. What we do have, however, are these basic yet scientific, evidence-based nutritional and naturopathic therapies. None of them hurt, none make the hair fall out and none adversely challenge the immune system. But they all nourish the body and allow it to work properly. What is required of course is a major commitment to health and healthy living and it is inevitable, for example, that one's diet will change before this book is finished! But then, living more healthily is exactly what we should all be doing to ensure a longer and more fulfilling life, as well as to avoid or recover from this modern-day scourge we call cancer.

Enjoy learning about different ways of cancer treatments from this book. You will find it informative, educational and inspiring.

Christine Burley B.Sc., ND, MRN
February 2011

TABLE OF CONTENTS

PART 1   INTRODUCTION AND BASIC CONCEPTS

The author's history, personal experience and approach.

Cancer is not a tumour. Cancer is a process, the Cancer Process. Phase One includes all the Predisposing Factors that increase your risk of developing cancer. Phase Two starts with permanent cancer cells. CAM therapies have multiple tools to offer.

An important difference between cancer and other diseases.

Arguably, over 90% of cancers are caused by diet and lifestyle. Being 'at cause' does not necessarily mean being 'at fault'. However, if your chosen lifestyle decisions can cause cancer, altering these decisions gives you the power to make positive and effective changes.

Defining cancer. Cancer is not 'having a tumour'. Cancer is being in Phase Two of the Cancer Process. Early testing. Biopsy-defined cancer. Cancer defined by early chemical changes indicating the earliest appearance of cancer cells.

PART 2   CAUSES AND ORIGIN OF CANCER

Trophoblast cells in the placenta are exactly the same as cancer cells. Cancer develops from stem cells. Cancer is not controlled when the pancreas output of enzymes is inadequate.

Cancer is not caused by genetic mutations and changes in the nucleus. Cancer is not caused by healthy adult differentiated cells suddenly changing behaviour abnormally. Cancer is caused by adult stem cells that behave aberrantly and grow out of control.

William Kelley's story. The use of pancreatic enzymes in breaking down tumour masses. Kelley's protocol, building on the previous chapters.

The need for essential fatty acids to restore cell membrane function and increase cellular uptake of oxygen.

Few cancers are entirely genetic. You can modify the activity of your genes by any lifestyle changes you may choose to make.

The Anthroposophical Approach and other mind-body connections.

Recap on the theories. Their synthesis into a coherent view of the development of cancer and the resulting logic behind an integrated approach to recovery.

<u>APPENDICES</u>

PART 1

INTRODUCTION and
BASIC CONCEPTS

CHAPTER 1

SYNOPSIS AND OVERVIEW

Synopsis

This is the second book of a series of linked books describing and explaining a logical and structured approach to the management of, and recovery from, cancer. This approach is based on an understanding of the origin of cancer that goes back over 150 years and has been supported and enhanced by a large number of eminent scientists and practitioners over the intervening decades. It is a biochemically-based approach to the use of complementary and alternative therapies, founded on recent and current research and clinical experience.

The overarching concept is that cancer is not merely the presence of a tumour. It is a process, the Cancer Process, the end result of which is the tumour. The Cancer Process starts many years before permanent cancer cells are present or a tumour is detected. The process is divided into two phases. Phase One includes the Predisposing Factors that, if not corrected, can lead up to the presence of permanent cancer cells. This phase, and prevention strategies, are discussed in detail in the previous book *'Vital Signs for Cancer'*. In this book, *'Cancer Concerns'*, the focus is on Phase Two. This phase starts once cancer cells, which are known to be formed and destroyed by the immune system daily, have somehow been allowed to survive and begin the process of building what will eventually become a detectable tumour. There are explanations of what is happening, how the various processes can be detected and what can be done to reverse the adverse changes, even before the detectable tumour has formed. This focus on the cause of cancer and the reasons for its development lays the foundation for a much more effective health care programme than is achieved by waiting for a tumour to form and then trying to remove or destroy it without addressing its cause.

How can cancer be feared if:

(a) there are tests you can do to make sure you are not heading in the direction of cancer, and strategies you can employ to reverse this pattern if it is detected;

(b) there is an early detection test that can warn you of the start of the development of cancer cells within a few weeks of their formation and up to as many as ten years before there is a detectable tumour;

(c) there are strategies you can employ to eliminate these cancer cells, if found, and reverse the process;

(d) there are additional lifestyle changes, protocols, supplements and remedies you can employ, building on the above, to aid your recovery if you already have a tumour;

(e) there are tests you can do to determine the detailed nature of your cancer cells and to help you select the most effective remedies and tools to correct your health and inhibit or destroy the cancer cells?

Early detection is your best safeguard. I hear so many patients say they do not want to do the early warning test, they fear cancer, and do not want to know if they do have it. This would, perhaps, be acceptable if there was nothing you could do to help yourself. But there is now a multiplicity of strategies you can adopt and, as described in this book, they build into a unified coherent whole once you have a basic understanding of the way cancers develop, wherever the tumour is finally located.

We are a long way toward the solution of cancer, but do not underestimate the disease. Do not be fooled by claims that you can *"cure cancer in 10 days with this simple remedy"* or *"drink your way out of cancer"* or *"11 easy steps to a cancer cure"* or *"burn cancer out of your body with this simple treatment"*. Cancer is a whole-body problem, not a local one, and, as such, the recovery has to involve your whole body and lifestyle. Recovering from cancer does require some effort and discipline on your part, yet people have accomplished this, and because it does involve your lifestyle, you have the power to make many positive changes yourself, you need not be at the mindless mercy of unknown drugs and machines with little or no idea of what is being done to you.

A few CAM (Complimentary, Alternative and Metabolic) therapists have incorporated at least some of these ideas into their practices over the past several decades. Their numbers are growing, though slowly. Those that do so are achieving convincing and positive outcomes, and doing so without toxic side effects or harm to the individual. Unfortunately, many such practitioners, in a number of countries, have been energetically attacked by modern medicine and its supporting industries, both legally and politically, to the serious detriment of all cancer sufferers. Fortunately, many of the strategies appropriate to these concepts can be practiced by you, the individual, on your own. The rest, once you know about them, you can discuss with an open-minded practitioner.

The aim, here, has been to bring together the various streams of research in a logical and integrated way. This leads to the basis of a sound and safe strategy for optimising general health and restoring homoeostasis. Each individual can then, in consultation with their practitioner, add the various supplements and therapies that seem appropriate to their particular cancer and situation. Large parts of this strategy can also be used, with great benefit, for prevention.

Many routes lead to the summit of Mount Everest, but eventually they must all come together. In this book I have endeavoured to show how the many concepts discussed can be brought together to form a coherent whole. The ease with which this can be accomplished supports the correctness of the component concepts.

The ideas expressed here also lead to, or suggest, many areas of development and research that could successfully convert cancer from being most people's worst health fear, to it being a chronic disease that could be generally avoided or, at the worst, managed in a similar manner to diabetes.

Overview

The first book, *'Vital Signs for Cancer'* is directed at the prevention of cancer, both the prevention of the process leading to a primary tumour and the prevention of a recurrence if you have once been declared in remission. In the nature of CAM (Complementary, Alternative and Metabolic) therapies, what is useful in prevention is frequently also useful in a recovery programme since the aim is to restore health, not attack or suppress disease.

In this second book the focus is on cancer itself. A coherent thesis is presented as to the way in which cancer develops. This leads on to general suggestions for the restoration of good health at all levels, from the body's basic chemistry, through cellular functions to overall metabolism. This then becomes the foundation for subsequent optimising strategies and a recovery programme you can create with the help of your supportive health care practitioner.

There is so much known, now, about the causes (as described here) and the prevention (as described in *'Vital Signs for Cancer'*) that cancer need no longer be the feared disease that many people feel it to be.

In Part One of this book you will find a brief look at some of the basic concepts behind this approach to cancer prevention. These same topics also form the foundation of a recovery programme. In Part Two you will learn about the causes and origin of cancer and of several key individuals who have contributed, over the past century (or more) to this comprehensive view. It is noteworthy that, although these views cover over a hundred years, they all build into a uniform, rational and simple theory and they all lead on to the same approach to a recovery programme.

Some chapters in Part Two are biographical and conceptual, and as such are relatively easy to read. Some are, necessarily, more technical and complex. I apologise for this and have tried to simplify things where I can. It would be easy to write a much more simplified book without the underlying biochemistry or the references to published research. However, cancer is a major disease and a serious business. It is my experience that many people who chose to 'step outside the box', people who do not wish to follow blindly the MDS (Medical, Drug, Surgery) route in relation to cancer, but who choose a CAM approach to the management of their health want to know the reasons that lie behind the advice they are being given. They are often highly motivated, intelligent, and keen to learn all they can. I have been struck by the depth of knowledge or reading evidenced by some of the questions I am asked in my practice. If you can follow all the discussions in the following pages well and good, if not, then skip the difficult bits. Even so, it is often comforting to know that there is a solid basis for the actions that you may decide to take. For many people, knowing that there is sound biochemistry underpinning the sometimes onerous lifestyle changes they are advised to make, may make it easier to follow and stick to these guidelines.

The first few chapters start with an explanation of the way your cells obtain energy. This understanding is helpful as a basis for what is to follow. Then we consider the various suggestions as to the causes of cancer. Dr. Warburg believes it is due to a lack of oxygen at the cellular level and that this results, among other things, from a lack of essential vitamins and minerals and from the presence of toxins. Dr. Fryda believes that cancer is due to stress and adrenal exhaustion, and that this in turn leads to a lack of cellular oxygen, as well as to other problems that have to be considered. A lack of oxygen is closely associated with mitochondrial damage. Dr. Abo also postulates that stress is a fundamental cause but focuses on the detrimental effect this has on the immune system.

The next few chapters focus on why, once certain cells have turned into cancer cells, they are not destroyed before they can develop further. Here it is time to go back over a century to the work of Dr. John Beard who relates cancer cells to the cells of the placenta. Two powerful concepts develop from this hypothesis. One is the role of the pancreas in prevention and recovery and the other is a test, built around the level of a hormone, HCG (Human Chorionic Gonadotropin). If you are not pregnant, then the presence of even the smallest amount of this hormone can indicate the start of the development of cancer cells. This test can indicate the start of cancer development many years before a tumour could possibly be large enough to detect. This then allows for an effective prevention programme to be put in place and the development of a full tumour to be avoided. This is also the time to explore several well-founded and well-evidenced approaches to recovery, based on the preceding concepts and following on from their further development.

Most of the ideas in Part Two can be tested and verified by readily available blood, urine and saliva tests.

A later book in the series will deal with the mental and emotional issues that lie behind the development of health problems, including cancer, and the resulting changes that can be made to resolve these issues as part of the therapy. However, it is appropriate that brief mention of these concepts is also made here.

In Part Three it is time to put these concepts into practice. Based on the solid foundation that has been developed to this point, a fundamental optimising strategy for the recovery of health can be established. This incorporates the need for improving the diet, alkalising the body, adding nutrients that may have been lacking in the past, and the removal of toxins. It is also important to address and remove any of the Predisposing Factors that are present, which are described and identified in *'Vital Signs for Cancer'*. A vital part of the strategy is to include the use of supplemental pancreatic enzymes, stress management and improving the function of the immune system, and all of this is based on many decades of successful clinical experience by many experienced practitioners.

The final programme, listed at the end, can form the basis for health recovery, whatever therapy path you decide to follow, as you and your health care team build your treatment programme. It can be the basis of your supplement and remedy programme if you choose to follow the CAM path. It can also improve your health and help in aiding your recovery if you choose to follow the MDS path. It lays the foundation for the application of some of the several hundred available therapeutic agents that are available and which your practitioner may suggest for you. The selection of these remedies, the ones that are uniquely appropriate for you, should be based on the results of the tests that can be done to indicate which ones are most needed. These tests, over the months ahead, will also indicate the progress that is being made and what adjustments may be necessary.

If you read this book through, from cover to cover, you will come across things you have already read. This repetition is intentional. Firstly, with so many new ideas, and with ideas and concepts that are particularly important, it is worthwhile to stress them. Secondly, you, or some other reader, may be dipping into the book at random, thus may not have read the earlier explanation for certain concepts.

CHAPTER 2

TRAINING AND PHILOSOPHY

I have always been a scientist, both by instinct and by training. I favoured arithmetic, maths, science, chemistry and biochemistry, in that progression, as I moved through eleven schools, two universities and one naturopathic college. It has never made sense to me to endeavour to try to heal the body by applying toxic drugs, be they aspirins or cancer chemotherapy agents.

To me it seemed much more logical to start from the assumptions that the body was inherently healthy and self-correcting, that ill health occurred because the body had either not been given all the nutrients it needed, or that it was poisoned or over-stressed in some way. The first step to health, therefore, had to be to correct both of these issues.

I have always been willing to think 'outside the box', on the basis of erecting and then testing any new hypothesis. This is the only way truly new ideas can bear fruit. However, I have also always wanted evidence-based proof or confirmation of the ideas put forward. This is why you will find over 400 references to technical papers at the end of this book. The ideas given in the following pages will be new to many readers, may be argued against by some and need the security of the tests and studies on which they are based.

Over the past several decades, as I have researched these ideas, particularly but not exclusively, in relation to cancer, one thing has become abundantly clear. On the one hand, there is a large body of medical, scientific, physiological, biochemical, nutritional and related research that has been done in relation to a wide variety of nutrients, diets and other therapies, generally now thought of as falling within the CAM field. Most of this has been written up in conventional peer-review literature, as will be obvious from the list of references at the end of the book. On the other hand, there are the clinical doctors, working at the 'coal face'. These appear to focus largely on what they are told by the various drug companies, and the purveyors of tests and physical treatments such as radiation, in the case of cancer, and by their professors and peers who have been similarly informed. There appears to be an immense wall between the two groups and never (or rarely) the twain shall meet. Those in clinical practice are frequently warned, at the risk of losing their medical licence, against applying any therapy that is not 'standard medical practice'; those in research have little contact with patients and the daily clinical application.

It is the aim here to try, at least in some small way, to help to bridge this gap. At least it is hoped that this book will help the people in need and will provide some of the tools and resources that will enable you to bridge the gap.

In this regard the Internet has become an invaluable resource. It has enabled anyone to put words into a search engine and be lead directly to appropriate and useful information. For instance, putting in the word 'cancer' and the name of any herb will lead you to a mine of information on many different and useful herbs, along with reasons why they are helpful and the results that have been achieved by their use. The same is true of using a food or nutrient and the word 'cancer'. The downside of this is not the paucity of information, but the often seemingly overwhelming abundance of information. This topic will be covered in a following book. Fortunately, many tests are now available that can help to target the remedies and supplements that are most relevant to your particular situation. There are, for instance, over 500 references in the research literature, as quoted by PUBMED[1] as to the benefits of curcumin in relation to cancer; there are many more that are quoted in other journals. However, it is almost unheard of for a doctor or oncologist to recommend this helpful yet harmless supplement to their patients.

This is clearly a vast and complex topic and if you have cancer, or are interested in making sure you do not develop cancer, I strongly recommend that your find yourself a suitably informed practitioner who is experienced in this field. They can then help you to find your way through this abundance of information and develop your own particular prevention or recovery programme. However, knowledge is power, and the more you can learn about the whole topic the better your outcome is likely to be. This is in part because you will better understand what is

---

[1] PUBMED, a service of the U.S. National Library of Medicine

being asked of you in the way of lifestyle changes and the taking of what may seem like just too many remedies. It is also because this knowledge can help to allay many anxieties, reduce stress and thus improve health in general. Finally, having a firm knowledge basis for what you are doing will help you when you are in discussions with the people who care about you but may have very different ideas as to what you should be doing.

If you have cancer and want to beat it with all the tools at your disposal, you have a lot of learning to do. Ultimately, the only person that can heal you is you. It is you that will either do or not do all that you are advised to do by whatever practitioner(s) you choose. It is you who will, or will not, follow the suggestions you receive from books, articles and the Internet. It is you and your own mental attitude that will have a major impact on the outcome, and for you to be successful you need to know as much as you are able to digest and utilise. It is my aim to help you in this process.

Disclaimer

I make no claim here to be defining a treatment or recovery programme for you to follow if you have cancer or any other health problem. Cancer is much too serious and complex a problem for you to deal with on your own, or simply with the help of a book. You are strongly advised to find a competent and appropriately qualified therapist in whom you have confidence and with whom you can work. The intention here is to provide you with an understanding of some of the fundamental concepts concerning cancer that underpin the CAM approach. When you know what is available, you are then in a position to look for a practitioner who can provide the support you want, and you will also be able to understand the reasons behind what they are advising you to do.

The aim here is to empower you, just at a time when many people feel most disempowered. Once diagnosed with cancer many people feel totally helpless. This is aggravated by the fact that many doctors will say there is nothing you can do for yourself. They may say that your diet doesn't matter, that there is nothing you can contribute to your recovery, that you should simply follow their instructions and then get on with the rest of your life, such as it is and as best as you can. This won't do. We know that the more positive you feel and the more actively you are involved the greater is your chance of recovery[2]. Numerous books and case reports attest to this[3].

CHAPTER 3

THE CANCER PROCESS

Other than blood and similar cancers, the medical profession generally regards cancer as being defined by the presence of a tumour or by a biopsy-identified mass of cancerous tissue. If you have a tumour that contains cancerous cells you have cancer. If you have no tumour, or no tumour that contains cancerous cells, you do not have cancer. Thus, all the medical efforts are based on detecting the presence of a tumour. Once found, the treatment is almost totally targeted on the tumour to (a) eliminate it and (b) stop its regrowth or its re-establishment either locally or elsewhere in your body.

From a CAM perspective, cancer is a process. The tumour is the end point of an extensive process, a complex sequence of biochemical and physiological activities. These can have been going on within your body for many years before there is any sign of a tumour. Phase One of this Cancer Process includes all the various small, and perhaps not so small, steps that have lead you up to the point where some cells turn cancerous and are not eliminated by your defences, but are permitted to remain and to multiply.

The way to deal with the activities of Phase Two, once cancer is established, is not to focus on a full frontal attack on the tumour. Destroying the tumour is not enough. If that is all you do you have failed to destroy or divert the activities that have been leading to its creation in the first place, and so you have done nothing to prevent a recurrence. It is more important to learn about the way in which the tumour has developed and to aim to reverse this process.

This is achieved by a two-pronged approach. It is important to remove the Predisposing Factors. It is also necessary to change the cancer biochemistry, the altered chemistry that is taking place in the cells that have turned cancerous. The aim should be to achieve this reversal by using lifestyle practices, compounds and remedies that support your body in its aim to restore itself to health, something of which it is eminently capable, if you will only provide it with all the tools that it needs and remove all the toxins that are harming it. It cannot be done, constructively or long term, with drugs that have harmful toxic effects on healthy cells, as well as on cancer cells, or by methods that damage your immune system, your endocrine or hormonal system, your nervous system, or that load your body with toxins and challenge your overburdened liver.

Anecdotally, there are individuals who will tell you that they had radiation and/or chemotherapy and that they survived and are cancer-free. Perhaps they would have been cancer-free anyway, perhaps it is more luck than judgement that they survived the ravages of radiation and chemotherapy. Individual anecdotal stories neither prove nor disprove either the medical or the CAM practices. We need to, and will, go further than that as we progress through this book.

You will also find references to 'optimising strategies' or 'recovery protocols' where you might expect to find the word 'treatments'. This is done partly to avoid making claims, actions which are frowned upon, particularly in relation to cancer. However, and very much more importantly, it is done to emphasise the fact that what CAM practitioners do is *not* treat a health problem. This cannot be emphasised enough as it affects the total way that you approach your own health care. What good CAM therapists *do* is focus on restoring the full health to the individual, from the molecular and cellular level up to the whole body and person. Thus, they are helping the individual to optimise their health and bring it to the best possible state it can achieve, given their age and present circumstances, and, as far as possible, to recover whatever health they have lost. The focus is entirely on supporting the individual in such a way that it can restore itself to, and rediscover, optimal healthy function. This is one of the reasons why, for instance, I have personally done every protocol I have ever recommended to my patients. Everything that will help them to restore their health will also help them and others to prevent disease. This is true of the CAM approach to health care in general, including its approach to people who have cancer. This is very much more than verbal pedantry, it is a fundamental difference between the medical approach and the CAM approach.

If you are concerned about preventing or recovering from cancer and looking for an appropriate CAM practitioner you may be surprised to find how difficult your search can become. That is because, in the UK, no one is allowed to claim or advertise that they treat cancer (British Cancer Act of 1939, plus developing legislation from European authorities) and advertisements or listings to this effect are banned.

If you are looking for such a practitioner and want a way to assess the extent to which they can help you, then check them out against this book. Make sure that they understand the concepts discussed here and recognise their relevance to the Cancer Process. There is a resource list in the Appendices.

Phase Two of the Cancer Process starts once persistent, transformed, mutated or cancer cells are present. There are many aspects to this phase and we will be discussing some of them in the chapters ahead.

This Phase Two includes, but is not limited to the following:

- **The development of cancer cells.** We will be exploring some of the suggestions as to what turns healthy cells into cancer cells. It is helpful to consider both the triggers that set the process off, and the mechanisms by which this occurs, and what facilitates this mechanism. Only by fully understanding the mechanism by which cancer comes about can we develop a fully effective recovery programme. Simply destroying the tumour is not sufficient to restore full health and prevent a recurrence.

- **Angiogenesis.** Clusters of cells need a blood supply to bring them oxygen and nourishment and to carry away their waste products. This process, known as angiogenesis, is needed for wound healing, tissue growth and for repair. This process is triggered by compounds such as Vascular Endothelial Growth Factor (VEGF). It is kept under control by another compound called Protein Kinase G (PKG) which inhibits a protein called beta-catenin that, if not inhibited, would continue to stimulate angiogenesis. It has been shown that cells with little or no PKG grow hard, aggressive and invasive tumours. Metastatic colon cancer cells, inoculated with PKG and then placed in mice who lacked an immune system produced soft, non-invasive tumours that readily fell apart. Possibly because of their own lack of angiogenesis, these soft tumours were clustered around existing blood vessels[4].

Cancer cells and growing tumours are no exception, they too need a readily accessible blood supply. In addition, they need this vascular system to facilitate the dispersal and spread of cancer cells to new (metastatic) sites. Tumours cannot grow any larger than approximately 1-2cu mm[5], and cannot metastasise without their own blood supply. It has been known for several decades that tumour cells produce an angiogenic diffusible factor that stimulates aberrant angiogenesis to fulfil their own needs[6]. A component of a successful recovery protocol should be focused at monitoring and controlling angiogenesis.

- **Apoptosis**. When healthy cells become old or damaged they are programmed to self-repair. If this fails they are programmed to self-destruct, a process known as apoptosis or voluntary suicide. Both processes are mediated by a tumour suppressor protein called p53. When cancer cells form there should be an appropriate increase in the level and activity of normal p53[7]. If the gene producing this is mutated and produces mutated p53 instead, as can happen in cancer, then apoptosis is not adequately triggered and the faulty cells are free to multiply endlessly. Apoptosis also depends on various activities within the mitochondria in the cells. Tests can indicate whether or not there is correct apoptosis; if it is not happening for you, it needs to be encouraged.

- **Metastasis.** A confined tumour is rarely life threatening, unless its space-occupying qualities are interfering with other bodily functions. Cancer becomes extremely dangerous once cancer cells move from the primary tumour and invade a new site, a process known as metastasising. Even the original tumour has to invade the tissue in which it is located. The invasion of cancer cells into areas of healthy cells depends on the health, the structure and the function of the extra-cellular matrix, the general material around the cells of your organs and tissues and the way they either do or do not hold together. As transport of the breakaway cancer cells is essential for metastases to occur, it is likely that angiogenic inhibitors can reduce the risk of this happening.

- **Protection of cancer cells.** From the start of the first formation of a cancer cell, it, and its subsequent progeny, face a hostile environment. Powerful though you may think cancer cells are, they are vulnerable to the full force of all your protective mechanisms. When they are first formed they are vulnerable to these mechanisms and are usually killed. In fact, it is estimated that we all develop cancer cells frequently, possibly on an almost daily basis, but that these cells are destroyed. When your health deteriorates, when the various Predisposing Factors become too much, then cancer cells can survive. They are able to attack your weakened defences in a variety of ways, one of which is to build up their defensive walls, such as by building a protective protein coating. If such a defence occurs, it can render cells resistant to both medical drugs and CAM remedies. The cells become MDR cells or medically drug resistant cells. The first focus must then be on removing this protective defence of the cancer cells.

Inevitably there is more, the devil is in the detail, and we will be discussing other contributing factors as we proceed through the following pages. This is all useful theoretical information, but the important outcome of this understanding is to learn more about any individual case of cancer and how it can best be overcome.

TESTS

Fortunately there are tests that can help us. There is one important set of tests, called the CA Profile[2] that indicates the presence of cancer cells, long before a tumour has formed. This gives us an enormous head start in relation to recovery. If you can both detect and start to eliminate cancer cells before there are even sufficient of them to form a detectable tumour, success is a lot more likely than if you wait until there is a tumour of significant size. This test can also be used to monitor your progress. If you do detect the early signs of cancer, and if you then adopt the healing strategies suggested in later chapters, you can then repeat the test. If this has improved you will know you are probably on the right track. If the results have not improved, or have got worse, you will know that further intervention is needed. The test is also useful to monitor the success of

---

[2] Test done by American Metabolic Laboratories. See www.caprofile,net for more details.

the Big Three of the MDS system, of surgery, chemotherapy and radiation. As you will discover, if your medical team think they have 'got it all', the results of this test should return to normal within six to eight weeks of the final anticipated beneficial effects of your treatment. If the results are not normal, then it is unlikely that they did 'get it all', and you almost certainly do still have more work to do to recover your health.

It is time to start. You may be reading this book simply because you are curious. However, it is more likely that you are reading this book either because you are concerned about cancer and want to do all you can to avoid it, or because you already have cancer. You may be reading it on your own behalf or because of people you care about, and the same two options exist.

1. If your aim is to prevent cancer:

(a) read *'Vital Signs for Cancer'*;
(b) correct any obvious lifestyle factors that could be increasing your risk;
(c) test for all the Predisposing Factors described in that book, particularly those that you may feel are particularly relevant to you;
(d) correct any errors that are found;
(e) finally, and possibly the most difficult, maintain all these positive changes and good resolutions, indefinitely.

2. If you are worried that you might have cancer:

(a) Follow steps (a) to (e) above. A solid recovery programme can only be based on the solid foundation of eliminating all the Predisposing Factors. You cannot repair an unstable building simply by adding ever stronger cement to fill in the cracks in the walls or papering them over. You have to ensure the foundations are sound. It is the same with cancer.
(b) Do the CA Profile test. This test is more fully discussed in Chapter14. It comprises eight tests including three for various segments of HCG (human chorionic gonadotropin) a hormone produced, with only very minor exceptions, either during pregnancy or by cancer cells. The next most important component of the Profile

is a test for PHI (phosphohexose isomerase). This provides an indication of the level of anaerobic activity within your cells, and increased anaerobic activity is suggestive of cancerous activity. The HCG hormone is thought by many to provide the best, first early warning sign of cancer. It can be detected as early as six weeks after the start of the development of a cancerous tumour (E.K. Schandl, American Metabolic Laboratories, pers. comm.). Your level of PHI not only provides indications as to your cellular use of oxygen, but can help to indicate useful optimising approaches when planning your recovery.

(c) If your HCG test results are normal, it is unlikely (though not impossible, few test are 100% infallible) that you have cancer and you can focus on prevention and the avoidance of Predisposing Factors to avoid the development of a possible cancer in the future.

(d) If your HCG test results are high, proceed as for (3) below, working on the assumption that you have some permanent cancerous or precancerous rogue cells, even if you have no detectable tumour.

3. If you have cancer, or if the results of your CA Profile suggest this:

(a) As in step 1 above, test for all the Predisposing Factors and correct any errors that are found until all your tests are normal.

(b) Apply the appropriate protocols based on the information in the following chapters, and as advised by your CAM practitioner, for they remain the foundation of good health. You can, if you choose, combine these with medical treatments.

(c) Continue with the strategies in (b) until all test results are back to normal.

(d) Continue with the strategies in (b) for another six months, doing regular testing throughout. During this time all test results should remain normal. If they do not, then reassess your protocol as in (a) and (b).

(e) Reduce your protocol slowly, doing repeat tests to make sure there is no relapse. Repeating the test every two or three months is suggested.

(f) Continue to test, possibly once or twice a year, and make sure there is no return of any indications either of cancer or any of the Predisposing Factors.

4. If you have had cancer but have been told you are now in remission:

(a) As in step 1 above, test for all the Predisposing Factors and correct any errors that are found.

(b) Do the CA Profile test for the three HCG levels described above.

(c) If the CA Profile shows raised levels of HCG, 'they' did not 'get it all', whatever treatment was applied. Move on to (d) below.

(d) Test for the characteristics of cancer cells.

(e) If any abnormalities are found in either (b) or (d) you may be technically in remission at the macro level, but are not in remission at the cellular level, revert to (3) above, and continue.

Cancer gives few warning signs

Many people with cancer can be heard to say, *"But I felt so well. I didn't realise anything was wrong. In fact I still feel well. There is just this lump, or unexpected bleed, or faulty blood test result. How can I have cancer when I feel fine?"* It is just because this is possible that you should consider the various aspects of Phase One of the Cancer Process and test for and correct any Predisposing Factors.

The other often heard type of common comment is, *"But I've never been ill.", "I don't get ill.", "Even if I get a cold or the flu I don't get a temperature."* Having the flu but not getting a raised temperature should, in fact, be recognised as an early warning sign that your immune system, far from being in control of things, is not responding adequately when faced with the flu virus, or any other type of virus or bacteria.

This is why it is so important to test for, and eradicate, Predisposing Factors.

Cancer may be a surprise

There is a very real probability that finding you have cancer has come as a surprise. It does for most people. What do you do now? You are probably in a state of shock. Many people think about avoiding heart disease, or diabetes, or arthritis or a host of other diseases or problems and what they would have to do in such an eventuality. Once such a problem is diagnosed they already have a head start, they have some idea as to what to do, even if they don't always do it. Fewer people have any idea as to what they can do for themselves if they are diagnosed with cancer.

I have known people refuse to do the CA Profile because they are afraid of the result, certain that a cancer diagnosis is a death sentence and unaware of the possibilities of limiting or reversing the process.

You may have read little, and know less, about helping yourself when faced with cancer. Perhaps, because the conventional treatment is so awful and the prognosis so poor, you too have found it more comfortable to ignore the topic of cancer altogether and hope it will not happen to you. The general instructions for prevention or self-help issued by the medical profession usually revolve round the somewhat hazy concept that about two thirds of cancers are diet and lifestyle related. Yet in practical terms no one pays much attention to this or tells you exactly how to improve your diet and lifestyle. Certainly the typical hospital diet, even if you have cancer, will do more to encourage the problem than to help resolve it. There is generally even less useful advice as to positive lifestyle changes, other than to exercise and reduce stress. Even then, relatively few useful details are generally provided.

All this means that you may be unaware of the extensive arsenal of CAM remedies, supplements and management options that are available and have proved to be beneficial in the fight against cancer. There are hundreds of them, and their number increases yearly as we learn more. Once you start to explore what is available you are more likely to become overwhelmed by the huge amount of information accessible to you, and the number of remedies you can choose from and purchase, than be concerned about your lack of choice. One of the aims of this book is to help you sort through this overload of information. As you learn more you should be able to select the remedies that will be most useful for you and to cut them down to a manageable protocol. If you are working with a CAM practitioner, and I strongly suggest that you should be, then the knowledge you have gleaned here will help you to understand the reasons behind the suggestions they are making to you.

A diagnosis of cancer may have come as a shock; it may have left you feeling helpless or overwhelmed, perhaps pole-axed into immobility. However, the moment to take action is now. The decisions you make, right at the start, can often have the most profound effect on the outcome. If you have been diagnosed with cancer, or if you have reason to think you may have cancer, you have some serious decisions to make, and, if you have a firm diagnosis, then you have to make them fast. Equally, this is not the time to rush into actions that may be irreversible. Surgery for tumour removal is not reversible. Biopsies, and their possible consequences, are not reversible. The damaging effects of chemotherapy and radiation are not reversible.

Remember, cancer, in the form of a tumour, does not suddenly appear overnight, even though the fully formed tumour may be your first warning or experience of it. Put simply, cancer starts when a single cell behaves incorrectly, with the characteristics we label as being 'cancerous', and is not destroyed by the normal mechanisms of your immune system and apoptosis. This cancerous cell then divides and multiplies. Over time the number of these cells increases, their chemistry changes, and they come together in a growing mass. Eventually, possibly several years later, this growing mass, stimulated or encouraged by a number of factors along the way, such as the various Predisposing Factors listed later, will develop into a full blown tumour. Eventually a detectable tumour may be felt, discomfort or bleeding may occur, or there may be an alert in the form of a raised blood marker such as a raised PSA (prostate specific antigen marker used to detect and monitor prostate cancer) or an increased level of alkaline phosphatase (a marker for bone and liver cancer for example), when blood tests are run, possibly for some other reason.

Yesterday you had no idea you had cancer. Today you know you have cancer. You might not have discovered it for another week, a month or more. Give yourself this time, or more or less, however long it takes, to research your options. You will know about the medical ones. It generally takes longer to discover the CAM options, yet they can be just as powerful as many studies and case histories have shown. Many people have, for instance, the belief that they cannot afford to take the risk of not having chemotherapy. Yet a well-researched Australian study has shown that cytotoxic chemotherapy increases five-year survival by no more than 2.1 per cent (USA) to 2.3 per cent (Australia); and this is a treatment that is generally accompanied by much more frequent and horrendous toxic side effects.[8]

Finally, many people who have decided to embrace CAM therapies, or incorporate them into whatever else they decide to do, quickly become very well informed on the subject. Thus I have aimed this book at the intelligent reader with some prior knowledge. Equally, I have tried to do this in such a way that even with no prior knowledge you can, hopefully, understand the explanations. If you find some parts difficult to understand, I apologise, but you will at least know what sort of questions to ask your practitioner. You will also know that there is a sound biochemical and physiological basis of what you are being advised to do. This is even true of the majority of the emotional material that is discussed, much of which is also based on experience with people who have had cancer.

CHAPTER 4

CANCER CELLS

In some respects cancer can be considered to be a collection of two hundred or more diseases, based essentially, but not entirely, on their location. It can equally be thought of as a single disease with many faces. The common feature of cancer is the nature of the individual cells.

In other health problems it is the tissue, the organ or the whole system that is the problem. In heart disease it is the heart itself that is malfunctioning, even though the heart cells are still trying to function as heart cells. In coronary artery disease there are problems with the structure and function of the arteries, even though the cells of the artery walls are still trying to function as normal artery wall cells. In kidney disease it is the kidney itself that is the problem, it is not that individual cells of the kidney have gone haywire and started to behave like a different type of cell. In arthritis it is the tissues of the bones and joints that are damaged, the individual cells are still trying to behave normally. In asthma it is the muscles of the bronchial tubes that are failing to relax appropriately, the muscles are still acting as muscle cells, and so on.

As a result, you treat heart problems with herbs and nutrients that support and help heart function, artery problems with diet and nutrients that help support healthy artery walls. If you have kidney problems, there are herbs that help to support kidney function, in arthritis there are dietary considerations that help, and in asthma there are minerals that help the muscles to relax. The story is somewhat similar even if you use medical drugs, your doctor would use drugs aimed at improving the function of the organ involved..

The focus is different if you have cancer. You do not, for instance, treat lung cancer with herbal remedies that help to improve lung function, or treat stomach cancer with nutrients that improve the digestion that normally occurs in the stomach. You may treat colon cancer with therapies designed to improve elimination via the colon and remove toxins, but no more so that you would if the cancer was in the breast, prostate or anywhere else in your body. Similarly, you do not treat ovarian cancer with remedies designed to improve ovary production.

It is not the function of the tissue in which the tumour is located that is faulty, it is the changed chemistry of the cells, and in general this chemical change is similar no matter where the cells are located. From this perspective it makes sense to treat almost all cancers as fundamentally one disease, with possible minor variations to the fine-tuning of the therapy. You may, for instance, add prostate herbs such as saw palmetto when treating prostate cancer or change the texture of the diet if you are dealing with partially obstructive stomach or colon cancer. By and large, however, the focus of a successful recovery programme should be to change the fundamental chemistry that is unique to cancer cells in general, wherever they occur in your body, and that does not occur in healthy cells.

When you are dealing with cancer it is individual cells that are faulty rather than the organ or tissue in which they reside. Eventually, of course, the tumour may damage local tissues or organs, but the tumour itself is not generally a functioning part of the tissue on or in which it resides. It is not, for instance, a failure of some aspect of liver function that leads to a liver tumour. The tumour is a cluster of cells that are behaving abnormally and are growing, invading and distorting the tissue in which they are located. These cells may have started out as healthy liver, breast, prostate, colon, pancreatic or lung cells, and then have changed their chemistry radically and in a way that is, at least to a first approximation, common to nearly all cancer cells. Equally, as you will learn [Chapter14] they may have started life as undifferentiated cells or mature stem cells, stem cells that have been located in the tissue in which the tumour has grown. This fact has a profound effect on the selection of therapies.

Cancer cells are genetically unstable. They have mutated from healthy cells, arguably stem cells, as we now know[9], into unstable cancer cells, and they continue to mutate as they divide and multiply. Mutation implies change. If a parent cell produces two mutated daughter cells these cells will be different to the parent cell. When these daughter cells subdivide they too may produce mutated, and so different, daughter cells.

Even cells within the same tumour may mutate differently. This makes it very difficult to treat cancer by using chemical warfare to attack the tumour, for the nature of the enemy is constantly changing.

A cytotoxic (cell killing) chemotherapeutic agent may be aimed at and kill the majority of cells in a tumour but it may leave behind some tumour cells that, because of their different nature, are resistant to the cytotoxic agent and so remain unscathed. Worse is to come. Some cells, following exposure, may develop resistance to the cytotoxic agent, possibly even to all drugs. These cells are known as MDR or multi drug resistant cells. One way or another, by inheritance or as a result of chemotherapy, these cells have changed in such a way as to be resistant to almost all drugs, possibly to all drugs. You will often hear it put another way: *"Cancer cells are very clever, they quickly learn how to change, and to alter their metabolism, so that they are not affected by specific cytotoxic agents to which they have been exposed. They learn to adapt to chemotherapy and change their nature so that the chemotherapy does not damage them."*

This is one of the reasons why the first time that chemotherapy is used it may seem to be successful. A tumour may be reduced drastically in size, possibly down to as little as one or two per cent of its original mass. This, of course, is seen as a reason for rejoicing. When there is a relapse and it grows again there is misplaced confidence that the same therapy will work as well the second time. In practice, it rarely does. There are a number of possible reasons for this. Firstly, not all the cells in a tumour mass are cancerous and it may have been mostly the non-cancerous cells that were killed off by the chemotherapy. Secondly, the residual cells may be residual simply because they are, or have become, MDR cells and so of course they were not affected by the chemotherapy treatment the first time, nor will they be if it is tried again[10]. If all the cells that were left behind the first time were MDR cells, it follows that the cancer cells in this resurgent tumour are now essentially all MDR cells and so of course they will not respond, in any measurable way, to the cytotoxic treatment. Even the nature of the individual MDR cells can vary from cell to cell and this further complicates and frustrates the treatments.

This is just one more reason why fighting the tumour is always going to be difficult, and may not be the best approach to overcoming cancer. On the other hand, working with the body to improve its own ability to resist the tumour (and all foreign, faulty or mutated cells, whatever their nature) and to change the cellular chemistry back to healthy chemistry, is much more likely to achieve a positive outcome.

Preventing a recurrence

There are two aspects to prevention. Firstly, there is primary prevention, the prevention of an initial experience of cancer. Then there is secondary prevention, the prevention of a recurrence after you have once had cancer. All the way through this book, you will be working with your body, supporting it in its own ability to heal itself and to avoid the various pathologies that can hinder your recovery. You will be endeavouring to reverse backwards through and out of Phase Two, and into and then backwards through Phase One to perfect health. The process of preventing a recurrence is similar to the process of preventing an original occurrence. However, you may have to do more to maintain the cancer-free state once you have developed cancer than you have to do to remain healthy if you have never had cancer. Prevention is a lot easier than recovery. There is the added challenge to secondary prevention in that you have already shown yourself to be eminently able to develop cancer. Your body has done it once, it can do it again. Care needs to be taken.

If you have once had measles you develop immunity to it and are unlikely to get it again. Cancer is not like that. If you have had cancer once, and have passed the five-year survival mark, and are symptom-free, you are generally considered to be in full remission. This is as close to 'cure' as is generally claimed for cancer. However, you are just as likely to develop a new cancer in the next ten years as the person beside you who has never had cancer. That is certainly true if you treated cancer last time purely by the MDS route, for in that case nothing was done within that system to cure, resolve, change or eliminate the initial causes, the Risk Factors and Predisposing Factors, and they are still there to start a new cancer.

If you have had cancer in the past and have followed the CAM path, then you are almost certainly at an advantage. By restoring your body back into better health you will have been removing and resolving many of the initiating triggers. So after all, if you have had cancer, followed the CAM therapies and now seem to be fully and totally cancer-free then you could be ahead, you are probably less likely to develop cancer than the person beside you who has never had cancer but has practised none of the preventive measures.

Some patients have said that having had cancer has been an advantage. It has triggered them into a better way of life. Not only has this helped their recovery from cancer, and probably reduced their risk of developing a cancer in the future, but it has also helped them to avoid other possible degenerative diseases.

A word about 'cure' is important here. When you have an infectious disease and recover from it you are said to have been cured. The same is true if you have a broken bone and it is repaired. Many other diseases can occur and then be treated, leading to a cure. In my own experience, I have known patients with sluggish thyroid glands to be stimulated back into full action with homoeopathic remedies and supplements. Migraine headaches have been reduced to a thing of the past with appropriate diet and lifestyle modifications. Poor arteries and stressed hearts have been brought back to improved health, with proper care. Other health problems can be cured when the contributing factors are removed. High blood pressure, for instance, can be returned to normal with appropriate diet management and supplements. For other diseases, particularly some of the more progressive degenerative diseases, and for some people, the aim is more usually to manage the situation. I have had patients with arthritis who have become pain free and who have slowed down, but not eradicated the developing stiffness of joints. Some of the time the best that can be achieved has been management, rather than cure, but even this is hugely positive. Patients who are diabetic, for instance, have been able to reduce or even come off their medication with the appropriate use of supplements such as chromium and vanadium, both of which are needed for glucose management. Yet, in this example, the need for careful diet management, supplements and remedies is ongoing and essential.

Some people have cancer once, recover from it, even return to some of their old ways, and remain healthy. However, they are the exceptions and you should not assume that you can take the same chances. For many people, once they have had cancer, the realistic aim is management. William Kelley, whose story you will read about in Chapter 16 managed his allegedly terminal pancreatic cancer. He was given weeks to live and told no treatment was possible. He successfully managed his situation for forty years and lived until he was nearly eighty.

CHAPTER 5

IS HAVING CANCER MY FAULT?

I recently listened to a radio debate. It followed yet another announcement that a large percentage of cancers, this time breast cancer, could be, or could have been, avoided if the individual had had a better diet and looked after themselves better. Much of the discussion then focused on the concept of fault and blame. I think this is an important issue to understand, particularly since it is recognised that the majority of cancers are diet and lifestyle related.

Doing something wrong or harmful, when you do not know that it is wrong or harmful, does not make you guilty. You may be 'at cause', but you did not know this and you are not 'at fault', you are not to blame. If, on the other hand, you continue to do it once you know it is wrong and harmful, then you are both at cause and, if you will, at fault. You are certainly responsible. An example will suffice.

In the eighteenth and nineteenth centuries most people smoked, there was little suggestion that you were actively harming your health and contributing to cancer. If you smoked then and developed cancer some time later you may have been at cause, but you were not necessarily at fault or to be blamed. You did not know there was a link. If, in the twentieth century, you smoked and developed lung cancer you might indeed have felt at least somewhat guilty. You were certainly at cause, there was increasing evidence that there was a real causative link, and so you were possibly at fault. You may feel like kicking yourself, recognising that there was already some suspicion that there was a connection, but you should not waste energy feeling excessively guilty. If, however, in the twenty first century, you choose to smoke then if you do develop cancer you will be both at cause and at fault as it is now well recognised that smoking significantly increases your risk of developing cancer.

Not all lifestyle challenges are so well within your control. Many people with cancer have experienced a period of severe stress two or three years prior to their diagnosis, stress that they felt was outside their control. The worst type of stress is of the type where you feel helpless and hopeless about things you cannot change. There is, obviously, something you have done that led to you being in that situation, but you may have found yourself in it without realising where you were heading. There are many examples. Such as the marriage that started out well and then became unendurable, but you can't leave because of the children; the highly paid job that you can't afford to lose but where you suddenly have a boss that is making your life intolerable; a small mistake you made that someone is now using to blackmail you; or a business partnership where your partner is cheating on you but you cannot run the business without them. While it is true that you did get into these situations intentionally, you did so in the expectation of a more positive outcome. You did not get into any of them in the expectation of experiencing the stress that led to cancer. Your actions put both you, and the other people involved, at cause but you are not at fault.

We are, ultimately, all responsible for our own actions, for the situations we cause, and for our responses to the situations in which we find ourselves. It is useless to blame other people, it is unproductive to keep beating yourself up. It is important to realise that spending energy, blaming yourself and feeling guilty will do nothing to improve your health and may well make it worse. There are many studies that show the health benefits of a positive mental attitude.

However, if you have developed cancer, then recognising that you may have been at cause does give you an enormous weapon in your fight back to good health. If the things you have been doing have contributed to your cancer, then by changing these things you can have a major impact on eliminating your cancer. These actions may not, on their own, be sufficient to recover your health, but they can contribute significantly to a positive outcome. Blaming yourself will achieve nothing; making positive changes based on what you recognise and learn could save your life.

Many people truly think they eat a good diet, not realising the existence of the many toxic food additives and processes that are allowed by our government and the food industry. You may be one of them. You may not realise how much sugar, refined carbohydrates and processed fats you are eating or how much danger they carry. The legislation allows these foods to flood the market place, and who are you to question that? However, once you do know what foods are bad for you it is then up to you to make the appropriate changes. Otherwise, any further worsening of your health that results will indeed be your fault.

Recognising that your choice of lifestyle has led to where you are can be empowering. After all, it is frequently something you can change, once you recognise the problem. You can change your diet, remove many toxic chemicals from your home or work place, ensure an adequate supply of all the essential nutrients, drink more water, breathe more deeply, do more exercise, take nutritional supplements. You can set about correcting any of the other Predisposing Factors. Even if it is difficult, you can generally get out of most stressful situations if you give serious thought as to what is really important to you. If you cannot change your situation you can always change your response to it, and you had better do so, or you may not recover your health.

So:

(a) recognise any past errors and use this knowledge to make positive changes;

(b) do not waste time berating yourself, this can be self-indulgent and is certainly unproductive;

(c) learn all you can and make use of this information;

(d) make appropriate corrections, and stick to them – and the good news is that there are many that you can make.

CHAPTER 6

DO I HAVE CANCER?
AND THE PROS AND CONS OF BIOPSIES

Do I have cancer? This is a common question in the minds of people who are ill. It is generally asked if they have symptoms without any other identified cause, or if there is cancer in the family. However, the question is ambiguous and before you answer it you have to define what you mean by 'having cancer'. It could mean either, *"Have I moved from Phase One to Phase Two of the Cancer Process?"* or *"Do I have a detectable tumour?"* For most people it is the latter question they are usually asking, yet the former is every bit as important.

The usual medical diagnosis of cancer is based on looking for a tumour. This is certainly true of the solid cancers which form by far the greatest majority of cancers, over 90 per cent. The search for a tumour is usually done by physical examination or by a variety of scans. If a particular type of cancer is suspected and if they are available for that type of cancer, tumour markers may also be tested for.

Once a tumour is detected or a possible site has been located, a biopsy may be done for final confirmation. There are several types of biopsy:

(a) a needle aspiration biopsy in which cells are removed for analysis but not the whole tissue structure;

(b) an incisional or core biopsy in which only a sample of the tissues is extracted and analysed;

(c) an excisional biopsy in which an entire lump or suspicious area is removed and then analysed.

The majority of biopsy samples are analysed under a microscope by a pathologist. Some are analysed chemically. There are advantages to doing a biopsy, but there are also many disadvantages, some of them serious, and it is worth considering the advantages and disadvantages before you embark on the procedure.

Biopsy Advantages	Biopsy Disadvantages	Advantages of the HCG Test and CA Profile
You can determine the type of malignancy.	Biopsies are impractical as a general screening tool. It would be impractical to do them on large numbers of people.	The test can be used as a screening tool as all that is needed is a simple blood sample and a urine sample.
You can determine the location of at least part of the tumour – the part that was extracted for biopsy.	Biopsies are location-specific, they are not a general guide as to whether or not you have cancerous cells anywhere else in your body.	The test is a general guide as to whether or not you have cancer cells anywhere in your body.
	Taking the tissue sample can be painful or inconvenient.	Drawing blood is simple and relatively painless. Collecting urine is completely painless.
If the biopsy has involved total removal of the tumour this may contribute to a 'cure'.	Waiting until there is the possibility of a biopsy means you have waited until there is a significant tumour present. This is leaving things too late.	You can detect the existence of only a few cancer cells within six to ten weeks of them forming, months or years before there is a tumour.
Testing a biopsied sample can indicate the degree of the malignancy at that location.	Biopsies can only tell you about the specific spot from which they were taken. They may even extract non-cancerous cells from a tumour and give a false negative result.	The test provides information in relation to your whole body.

Biopsy Advantages	Biopsy Disadvantages	Advantages of the HCG Test and CA Profile
	When tissue is taken for biopsy, cancer cells can be released from the local site and metastasise to another tissue.	Drawing blood does not increase the risk of metastasis.
	You cannot use a biopsy, after surgery, to tell you if they 'got it all'.	If the surgeon 'got it all' the HCG level should return to normal within 6 weeks.
	You cannot use biopsies to monitor treatment.	The test is excellent for monitoring your progress.
	Biopsies cannot warn you of a recurrence until it is well advanced.	An increase in HCG can provide very early warning of a recurrence.

From a CAM perspective, and for practical and therapeutic purposes, it is more important to know whether or not you are in Phase Two of the Cancer Process rather than whether or not you yet have a cancerous mass large enough to constitute a tumour. After all, you may not yet have a tumour, but still have many, and a growing number of, cancer cells in your body. The sooner you can learn about this the better. One of the most useful tests to do to determine this involves testing for the HCG hormone already mentioned and it is instructional to compare the risks and benefits of a biopsy against this non-invasive chemical blood and urine test.

Doctors need biopsies because their treatments are focused on the tumour, and for that they have to know where the tumour is. CAM therapies are systemic, not based on the location of the tumour, and so the HCG test is valuable and can help you make decisions about optimal recovery programmes very early in the process.

People operating solely within the MDS model will say that the lack of location specificity is a disadvantage of the HCG test. However, keep in mind:

(a) that in many instances a positive HCG test will be detecting cancer cells before there are sufficient even to form a tumour of a size that could be detected by physical means;

(b) the CAM recovery approach is to work systemically, helping the body to heal itself, not to focus solely on tumour-targeted destruction by means that apply to the specific location at or within a tissue type; and

(c) that, once a tumour is present of sufficient size to be detected by other means, any recovery protocol can be adapted accordingly.

Medical treatments for cancer all have adverse toxic side effects. Therefore, doctors have to be absolutely certain that you have cancer before applying a treatment, as the treatment is a trade-off between perceived benefits and the dangerous toxic effects for the whole body of cytotoxic chemotherapy or radiation, or the physiological and emotional stress of surgery. For this reason doctors generally want a biopsy-proven cancer before they introduce any of their treatments.

CAM procedures in relation to cancer have no adverse toxic effects. This is true of all the early stage treatments which are also generally relatively inexpensive. Some of the more advanced or technological treatments, such as hyperthermia, regular intravenous vitamin treatments, hyperbaric oxygen and others may stretch the budget and make demands on time and travel that are a challenge; but they are not harmful. This means that if cancer is suspected then all the basic and beneficial diet and lifestyle changes should be put into place immediately. Whether or not cancer is present, there will almost certainly be an improvement in overall health, and if cancer is present you will have made a head start in your recovery plan. You do not need, therefore, to have biopsy proof of malignancy. A raised HCG should be sufficient of a trigger to start you on some positive changes.

In this book you will also learn of other tests for the presence of cancerous cells, such as Kelley's self test using pancreatic enzymes [Chapter16]. These are tests that you can do instead of biopsies.

With what you will learn here you will learn to change the question from, *"Do I have a (detectable) tumour?"* to *"Do I have any cancer cells, am I in Phase Two of the Cancer Process, and should I be taking action now to reverse the process and avoid the development of a tumour?"*

PART 2

CAUSES AND ORIGIN OF CANCER

INTRODUCTION TO PART 2

Overcoming cancer necessitates reversing the conditions that allowed the cancer to develop – but more is required.

In Part 2 we will be looking at some of the most plausible and scientifically sound theories relating to the causes of cancer. Over the past one hundred years a number of valuable suggestions have been made by eminent scientists and, by and large, they have all been virtually ignored by the general medical profession.

They have several things in common. They do not fit into the accepted medical model of the day. They do not lend themselves logically to endorsing the three medical therapies of our day, surgery, cytotoxic drugs and radioactive radiation, nor do they endorse the claim that all treatment efforts should be aimed dominantly at destroying the tumour, by whatever means are available.

On the other hand, they have all been utilised, endorsed, and found to be successful by CAM therapists. Many of these practitioners and researchers have been equally eminent scientists, including one Nobel prize winner (Dr. Otto Warburg) and two nominees for a Nobel Prize (Dr. Johanna Budwig and Dr. John Beard). Some of them were the top people in their field until they had the temerity to suggest that the current medical approach to, and theories about, cancer were incorrect (e.g. Dr. John Beard). All of them have been excellent and effective clinicians or researchers and have offered highly effective inputs into clinical practices. Countless numbers of them have been harassed by their governments or forced to relocate to different countries to continue in their work. All of them have saved countless lives of people who had been told they had terminal cancer, and helped other people to avoid a recurrence.

As we go through the various theories you will discover that they all feed easily and logically into and endorse each other and that they come together to create a coherent whole. They do not contradict each other, nor are they alternatives, they are all aspects of this one coherent whole. This, in addition to the soundness of the underlying theoretical base and the positive results that have been obtained in practice, can give us confidence that there is merit in paying attention to these views and applying them in practice.

To explore these ideas we will be considering, at the fundamental cellular and chemical level, the factors that change within the cells when they turn from healthy to cancerous cells. Based on this understanding you and your practitioner, for keep in mind that you do need one, will be able to build a rational programme for optimising your health. This will consist, as appropriate, of:

(a) assisting you in the prevention of cancer;
(b) the (healthy) reduction of your tumour in ways that are not harmful to healthy cells;
(c) the prevention of a tumour recurrence;
(d) correction of the faulty cellular chemistry, as defined by a variety of blood and urine tests, that are indicative of Phase Two of the Cancer Process, thus further reducing the possibility of either a primary or a secondary occurrence.

It is important to stress, and that you understand, that these theories are all based on well understood biochemistry and physiology. They lead on, logically, to useful and generally available tests so that you can determine whether or not you have cancerous cells, and they can help you in planning your recovery programme. Some of the later tests, described below, will tell you about specific strengths and weaknesses of any cancer cells that may be present, and this will then guide you as to the detailed nature of the supplements and remedies you can use and the therapies you can follow to give you the best chance of success.

The MDS system and genetic mutations

In general terms, the MDS system focuses, in relation to cancer, on the nucleus within cells. Anything that alters the DNA of a cell and leads to the production of a cell that is different to the parent cell is a mutagen and the resulting faulty cell is a mutation. Anything that causes cancer is a carcinogen. In the medical model, nearly all carcinogens are mutagens. However not all mutagens are carcinogens.

Cells, as we shall see, replicate by doubling up on themselves and then dividing in half. Every time they do this there is the possibility of an error occurring. In the vast majority of cases, if such an error does occur, the offspring, the mutant daughter cells, are unsuccessful and do not survive.

The faulty or mutated cells may fail to survive for a number of reasons. Faulty cells may simply not be viable. In general, faulty or old cells commonly, and of their own doing, self-destruct, in the process known as apoptosis. This is brought about by mechanisms that exist within all cells and normally operates when the cell has become old or damaged, but it can also operate at the birth of a new, but faulty cell. Faulty cells may be recognised as faulty by other cells, such as those of the immune system, and so destroyed. However, if the mutated cell does survive then it can reproduce and create either more similar mutant cells or it can produce newer and different mutations.

Either the original mutation or the survival of the mutant cell can be caused by a wide range of factors that, collectively, are called carcinogens. These carcinogens include a wide range of toxic chemicals and viruses, plus physical factors such as physical damage or injury, exposure to many different types of radiation and electro-magnetic fields, or lack of oxygen.

The most successful mutations, and so to us the most harmful, are those that amplify themselves until eventually these mutated cells are multiplying at an exponential rate and build into a tumour. An obvious possibility is a mutation that increases the rate of division of the cells, but another is the possibility that the cell becomes immortal and refuses to die, ever. Or the cell may be sending out faulty messages to the surrounding cells. It might, for instance, block the action of cells of the immune system, destroy or damage surrounding healthy cells, or it may build up a protective layer or mechanism such that it is impervious to outside factors that would normally control or destroy it. Even more importantly, the faulty cell may be programmed to create newer varieties of cells that have even more errors, and so the whole process is again compounded.

It is important to keep this in mind. It is one of the reasons that you cannot simply remove the cause and get rid of the cancer. You cannot simply reverse back out of Phase Two and then into Phase One of the Cancer Process, though you do need to do that. You may have developed cancer because of excessive stress and adrenal exhaustion [Chapter11], but simply recognising this and removing the stress will not necessarily solve the problem once you have these faulty cells, they do not simply disappear in the absence of the causative stress. There is more work to do for you to achieve a recovery.

Medically, cancer is seen as a problem that is localised to the specific tissues and cells which constitute the tumour, not as a more generalised systemic problem. It is also seen as one that is focused on the nucleus of the cells and not elsewhere in the cell. It is time to ask whether or not this is true or if there is evidence to the contrary.

In fact, many attempts have been made to convert healthy cells into cancerous cells by injecting the nucleus from cancer cells into the healthy cells. For instance, researchers replaced the nucleus of a healthy fertilised mouse egg with the nucleus taken from a cancer cell. If the fault derived from damaged nuclear DNA, the recipient, in this case the resultant mouse, should develop cancer. Repeatedly, this and similar tests have failed to produce cancerous offspring, or even offspring that developed cancer[11]. Thus, it seems clear that it is not necessarily the damaged DNA in the nucleus of the cancer cell that is the original cause of the problem. It is therefore appropriate to look elsewhere for the cause, somewhere outside the nucleus of the cell.

The CAM system and the systemic approach

This view, that of mutations of healthy tissue cells as being the prime cause of cancer, is very different to the view held by many CAM practitioners, and to the thesis propounded here. In this view cancer is a systemic problem, it involves the whole person and all the tissues and systems. The tumour is merely the end symptom, the tip of the iceberg of a much greater problem. This view, as we shall discover, leads to the possibility of many more useful therapies.

It is proposed by the theories discussed in the following chapters that, in the majority of cancers, it is not a genetic mutation in the nucleus that is the cause of cancer. Instead, it is proposed that the cause is metabolic errors in the cytosol or general matrix inside the cells, plus problems involving the mitochondria and the cell membrane (wall). The mitochondria are the energy-producing organelles within the cytosol, they also play a major role in initiating apoptosis and thus curtailing the survival of damaged or mutant cells. These factors are affected in turn by the chemistry of the membrane of the cell and the way it both communicates with the outside environment, and permits, or does not permit, transit of substances across the membrane. The mitochondrial membrane chemistry is also relevant, as we shall see.

If this latter view is correct, then chemotherapy that focuses solely on eradicating the tumour is not the most appropriate treatment and carries a high risk of failure. When you cut through all the claims and counter claims, it is clear that modern medicine has made very little impact on the recovery and survival of people with solid tumour cancers, a mere increase of less than 2.3 per cent in five-year survival, in the case of chemotherapy[12]. This should be no surprise if it is the Cancer Process that is the problem, rather than the end product, the tumour. In fact we know that many chemotherapy drugs can cause cancer, as can radiation [Chapters 22 and 23], so that a long-term positive outcome from following this MDS approach is unlikely.

CHAPTER 7

YOUR CELLS

To understand much of the reasoning in the following chapters, it will help if you know something about the structure of a typical cell. There isn't actually a typical cell of course. A nerve cell, for instance, is long and thin and may be up to a foot or more in length. Conversely, a red blood cell is a tiny doughnut-shaped disc of about seven microns in diameter and only visible under a microscope. Liver cells contain between 1,000 and 2,000 mitochondria, red blood cells contain none, nor do they contain nuclei. However, we will consider a compromise, if mythical, typical cell.

Cell membrane

Every cell is surrounded by a membrane or wall made up of a lipid (fat) bi-layer. It will be important later to understand something of the nature of this membrane, so here is the description.

Most of the fats that you eat are in the form of triglycerides. Triglycerides consist of three fatty acids, lying parallel to each other and attached to a single glycerol molecule. Fatty acids vary in length from short through medium to long chains. They can be saturated, or have double or unsaturated bonds. When one of the fatty acids is removed and replaced by a phosphate group you have a compound called phosphatidic acid. When an additional molecule such as choline or inositol, is attached to the phosphate group, you have a phosphatide. It is these phosphatides, or phospholipids, that are the major component of the cell wall. The phospholipids line up with all the phosphate heads adjacent to each other and the fatty acid tails all pointing away from the heads. When two of these phospholipid layers come together, making a sandwich, the long tails of each layer line up and point towards each other. The phosphate ends sit side by side and this surface forms either the external surface of the cell membrane, which faces outwards towards the bloodstream, or adjacent towards a neighbouring cell on the one hand, or else inwards facing towards the centre of the cell on the other. This double row of tails-to-tails creates an effective and dynamic boundary and a framework for the cell and for cell organelles inside the cells.

Cholesterol molecules are wedged in between the tails of the fatty acids, in the centre of the membrane, where they have important roles to play. Although this is not relevant to the current topic, it is timely to point out that in spite of the bad press cholesterol generally receives, it is essential for the function of cell membranes in general and for specific actions in a variety of issues.

Protein molecules, generally somewhat globular or sausage-like in shape, though this can vary enormously, sit on either the outside or the inside of the membrane. They extend either only a small way into it, or else penetrate the whole way through the membrane and emerge on the other side. The surface proteins act as receptor sites. Because of their shape and electrical charges they are able to receive specific chemical messages from outside the cell or from the internal activity of the cell respectively. Receptor sites on the outer membrane, once triggered, act by passing a chemical message on to the internal workings of the cell, triggering a sequence of chemical reactions that, in effect, tell the cell that certain actions are required. This action may be the synthesis of a specific compound, usually though not always a protein, or to start a specific sequence of reactions within the cell. Receptor sites on the inner wall of the membrane receive information from elsewhere in the cell and can pass signals to the outside. In this way information or instructions are passed on to other cells. Larger protein molecules that extend from the outside, all the way through the membrane, can act as channels for the absorption of nutrients and incoming messenger molecules, or for the expulsion of waste products, outgoing messenger molecules or functional compounds, such as hormones, that have been produced within the cell.

Cytosol

Inside the cell surrounded by its membrane is the cytosol, the matrix that fills the cell. It was once thought that this was an amorphous jelly-like substance in which the various organelles floated. We now know that it is a lot more structured than this. However it remains, in essence, the continuous matrix in which all the organelles are placed. The organelles of the cells are somewhat analogous to the organs of the human body.

They include the nucleus that carries the genetic material, ribosomes where proteins are made and mitochondria where most of the energy is released from the fats and carbohydrates that you eat. Other organelles deal with waste materials and perform a variety of other individual functions.

Nucleus

The nucleus of the cell contains the genetic material, the DNA that makes up the genes that in turn make up the chromosomes that constitute your genetic make-up. It was once thought that the nucleus of the cell was the brain of the cell. However, it can now be argued, following the work of Candace Pert[13] and Bruce Lipton[14], that the most 'intelligent' part of the cell is the membrane. The nucleus, like the hard disk on a computer, stores the information, but it makes no decisions, it does not run the cell. In fact, a cell can live for one or two months without its nucleus[15], only dying for lack of essential proteins when replacements are needed and the blueprint (gene) is not available from the missing nucleus. It is true that certain activities cannot happen unless the data (the correct and healthy genetic material) is in place in the nucleus; this consists mainly of the 'blueprints' for making new proteins, when they are required. But it is the cell's membrane that 'decides' what the cell will do, that operates the cell via the messages it allows (or does not allow) to enter and leave the cell, and so decides what proteins are needed. The way that the membrane receives (or fails to receive) information from the outside world and acts (or fails to act) on it dictates how the cell will function. Thus the membrane's function is analogous to the function of the human being that decides what information to input and draw out of the computer's hard disk (the nucleus). The nucleus merely carries the genes that code for the production of the proteins that facilitate the thousands of actions that may be required. But unless it is triggered into action by messages coming to it, via the cell's membrane, very little happens.

Mitochondria

Mitochondria are often, and rightly, called the power-houses of the cell as the majority of the cell's energy production occurs in them in a series of reactions that require large quantities of oxygen. They are interesting organelles, and it is thought that at one time our cells (or those of our very far distant ancestors back along the evolutionary scale) did not contain mitochondria. It is thought that these very primitive ancestors functioned entirely anaerobically and that the mitochondria were once some type of independent organism, possibly a bacteria, that was then entrapped and made use of by the anaerobic cells. The resultant combination of these two organisms was able to utilise oxygen and set off on an entirely new evolutionary sequence of changes which eventually led to the majority of the animal kingdom, including us human beings.

These mitochondria are not only the seat of most of our energy production. They have many additional functions including some in relation to cell signalling, cell differentiation, control of the cell cycle and cell growth, and cell death or apoptosis, all of which can have a profound effect on the occurrence and development of cancer. This will be discussed in more detail in the third book in this series.

Other organelles

There are many other organelles within the cell. Proteins, you will recall, are made on the ribosomes. Another part of your cells, the Golgi apparatus, packages these proteins and some lipids in preparation for their transport out of the cell and to their destination. Lysosomes 'digest' or break down some of the larger molecules that enter the cell. There are more, but none of these other organelles will concern us here. Many of these organelles are surrounded by a membrane or wall, analogous to that of the cell itself. Although we have little to say about them directly, these membranes, just like the cell's other membranes, are important to cell function, and we will have more to say about the health of cell membranes in Chapter 17.

If you could 'see' down to the level of molecular activity within the cell all you would see would be a blur of activity. You would have to slow the action down by an indescribable amount to be able to see what was going on, reaction by reaction. Many thousands of different types of reactions take place within your cells, and they are happening many times a second. A large number of the reactions will be common to all your cells. They all, for instance, have to produce energy, synthesise proteins, eliminate waste products and communicate with the outside world via the activity of their cellular membrane. Not only are there thousands of different types of such reactions, but each one is happening dozens or hundreds of times a second.

Mature red blood cells constitute an interesting exception. They do not contain mitochondria. They have little need for energy and are simply swept along by the flow of the circulation system. They get sufficient energy for their very basic needs from glycolysis in the cytosol [Chapter 8]. This has the benefit that they do not use up the oxygen they are carrying but deliver all of it to the various target cells. In fact, red blood cells contain very few organelles, no ribosomes, no Golgi apparatus and no endoplasmic reticulum. Once they have matured they do not even have nuclei as they do not reproduce. New red blood cells develop in the bone marrow, then jettison their organelles, effectively making room for the huge amounts of oxygen they must collect from your lungs, transport through your body and deliver to the individual target cells in all your various tissues.

In addition to this basic cellular physiology there are the chemical reactions that are unique to individual cell types. Bone cells will be building or breaking down bone structures, the calcium phosphate matrix that gives strength to your bones; nerve cells will be making, sending and receiving neurotransmitters (chemicals that carry messages from nerve cells); endocrine cells will be making and exporting hormones, and so on.

The life of the cell is a fascinating story and worth reading about, but that is for another time. This view of the cell is sufficient for our needs. It is now time to consider how energy is produced within the cells, as when this does not occur correctly it will have a direct bearing on the development of cancer.

CHAPTER 8

CELLULAR ENERGY PRODUCTION

Cellular energy production and the way this is accomplished by healthy cells, versus the way cancer cells do it, is a key consideration in the development of cancer. This is a fairly technical chapter, I make no apologies for this, though I have tried to simplify it as much as possible. It is necessary for an understanding of what happens when a cell turns from a healthy cell to a cancerous cell. If you do not read it now you may want to come back to it later. Otherwise you have several options:

- You may decide it is too technical for you and skip it altogether.

- You may be keen to understand it and do your best to work through it. At the very least, by the end, you will have come to realise there is some very solid biochemistry behind many of the suggestions you will almost certainly receive from your practitioner. If you do not have a practitioner, you will still have a better understanding of the implications behind the dietary and supplement suggestions you will be building into your protocol, based, possibly, on other books and papers you have read as well as this one.

- You may have an interest in the underlying science and be able to follow all the details.

- You may be a biochemist or practitioner and already understand the basics, in which case this chapter will serve to blend them into a fundamental understanding of the basis behind the CAM therapies for cancer.

One thing I have learnt, after many years of writing and lecturing in this field, is just how intelligent, knowledgeable and well-informed many of the people are who are seriously interested in the CAM therapies and in using them for themselves, particularly when the health problem is cancer and their need to fully understand what they can do is high. I have also learnt that, even if they do not fully understand the chemical details and their full ramifications, they want to know about them. They want to know the details which exist and that, with a bit of effort on their part, they could eventually get to grips with them. This generally gives people confidence in the procedures they are advised to follow. This further underlies my decision to include these details here.

One of my first articles in a health magazine was written in Australia in 1980[16]. It was on the different forms of vitamin D, with explanations as to their chemical structures and differences. The publisher of the magazine insisted the article was too technical and should be withdrawn. The editor insisted on publishing it, and he won the day. He later reported, with obvious glee, that although it was only a short article they had had more positive feedback from it than almost any of their previous articles. People wanted to know then. I hope you do now.

So in spite of publishers' exhortations to 'keep it simple', I am including this chapter in all its details. An understanding, at whatever level, of the mechanisms described here will help you to understand the following chapters and the theories of cancer development described in them by Dr. Warburg [Chapter 9], Dr. Fryda [Chapter 11] and others. It will reassure you that there is a firm foundation and rationale for the protocol you will probably be advised to follow if you have cancer.

Cancer cells are unstable

Whatever view you take of the cause or origin of cancer, it is clear that cancer cells do not behave like healthy cells. If they did they would not be cancer cells. From the start of Phase Two of the Cancer Process some of your cells are changing and behaving abnormally. They are changing their cellular chemistry and their cellular activity. As the activity and effect of the cancer cells spreads, these chemical changes become progressively more apparent and can be detected and measured by analysing for specific compounds in blood or urine. By measuring these changes you can pick up some early warning signs that indicate that you are at increasing risk of developing cancer, even before the cells have finally turned cancerous. You can tell that you are moving along Phase One of the Cancer Process to Phase Two [See the ONE test in Chapter 9]. You can also detect the early development of cancer, before a tumour is formed or becomes detectable, the early stages of Phase Two of the Cancer Process.

One of the major differences between healthy cells and cancer cells is the way they get their energy, and this has a profound effect on the way we can help to restore sick cells to healthy cells.

Methods of energy production

When considering energy production we are concerned with what is happening in both the cells and the cells' mitochondria. In broad sweeping terms we will find that:

(a) healthy cells produce a very small amount of their energy by anaerobic (without oxygen) chemical changes in their cytosol and almost all of their energy by aerobic oxidation in their mitochondria, and they do this from compounds derived from the breakdown of glucose, fats and amino acids;

(b) cancerous cells produce almost all their energy by anaerobic fermentation in the cytosol, and they do so only from glucose or from a compound derived from the breakdown of glucose.

Here is what happens:

Carbohydrates

Grains, vegetables, legumes, fruits and sugars all contain carbohydrates. Some of these are non-digestible carbohydrates (colloquially called 'fibre') and these are not digested or absorbed but remain within your digestive tract and pass out of your body in your stool. Much of this 'fibre' is in the form of cellulose, hemi-cellulose, or related compounds and contains long chains of glucose units, but they are joined together by a type of bond for which the human digestive tract has no enzyme and so these bonds remain undigested, or unbroken. You should consume large amounts of fibre-rich foods, the best of which are vegetables. They help you to maintain intestinal health and prevent constipation and the absorption of toxins. But that is another story.

The rest of the carbohydrates in your diet are composed largely of glucose molecules joined together by bonds that are broken within the human digestive tract. This glucose comes as the component of several larger molecules. In starches it is in the form of large molecules made up of chains of glucose molecules joined together, and called amylose and amylopectin. In oligosaccharides it is in the form of several glucose molecules (up to about eleven) joined together in the form of dextrins. In disaccharides it is in the form of one glucose molecule (a monosaccharide) attached either to another glucose molecule (as in maltose), attached to a fructose molecule (as in sucrose or table sugar), or attached to a galactose molecule (as in lactose or milk sugar). Some of it is present as individual monosaccharides, such as glucose and fructose (not joined together) in honey and fructose on its own, found in many fruits.

The digestive process that occurs in your small intestine reduces all these carbohydrates to monosaccharides and once they reach your liver the fructose and galactose are converted into glucose, so from there on, when we talk of sugar, we are talking about glucose. Your cells need glucose for energy. They cannot live without it. You cannot, for instance, live on a diet that is composed entirely of fats and proteins, as we shall see. You need some glucose, not a lot, but you do need a small amount, the amount you would get, for instance, from a healthy plate of salad vegetables.

Once you have eaten and the food components, including the glucose, have been absorbed, your blood glucose level will rise. This is normal, but the level should not remain high and should rapidly return to normal. There are three basic ways that this is achieved. The glucose can be taken up by a number of cells that can burn it up (oxidise it) for immediate energy. It can be built back up into and stored as complex carbohydrate molecules called glycogen (also known as 'animal starch') in your liver or muscles. Or it can be converted into fat and stored in your fat deposits until the energy locked up in it is needed.

Cancer cells thrive on glucose

Healthy cells obtain most of their energy from fats and carbohydrates; small amounts may be obtained from any spare protein that is available or left over from the normal protein building requirements. Cancer cells, on the other hand, depend almost entirely on glucose for energy, but they use it very inefficiently. To overcome this defect they have many more receptor sites for glucose than do healthy cells. If you do not want to feed your cancer cells it is important that you do not supply them with a steady diet of glucose. You cannot achieve this aim by refusing to eat any carbohydrates because your healthy cells also need glucose. The way to do it is to avoid anything that causes a rapid or prolonged surge in your blood glucose to a level that is significantly above normal, and to do all you can to return your blood glucose level back to normal as soon after eating as possible.

Diabetics typically have prolonged periods of high blood glucose level and this is one of the reasons that they are particularly prone to cancer and why I list diabetes as a Predisposing Factor. If you are diabetic and have been told by your doctor that a moderately high level of glucose is, *"all right, to be expected, and is manageable,"* don't believe him or her, but do everything you possibly can to maintain it as near normal as possible. How do you do this? You need to do all you can to normalise your insulin output and its effectiveness.

When you eat vegetables, other than potatoes or parsnips, the starches they contain are released only very slowly because of the very high fibre content. When you eat whole grains, legumes or foods containing other complex carbohydrates, the starches they contain are broken down only slowly in your digestive tract. The released glucose molecules trickle slowly into your bloodstream, over an extended period of time, usually a few hours. There is then a slight rise in your blood glucose level and the incoming glucose is disposed of (as described above) at a steady state. On the other hand, when you eat fruit or eat refined grains, such as white flour, white pasta, white rice etc, there is a more rapid surge in your blood glucose level. When you drink fruit juice, eat bananas, potatoes or parsnips the surge is more rapid, and when you eat sweets and foods laden with sugar (sucrose), the surge is very high indeed. The higher your blood glucose the more food or fuel you are providing for your cancer cells. Clearly the best foods for you to eat, if you want to 'starve' these cancer cells of glucose, are vegetables.

You may be wondering why glucose trickling into your bloodstream 'little and often' is better for you than the same amount entering your bloodstream in a large surge. Consider two groups of people. In one group the people have small stomachs and in the other group they have large stomachs. If food is provided only once a day the people with small stomachs (healthy cells) are soon full and stop eating, and all the excess food is available to feed the people with large stomachs (cancer cells). If only small meals are provided at any one time, even if it is little and often, then it is taken up more equally by all the cells and the people with large stomachs get a lesser share than before. Furthermore, if the total amount of carbohydrate available (eaten) in any one day is limited to the small amount the small stomachs (healthy cells) need, the large stomachs (cancer cells) will be starved. This is the best you can do. Even so, as cancer cells have many more receptor sites for glucose than do healthy cells they are always going to win out and get at least somewhat more glucose than the healthy cells, but you will have done the best you can.

Whenever your blood glucose level rises, insulin is, or should be, produced and called into play. This insulin then assists the glucose to enter the various cells that need or can use it. Insulin is a hormone produced by your pancreas. The exocrine (outside) activity of your pancreas deals with digestion, squirting digestive juices out of your tissues and into your digestive tract. This is considered to be exocrine or external as your digestive tract is continuous with the outside world. If your exocrine pancreas is under-performing you are at increased risk of cancer, (as you will learn in Chapter 14 and Chapter 16) because you need the protein-splitting enzymes, trypsin and chymotrypsin, that it produces. The endocrine (internal) activity of your pancreas involves excreting compounds, in particular the hormone insulin, into your bloodstream. Here it deals with what is going on inside your body, in particular it is a major player in controlling and normalising your blood glucose level and in this way, again, your pancreas helps to prevent cancer. In other words: if your exocrine pancreas is compromised, not only will your digestion be poor but you will not have sufficient levels of the trypsin and chymotrypsin you need to break down cancer cells. If your endocrine pancreas is under-performing you are at increased risk of diabetes, and, since your blood glucose level then remains high, you are also at increased risk of feeding cancer cells. Clearly both the exocrine and endocrine aspects of your pancreas are important. Thus your pancreas, overall, is a very important organ in preventing and, as we shall see, in treating cancer. From this it should be no surprise to find that pancreatic cancer is one of the fastest growing and one of the most difficult to treat. It is destroying the organ that is vitally important to recovery.

Insulin production requires zinc, so it is important that you make sure you are not zinc deficient. Insulin function requires chromium and vitamin B3. Chromium in combination with vitamin B3 is part of a complex called glucose tolerance factor or GTF, and GTF plays a critical role in the management of normal blood glucose levels by increasing the cellular response to insulin and hence the cellular uptake of glucose. Without GTF the cells do not respond to insulin, they become 'insulin resistant' and the glucose remains in your bloodstream and available to feed any cancer cells[17].

Both the insulin function and blood glucose levels are improved by vanadium. Vanadium has been shown to mimic many of the metabolic actions of insulin both *in vivo* (animals) and *in vitro* (test tubes), though the exact mechanism is not clear. Vanadium has been shown to decrease blood glucose levels, appetite, body fat and body weight in experimental animals[18].

Thus, for the efficient and appropriate entry of glucose into your cells, for the maintenance of a normal blood glucose level, and to avoid over feeding any cancer cells that may be present, an adequate supply of these three minerals, zinc, chromium and vanadium, is important.

Energy release

Once the glucose molecule is inside the cell it is broken down by two sequential pathways, occurring in two distinct parts of the cell. The first pathway involves essentially a rearrangement of the glucose molecule and preparing it for entry into the second pathway. The second pathway releases the glucose-stored energy and repackages it into smaller, more manageable, units stored as ATP-energy.

E-M pathway

The first and most common glucose-converting pathway is the E-M or Embden-Meyerhof pathway. This takes place in the anaerobic cytosol of the cell. In this pathway, of several steps, the six-carbon glucose molecule is first rearranged and then broken in half to form two molecules of (three-carbon) pyruvic acid. One of the steps in this pathway is catalysed by an enzyme called phosphohexose isomerase, or

PHI, about which you will read more later. The level of this enzyme is a very useful diagnostic tool, as you will discover. In the process of the rearranging that takes place in the pathway a small, but only a relatively small, amount of energy is released and used to produce the high energy molecule, ATP. No oxygen is present in this cytosol and so no carbon dioxide is produced.

Pivotal Step

Then comes a critical and pivotal step. The proper pathway from here is for the three-carbon pyruvic acid to turn into a two-carbon acetyl group and release one molecule of carbon dioxide. The acetyl group then enters one of the mitochondria. Although I have labelled this a single pivotal step it is in fact a sequence of interconnected chemical changes and it requires many nutrients including vitamin B1, vitamin B3, vitamin B5, magnesium, manganese, lipoic acid and, indirectly, biotin.

If there is any block at this pivotal point, if the various co-factors are not present in sufficient quantity, or if the mitochondrion is not working properly, the pyruvic acid will remain in the cytosol and be converted into lactic acid. This creates a serious and major problem, one to which we will return [Chapter 11].

Krebs Cycle, or Citric Acid Cycle

The Krebs Cycle, Citric Acid Cycle, or Tricarboxylic Acid Cycle is a series of nine biochemical reactions that occur in the matrix of the mitochondria. During this cycle of reactions the acetyl group is converted into carbon dioxide and water with the release of energy, using oxygen from respiration to govern the cycle's activity.

In more detail, once the acetyl group is produced and enters the mitochondrion it is taken up, rather like the rider on a merry-go-round, by a larger molecule in the Krebs Cycle. Then follows a sequence of reactions that progressively break down the acetyl group and release its two carbon atoms. These carbon atoms are oxidised to carbon dioxide, and the hydrogen atoms to water. As these reactions are occurring, small quanta of energy contained in the original acetyl groups are released. These small energy quanta are taken up by low-energy molecules called

ADP (adenosine diphosphate) which are thereby recharged, rather like a rechargeable battery, with another phosphate group, up into high energy compounds called ATP (adenosine triphosphate). If there is any block at this point, if the mitochondrion is not working properly, the pyruvic acid remains in the cytosol and is converted into lactic acid. This is a problem, one to which we will return [Chapter 11].

The Krebs Cycle does not operate entirely on its own. From time to time it needs to be primed. If this was a merry-go-round it would be analogous to having to replace one starting horse for the riders to get onto. For this, some carbohydrate intake is needed. This is one of the reasons why you cannot live on an entirely carbohydrate-free diet, but you can get an ample amount of carbohydrate for this purpose from the vegetables you are encouraged to eat. On average, a carbohydrate intake of around sixty grams (or just over two ounces) will usually satisfy this requirement. Other than that, strictly speaking, you have no absolute requirement for dietary carbohydrate other than fibre. You could derive the rest of your energy from fats and protein. This is an important consideration when you are being advised to follow a diet with very limited carbohydrate intake. Remember that sugar feeds cancer cells far more beneficially than it feeds healthy cells as cancer cells absolutely have to have glucose to survive, whereas healthy cells can get their energy from fats. You will read more about this below.

Fats

Most fats are taken into the body as triglycerides. These are made up of three long-chain fatty acids attached to a single three-carbon molecule of glycerol (hence the name) rather like a three-pronged fork without the handle and as we discussed when talking of the phospholipids of the cell membranes. During digestion these triglycerides are broken down into their components and carried through the bloodstream attached to proteins in complexes called chylomicrons. When they reach the liver they are converted into smaller and more manageable packages called lipoproteins.

These lipoproteins contain cholesterol, triglycerides and proteins and form three categories. VLDLs or Very Low Density Lipoproteins contain proteins, cholesterol and a high proportion of fatty acids. It is these fats that keep their density low (fats float on, and so are less dense than, water). The VLDLs deliver fatty acids to the tissues that need them for energy and any excess is delivered to the adipose tissue cells for storage. In the process, and after a pass through the liver where they are rearranged, they become LDLs or Low Density Lipoproteins. They are less dense because of their loss of some of their triglycerides, and they are now relatively concentrated in cholesterol. The LDLs' cholesterol is then delivered to all the tissues that need it such as the brain and nerve cells, skin (for vitamin D), adrenal glands (to make steroid hormones), liver (for bile acids and salts) and to cells (for the membranes, where it is stored). In the process, and after another pass through the liver for further rearrangement, they become HDLs or High Density Lipoproteins. These HDLs can then travel round your system gathering up old, used cholesterol which they take to the liver where it is dispatched from your body in the bile. HDLs are the so-called 'good' cholesterol and LDLs the so-called 'bad', though both have their uses and their appropriate roles to play. Since cholesterol is essential for health in a variety of tissues, 'bad' is really a misnomer. The problems occur when there is a blockage in the sequence and hence an excessively high ratio of LDLs to HDLs. This is one ratio to monitor in any health problem as it also reflects on the healthy function of your liver (where the proper rearranging should take place) which is a vital organ in both the prevention of heart disease and the prevention of and the fight against cancer.

As a result of these activities the fatty acids are delivered into the cells. Their next step is to find a way into a mitochondrion. To achieve this they need to be activated. This is accomplished with the help of the high energy molecule, ATP, aided by vitamin B2, vitamin B3, and vitamin B5 plus carnitine. Carnitine is a dipeptide made from two essential amino acids, lysine and methionine, in a process for which the presence of vitamin C is essential.

The activated fatty acid, attached to carnitine, is then able to enter the mitochondrion. Here it is broken down by a process called beta lipid peroxidation. In this process each step chops the next two carbon segments off the main chain and each is thus transformed into an acetyl group the same as those that come in from the break down of glucose via the Pivotal Step. As, essentially, all dietary fats consist of even numbers of carbon atoms, this process finally completes the breakdown of the original long fatty acid chain. The acetyl groups now join into the Krebs Cycle in the same way as do the ones that come from glucose.

As you will learn later, it is now thought that a significant problem in cancer cells is that the mitochondria are no longer functioning. This means that the majority of cancer cells can derive little, if any, of their energy from fats, so whereas it is safe to say that 'sugar feeds cancer', it is a reasonable generalisation to say that 'fats do not feed cancer cells'.

Protein

Dietary proteins are broken down, by the various digestive processes that occur within your digestive tract, mostly into individual amino acids. Most of these amino acids are then transported to your liver where a multitude of reactions can occur. There are twenty amino acids that are essential for good health. Of these, ten absolutely must be derived from your diet, you cannot make them yourself, even if you have all the components. Thus, they are the ones that are generally referred to as 'essential amino acids' meaning that they are 'essential in the diet'. The other ten amino acids can be made, usually by your liver, provided that you have all the necessary components. The critical component is the amino group and this has to come from another amino acid. So if you have an excess of one type of amino acid, over and above the amount you need for protein building and other uses, then this can be broken down and the amino group that is released can be used to build the amino acid that is in short supply.

Amino acids have many uses. A large proportion of them are rebuilt into large protein molecules, but this time into human proteins, not beef, egg or lentil proteins. These proteins may be used for structural purposes, such as building the myo-proteins of your muscles, the collagen of your connective tissues or other protein-rich tissues such as your various organs. Some are functional proteins, of which enzymes are an important example. All enzymes are proteins, and the blueprint for their formation comes from information in your genes, in the DNA of the nuclei in your cells. Enzymes catalyse a multitude of reactions within your body. In fact, most such reactions simply would not happen without the facilitation of their respective enzymes. These enzymes are helped in turn by coenzymes, the essential nutrients that come from your diet. Most, but not all, of these coenzymes are vitamins and minerals. Some amino acids are used to build hormones. Some of your hormones are steroids, and so technically are lipids, the others, such as the thyroid hormones or adrenalin are based on individual amino acids; others still, such as insulin, are larger protein molecules. A third role for amino acids is as sources of neurotransmitters, such as adrenalin, which send chemical signals to other cells and tissues.

If you have consumed more protein than you need for your specific protein requirements, the remainder, in the form of the various amino acids, is then broken down into ammonia, carbon dioxide and water and the energy contained within the amino acid is released. Some of these amino acids, once the amino group has been removed, break down to produce acetyl groups, others enter the Krebs Cycle at various stages around the circuit.

A Brief Summary of Energy Production from Food

- Nearly all **carbohydrates** are eventually converted to glucose (xylitol is an exception).

- Glucose is process in the anaerobic cytosol by the E-M pathway and becomes acetyl groups with a small release of energy.

- Acetyl groups are broken down in the aerobic mitochondria via the Krebs Cycle, to carbon dioxide and water with a large release of energy.

- The major components of **lipids** are the fatty acids.

- Fatty acids are processed in the mitochondria by beta-oxidation and then via the Krebs Cycle with a large release of energy.

- **Proteins** break down to amino acids. Amino acids that are not wanted for protein building are broken down in the aerobic mitochondria via the Krebs Cycle, into which they slot in different positions with the release of varying relatively small amounts of energy.

Thus it is in the mitochondria that the majority of the energy is released from glucose and lipids and a small amount is obtained from any spare amino acids. Some cells, those with little to do, have only a few mitochondria, others can have many thousands of mitochondria. Energy release in the cytosol comes almost entirely from glucose. This is an important fact to keep in mind.

High Energy Compounds

Energy is powerful stuff, and it has to be handled gently. You cannot simply release the energy from foods in a burst and then hope to be able to use it in exactly the way that you want, any more than you can set off a nuclear explosion and expect to be able to harness that energy for the production of useable electricity. We saw above that the ultimate, and most useful, quanta of energy is that contained in a molecule called ATP. This is equivalent to your domestic rechargeable batteries, and ATP can deliver its energy to any reaction site where energy is required for the reaction to take place. However, all the energy produced by the Krebs Cycle is not in this form, some of it is in the form of higher energy compounds, containing amounts of energy intermediate between that of the acetyl group at the start and the ultimate ATP group.

During the reactions within the Krebs Cycle:

- low energy NAD is charged up, by the energy that is being released, stepwise, from the starting acetyl group, to high energy $NADH_2$;
- this then goes through a series of reactions known as oxidative phosphorylation and the electron transport system, and as a result of this three molecules of low energy ADP are converted to three molecules of high energy ATP. This, at last, is a manageable amount of energy that can be put to general use;
- low energy FAD is converted into high energy $FADH_2$;
- this converts two molecules of ADP into two of ATP, also by oxidative phosphorylation.

The reason for discussing these complex reaction sequences in detail is to emphasise the need for certain trace nutrients. Oxidative phosphorylation has an absolute requirement for the trace minerals, iron and copper, for vitamins B2 (in FAD) and B3 (in NAD), and for oxygen, needed to convert the released hydrogen (H) to water, the final chemical end product.

So when you are told to make sure you get significant amounts of the B group vitamins to avoid fatigue and to breathe more deeply and to exercise, to inhale more oxygen, you will now know at least part of the reason why these actions are important. Further nutrient needs are described in the rest of this chapter.

More on the Pivotal Step

It is time now to explore the Pivotal Step (above) in further detail. Even in healthy non-cancerous cells, this step can be blocked or slowed down by a number of different factors.

The first blockage can occur at the Pivotal Step itself. It can happen when the essential cofactors, vitamin B1, vitamin B3, vitamin B5, magnesium, manganese and lipoic acid are unavailable in fully adequate amounts. This is one of the reasons you may have been advised to take a good B complex supplement when you feel tired, although on its own it may not be sufficient as other nutrients are also needed. It is also why you have been advised to ensure that you have a healthy digestion system and that you are absorbing all the nutrients you obtain, both from your food and from supplements. Toxins can interfere here too, such as the toxic elements, antimony, arsenic and mercury. Arsenic, for instance, combines with lipoic acid and renders it out of action[19]. This Pivotal Step can also be inhibited by anything that slows down the Krebs Cycle as the entire reaction sequence is then backed up.

For those that are interested in the details the steps in the cycle are as follows:

(Acetyl +) oxaloacetate → citric acid → cis-aconitic acid → isocitric acid → oxalosuccinic acid → alpha-ketoglutaric acid → succinyl CoA → succinic acid → fumaric acid → malic acid → oxaloacetic acid.

There can be blockages in the mitochondrial reactions in the Krebs Cycle itself. You need biotin, also known as vitamin B7 or vitamin H, to ensure there is an adequate supply of oxaloacetate[20]. Not every cycle is perfect and sometimes the oxaloacetic acid is not returned to the start, so replacement is needed. This is produced from some of the pyruvic acid in a reaction catalysed by biotin-dependent pyruvate carboxylase. Without an adequate availability of oxaloacetate, the acetyl groups cannot even get started on the cycle. Unless there are inherited metabolic disorders, you derive almost all of your biotin from the beneficial organisms in your digestive tract, but if you take antibiotics you kill off most of these.

The full process of the cycle is one of oxidation. Oxygen has to be available to be added to the carbon atoms in the acetyl groups and convert them into carbon dioxide, and you need more oxygen to add to the hydrogen atoms in the acetyl groups and convert them into water. This is one of the reasons that exercise is so important, as is regular deep rather than shallow breathing.

More trace nutrients are needed, for two major reasons. Some are needed for the cycle itself to function, others are needed for the various steps round the cycle in which the energy from that particular step is being used to convert low energy ADP (see above) into high energy ATP, as in oxidative phosphorylation described above. The cycle itself needs several trace nutrients such as vitamin B1, B2, B3, B5, and manganese.

A large number of toxins can inhibit the cycle. A few examples will suffice. Fluorocitrate, a rodent poison can block the cycle completely, hence its use as a poison. It inhibits the enzyme that catalyses the step from citric acid to cis-aconitic acid. Antimony, arsenic and mercury also interfere with this step, and with the step from alpha-ketoglutaric acid to succinic acid. Aluminium hinders the step from iso-citric acid to alpha-ketoglutaric acid. Tartaric acid inhibits the cycle at the malic acid point. Many fungicides inhibit succinic dehydrogenase that catalyses the conversion of succinic acid to fumaric acid.

These few examples should be enough to alert you to the vital need to both avoid taking in toxins, and incorporate detox procedures into your life so as to eliminate toxins that are already present. The fact that many pesticides can interfere with the Krebs Cycle should encourage you to choose organically grown and produced foods.

If any of the following occurs if:

(a) you are deficient in the nutrients needed for the Krebs Cycle;
(b) the cycle is blocked by toxins;
(c) you do heavy (anaerobic) exercise and use up all your cellular oxygen, faster than your blood can deliver a new supply from your lungs,

then several things happen:

(a) mitochondrial aerobic oxidation stops;
(b) glucose breakdown does not go past the Pivotal Point;
(c) instead the pyruvic acid is converted into lactic acid.

This build up of lactic acid:

(a) means you have to stop moving your muscle;
(b) generates the state which runners talk of, for instance, when they have 'hit the wall'. They simply cannot keep moving, not, at least, until they 'get their breath back' (restore their oxygen supply) at the cellular level;
(c) cannot be metabolised within the cell in which it was produced. It has to be transported out of the cell and via the bloodstream to the liver where it is reconverted into glucose by a process that requires the input of energy;
(d) if it is the l-lactic acid form, stimulates mitosis (cellular division and reproduction) in cancer cells and so increases the speed of tumour growth.

It is common to find in cancerous tissue that the mitochondria are damaged[21, 22], not working properly[23], or not working at all. This has several consequences including:

(a) glucose becomes the cell's only energy source;
(b) only a very small amount of energy is produced (around 5-10% of that contained in glucose);

(c) the energy comes from the cytosol conversion of glucose to pyruvic acid. This greatly reduces the amount of energy the cells can produce, and this is why fatigue and exhaustion are so often a devastating part of the disease, particularly in the latter stages when the ever-increasing number of cancer cells is gobbling up all the available glucose and using it inefficiently, while all the healthy cells are being starved;

(d) the cancer cells are constantly 'sugar hungry';

(e) without functioning mitochondria, cancer cells can derive almost no energy from fats and proteins, thus further focusing their requirements on the availability of glucose.

Lactic acid itself poses a problem in that it:

(a) provides cancer cells with a form of fuel they can use;

(b) encourages the process of mitosis (see below) and the formation of more cancer cells.

There are different types of lactic acid, the dextrorotatory or normal lactic acid (d-lactic acid) and the levorotatory (l-lactic acid) or bad lactic acid, and we will be discussing these further, in a later chapter [Chapter 11]. The d-lactic acid is produced during anaerobic exercise when oxygen intake is insufficient for the production of the energy demanded by the activity. It can be converted back into glucose in the liver relatively easily. The harmful l- form of lactic acid is produced by cancer cells and encourages mitosis, part of the process by which the DNA in the nuclei of the cell divides into single strands, each of which can then make a new partner for themselves. Following this, the nucleus and then the cell can divide into two new daughter cells. If these are cancer cells then increased mitosis encourages the rapid production of more of these unwelcome biochemical problems, and more cancer cells.

A discussion of tests and corrections follows at the end of the next chapter as there is more to discuss on this topic first.

CHAPTER 9

OXYGEN DEPRIVATION AND DR. OTTO WARBURG

The ultimate cause of cancer and of all its manifestation was, for Nobel Prize winner and physiologist Dr. Otto Warburg, back in 1931, a lack of oxygen at the cellular level[24]. Healthy human cells absolutely have to have oxygen to survive. Cancer cells can live without *any* oxygen and actually prefer, or thrive best, in an anaerobic environment. For Dr. Warburg this was a critical distinction between healthy cells and cancer cells.

Dr. Warburg was arguably one of the best cell biologists of the last century. He was among the first to suggest that the development of cancer cells and their evolution into a tumour are a consequence of the fact that cancer cells derive their energy, their ATP units, from the anaerobic (or, as he called it, fermenting) breakdown of glucose along the E-M pathway, whereas healthy cells, as we have seen, get almost all of their ATP units from the aerobic Krebs Cycle.

He then postulated it was the lack of oxygen that caused the healthy cells, which utilised both the anaerobic E-M pathway *and* the aerobic Krebs Cycle for energy, to revert to using only the E-M pathway[25]. He stated that, "*…the cause of cancer is no longer a mystery, we know it occurs whenever any cell is denied 60% of its oxygen requirements,*" [26] and "*Cancer, above all other diseases, has countless secondary causes. But, even for cancer, there is only one prime cause… the prime cause of cancer is the replacement of the respiration of oxygen in normal body cells by a fermentation of sugar.*" [27]

Every time Dr. Warburg took healthy cells, put them in a controlled laboratory environment and totally deprived them of oxygen he found that they had turned into cancer cells. They reverted back to being primitive or undifferentiated cells [Chapter 14], eminently capable of multiplying to form a tumour. Warburg then went a step further and suggested that cancer was the result of poor or failed activity of the mitochondria, as a consequence of the oxygen deprivation. Modern research is proving Warburg's theory[28]. An alternative theory is that it is fundamentally mitochondrial damage, rather than oxygen deprivation, that leads to cancer[29]. However, it is known that if mitochondria of any cells are deprived of oxygen for an extended period of time they suffer irreversible damage[30]. In fact, the two are almost inextricably linked, and the solution to the two problems is similar. You should aim to improve mitochondrial functions and increase the oxygen availability within the cells. Whichever comes first, mitochondrial damage or oxygen deprivation, there is also evidence that a high level of oxygen inhibits the growth of cancer cells[31].

While reverting to fermentation and the E-M pathway may allow these cells to survive, it disables many of their functions including their ability to communicate with other cells or receive communications (or restrictions) from other cells. Thus, they are free and able to multiply without restriction, according to their own nature, and they become cancer cells.

There are many reasons why cells become oxygen deficient. In Chapter 11 we will learn of Dr. Fryda's theory that cancer is the result of adrenal stress, adrenalin deficiency and so reduced oxygen delivery to cells.

Many toxins (a Predisposing Factor), and carcinogens, inhibit mitochondrial oxidation enzymes[32]. If these substances are present, the cell's ability to utilise oxygen is reduced. Such toxins may also adversely affect receptor sites on cell membranes so that the oxygen cannot be received or enter the cells, or they may damage the cell membranes. This latter can come about if your diet is deficient in lecithin (as found in egg yolk) and the essential fatty acids within it, especially ALA (alpha-linolenic acid) the omega-3 fatty acid (essential fatty acid deficiencies are a Predisposing Factor). Alternatively, there may be a lack of the nutrients needed for cellular respiration (nutrient deficiencies are another Predisposing Factor). Lack of exercise and poor breathing habits can reduce the fundamental availability of oxygen in the bloodstream, as can anaemia and a lack of haemoglobin.

Once cells have turned cancerous and produced lactic acid it is the l-lactic acid form. This in turn tends to prevent the transport of oxygen into nearby healthy cells.

Based on his own ideas, Warburg suggested that the appropriate treatment for cancer should consist of 3 steps.

Firstly, all the cells should be saturated with oxygen.

This can be helped by aerobic exercise which offers several benefits:

- it increases the breathing rate and hence the intake of oxygen;
- it increases the amount of oxygen attached to the haemoglobin in the red blood cells;
- it stimulates the flow of blood around the body;
- it opens up the fine capillaries so that oxygen-rich blood reaches all the cells, not just those adjacent to the larger blood vessels.

He stated that it was important, *"...to keep the speed of the bloodstream so high that the venous blood still contains SUFFICIENT OXYGEN."*[33]

The second step should be the removal of all toxins.

There are several levels of toxins.

(a) some toxins are identified as direct carcinogens;
(b) some toxins interfere with reactions and, as a result, cells can turn cancerous, e.g. those that interfere with the Krebs Cycle;
(c) some toxins interfere with the liver and inhibit its ability to deal with both the active metabolism required of it and its ability to deal with toxins in general.

All these, and other effects of toxins can have knock-on effects in relation to physical health and mental and emotional states, decisions and actions.

Warburg believed that such toxins reduced cellular respiration either directly or indirectly by deranging capillary circulation and blocking mitochondrial function. We have learnt more since Warburg's day and now know that the mitochondria are even more important than he postulated in controlling both cell behaviours and preventing or reversing cancer.

His third step involved providing the body with the 'active groups' needed by the mitochondria.

What Warburg called 'active groups' would today be recognised as the various vitamins and trace elements that are now known as the coenzymes required for a number of the enzyme-catalysed steps in the Pivotal Step and the Krebs Cycle. Warburg was working and writing in the 1930s and the various vitamins were being discovered during that decade and beyond. 'Active fractions' derived from rice bran and other food sources had been recognised for some years, but the individual vitamins were being isolated and their chemical structures determined while Warburg was working and putting forward his theory on cancer causation (e.g. vitamin B1 in 1926 up to vitamin B12 in 1948).

Warburg was of the opinion that increasing the consumption of these active groups, these trace nutrients, would benefit the healthy cells, particularly their mitochondria, and reduce the conversion of healthy cells into cancer cells. However, he thought it was unlikely that they would help fight a tumour once it was formed as the tumour would be almost entirely anaerobic and function well in spite of their absence. He therefore suggested the surgical removal of all detected major tumours.

Not all tumour cells function anaerobically. Those that are adjacent to blood capillaries generally have sufficient oxygen that they can both metabolise glucose normally, like healthy cells, and metabolise lactate, like cancer cells. This means that early, or small, metastatic clusters can function aerobically as the majority of their cells are able to be close to the surface. Warburg therefore felt that they could be treated by taking the largest possible amounts of the active groups, the vitamins and minerals, for many years, maybe for ever. Keep in mind that the concentrated supplements, whether synthetic or food based, available today were not available then.

Following on from this concept, we can come to understand possible reasons for the increasing incidence of cancer over recent decades. The high level of air pollution, resulting from traffic fumes, cigarette smoke, industrial gases and more, leads to increased levels of carbon monoxide in the air. This gas cannot be smelled but can be lethal. It combines with the haemoglobin in your red blood cells more readily than does oxygen and so, even when present in small quantities, decreases the amount of oxygen that can be carried through your body and to the cells, and thus reduces the activity of the mitochondrial Krebs Cycle, but not the cytoplasmic E-M pathway. Further problems are caused when you do not do regular aerobic exercise, and fail to breathe deeply or use your full lung capacity. In addition, we are daily exposed to the toxins that inhibit mitochondrial function and the modern diet is woefully deficient in the active groups, or vitamins and minerals, needed by the mitochondria. No wonder cancer is becoming increasingly common.

We can also come to a better understanding of the poor results obtained by the common medical cancer treatments. Low oxygen levels in cells not only make the cancer more aggressive, they cause resistance to radiation therapy, and make many forms of chemotherapy less effective. Thus, the treatments act more powerfully, and damagingly, on healthy cells than on cancer cells[34].

As a result of their reliance on the E-M pathway and the resulting production of lactic acid as the end product of their energy production, cancer cells are more acidic and so have a lower pH than healthy cells.

Reducing the glucose available to cancer cells

As we have seen, the E-M pathway, on its own, is a hugely inefficient method of generating the energy that cancer cells need and, as a result, they are desperate for glucose. Remember, to help them get it they have many more times the number of receptor sites for it compared to healthy cells, so they can take it in from the blood faster than can the healthy cells as they all, in a sense, compete for the glucose flowing past them in the bloodstream. So every time you are tempted to eat sugar, or refined carbohydrates such as white flour, pasta or rice, or to drink soft drinks or fruit juices, or (if you already have cancer) eat fruits, other than the berries, which are rich in protective nutrients and low in sugar[35], keep this in mind as all this glucose, no matter where it comes from, feeds cancer cells. As cancer cells become more active and as more of them are formed, they take an increasing proportion of the glucose and there is less and less glucose available for energy production in the cells of the rest of your body. Eating more sugar or glucose is not the answer to your fatigue as this simply feeds the cancer cells; starving your body of glucose is not the answer either as healthy cells do need some glucose for energy[36].

So remember, the solution is to eat large amounts of vegetables, especially above ground, low-starch vegetables, and drink the same vegetables, juiced. This will provide sufficient glucose to keep the Krebs Cycle going in your healthy cells. It will also provide you with the maximum amounts of vitamins, minerals and other valuable phytonutrients for a minimum intake of glucose. Then, get the rest of your energy from the fat-rich foods already listed in Chapter 25 such as nuts and avocados.

Keep in mind that the optimum solution, if you have cancer, or to assist in the prevention of cancer, is to eat in such a way that there is a steady supply of a small amount of glucose into your bloodstream, as indicated by a normal blood glucose level (BSL), and that this level never rises much above normal or drops too far below the normal level. This is why you are advised to eat foods with a low glycemic index. There are many lists of the glycemic index of foods, and many are contradictory. The concept is good, the details may be confusing. The best answer is to follow the suggestions already given here.

Foods with a low glycemic index break down slowly in the digestive tract into glucose which then trickles, over an extended period of time, into the bloodstream. This is the scenario that gives the healthy cells their best chance to grab their share of the glucose that is temporarily available and prevents a sudden glut of glucose which would continue to feed the ever-hungry cancer cells.

Even if you are a sugarholic, these guidelines do not translate into eating a small piece of a candy bar at spaced intervals rather than eating a whole candy bar in one sitting. Keep your permitted carbohydrate intake to those that you obtain from vegetables and berries. You can achieve the desired outcome by eating no sugar but concentrating instead on complex carbohydrates, particularly those found in vegetables. You have absolutely no nutritional requirement for sugar. You can live perfectly well without it. The instruction to eat no sugar means that you should eat no six-carbon sugars, whether singly, like glucose (or dextrose), fructose (or levulose), mannose or galactose, or as dimers such as sucrose (table sugar), lactose (milk sugar) or maltose (from grains). It also means you should avoid sugars that hide behind the various safe-sounding names dreamt up by the ever-inventive food industry. These include evaporated cane juice, corn syrup, malt, maltodextrin, agave, brown rice syrup (brown or white rice, it is the starch that is used to produce the glucose), fruit syrups, fruit sugar (the word fruit does not make the sugar any safer) maltodextrins, or as many of the other clever ways that food manufacturers have evolved of sweetening foods with dangerous sugars yet calling them 'sugar-free'.

Five-carbon sugars are permitted and these include the monosaccharides ribose and xylitol. They are metabolised very differently to six-carbon sugars. They are not converted into glucose within the body, they do not depend on insulin for their metabolism, and they do not feed cancer cells. Xylitol is made from the fibre found in many fruits and vegetables, including berries, corn husks, oats and mushrooms. It can now be bought at many health food shops. It looks and tastes almost exactly like sucrose, so if you must have 'something sweet' use it. However, it still provides 'empty calories', providing no beneficial nutrients and replacing some other nutrient-rich food in your diet, so use it sparingly. A few people find, that in large quantities, it may cause diarrhoea. On the plus side, xylitol both improves your calcium absorption and does not lead to acid production in the mouth, as sucrose does, thus benefiting your teeth in two ways[37, 38]. Ribose can also be used and can help to give you energy. It is part of RNA and the high energy compound ATP.

Remember, complex carbohydrates such as those found in vegetables break down slowly in the digestive system and lead to the desired slow trickle of glucose into your bloodstream. Potatoes and parsnips are an exception to this and they have a high glycemic index. The starch found in whole grains is broken down fairly slowly. However, the starch in refined grains such as white rice and white flour breaks down much more rapidly and can lead to a surge in your blood sugar level. Thus, if you have cancer, or if it is suspected, vegetables and whole(meal) grains become the most desirable carbohydrate food. However, vegetables win out handsomely over the grains in that they also provide a wide range of phytonutrients such as vitamins, minerals and bioflavonoids, far more than are found in grains. This may sound repetitious, however it is an important point to drive home, and I have found that it can be some time, and only after many tellings, that patients pay full attention to this and recognise its absolute importance.

TESTS

Following on from this and the previous chapter, it is time to consider which tests you can use to assess the situation in relation to mitochondrial function and the degree of anaerobic activity of your cells. Several tests are helpful:

Optimal Nutritional Evaluation or the ONE Test.

One of the early tests you should do involves checking on your fundamental, normal cellular activity as it pertains to energy production. You need to know whether or not the various pathways are all working and are doing so to their optimal best. For that to happen you need to have all the nutrients you need to ensure that all the transformations of compound A to compound B to compound C etc., are working correctly. You also need to check for any evidence of possible toxins that could be causing problems. An excellent test that provides this information is the Optimum Nutrition Evaluation or the ONE Test. This test is offered by Genova Diagnostics Laboratory.

Lactic acid (d- and l- forms)

You can test for your levels of both d-lactic acid and l-lactic acid. A raised level of d-lactic acid will warn you that there may be a blockage at the Pivotal Point. If this is the case, the results you obtained from the ONE Test could help to pinpoint the problem.

A raised level of l-lactic acid is more dangerous and should warn you that there could be the start of the development of cancer cells and that whatever you are doing it is encouraging their further development.

Neuro-Lab offers you both of these tests as do some other laboratories, so ask around or listen to your therapist's advice.

PHI

In general, as we have seen, when cancer is developing there is a gradual failure of mitochondrial activity and increased energy reliance on the E-M pathway, at least in the affected cells. In their effort to deal with this increasing demand for, or activity of, the E-M pathway, the cells produce more of the enzymes that facilitate the reactions along this pathway. One of these enzymes is phosphohexose isomerase or PHI. This enzyme catalyses one of the rearrangements steps in the E-M pathway.

The transformed cells or trophoblastic cells, cells with increased anaerobic activity, contain increased amounts of this enzyme and in addition they secrete increased amounts into the bloodstream. Thus, if the blood level of PHI rises this is suggestive of anaerobic activity and the probable development of cancerous cells. It can readily be measured in the blood.

The level of PHI can be elevated when cancer is first developing or when an active tumour is present. However, it can also be elevated in some other conditions, and it is important to remember this. It can be raised immediately following a heart attack or severe muscular trauma or in severe hypothyroidism (not low-grade chronic hypothyroidism), AIDS[39] or viral hepatitis[40]. In relation to the latter it has been compared to other enzymes including aldolase, isocitric dehydrogenase and pyruvic transaminase[41] and used in the differential diagnosis of liver disease[42].

If none of these conditions apply and if your PHI level is high then it could be caused by the Cancer Process[43, 44, 45, 46, 47]. PHI, for instance, was found to be more useful than two other enzymes, alkaline phosphatase or glutamic oxaloacetic transaminase, in detecting early lung cancer[48].

Take Your Time

The first thought many people have when they hear the diagnosis of cancer is, *"Cut it out, get it out of me, stop it spreading."* There is the fear that every moment longer that the tumour is *in situ* increases the risk of it spreading to other sites and that once it has been surgically removed, especially if they 'got it all', the risk of any future metastasis has been stopped. However, there is now evidence that this may not be true. In fact, there is growing evidence that by the time the tumour has been detected cancer cells may already have spread to other sites where they may be lying dormant until such time as they are triggered, by whatever mechanism, into reproduction and growth[49].

Conventional wisdom has it that the dispersion and spread of cancer cells to other sites, at a distance from the primary tumour location, occurs relatively late in the disease progression. However, the results of recent research[50] suggest that cancer cells may spread around the body much earlier than was previously thought[51]. It is now thought possible that normal cells can carry cancer cells to new sites and lie dormant until the key genes are activated. These findings help to explain why some metastatic tumours can develop long after the original one has been removed together with a wide margin of clear or healthy tissue surrounding it.

If this was more widely known, then perhaps people would take a little time to consider their options, and come to a more rational decision as to which course of action they would follow, instead of rushing, or allowing themselves to be rushed, headlong by the medical system, into actions they might later regret.

More on PHI

Clearly these findings reduce the value of rushing into surgery. They also increase the value of prevention and of testing and monitoring your health. There is good news, and this relates to PHI and the importance of testing for it, in a prevention panel. The level of PHI in the blood can rise as much as fourteen years before a conventional tumour diagnosis[52]. This means that if you have this test done at regular intervals you can 'nip the problem in the bud', or set about restoring your health, many years before any tumour is detected.

There is more to know about PHI. Not only is it indicative of increased E-M pathway activity in the cell's cytosol, and so of the possibility that the cell is turning cancerous, raised levels actually have further negative consequences. In 1996 the structure of a compound known as tumour cell autocrine motility factor (AMF) was determined. Autocrine substances are ones that act on the cells that produced them. AMF was found to be the same thing as PHI[53]. The authors also state that, *"AMF was detected in a major proportion of lung carcinomas, and may play a part not only in proliferation and/or progression of the tumours, but also, possibly, in the differentiation of squamous cell carcinoma."*

It is now clear that PHI, once it is present in excess, is not only an indicator of faulty or cancerous cells, but that it also creates or exacerbates further problems. It (usually referred to in research papers as AMF) inhibits apoptosis, the voluntary suicide of unhealthy or faulty cells, including cancer cells.

Many substances are needed to turn healthy cells into unhealthy ones and to protect them from harm and facilitate their survival. These substances include hepatocyte growth factor (HGF)[54], fibroblast growth factor (FGF)[55], insulin growth factor (IGF)[56], nerve growth factor (NGF)[57], and specific cytokines[58]. It is now suggested that PHI/AMF also contributes to this process, in part by increasing the cell's resistance to apoptosis. When AMF-affected cells were inoculated into mice, tumours formed, the cell proliferation rate doubled and there was increased resistance to apoptotic agents[59]. There have been other reports of AMF (PHI) induced resistance to apoptosis. When, for instance, the anticancer apoptotic drug mitomycin C was used, the AMF-affected cells were found to be resistant to it[60].

Many compounds lead to, or stimulate angiogenesis, or the building of new blood vessels. This process is needed not only for wound healing and repair, but for the growth of the additional blood vessels that are needed by a tumour to feed the individual cells within it. Angiogenic factors include fibroblast growth factor (FGF), tumour necrosis factor (TNF-alpha), transforming growth factor (TGF-beta) and vascular endothelial growth factor (VEGF)[61, 62, 63]. The most important of these is VEGF[64, 65]. AMF has been found to increase the production and activity of VEGF[66].

PHI, or AMF, causes a further problem. Either directly or indirectly it increases permeability and thus increases the accumulation of ascites[67], leading to a build up of fluid in the abdomen. Thus, an increased level of PHI both suggests that cells have turned cancerous, and contributes to the further development of cancer by inhibiting apoptosis and increasing angiogenesis and inducing ascites.

Dr. Schandl of American Metabolic Laboratories has suggested that the biochemical initiator of metastasis is PHI or autocrine motility factor (AMF), and that elevated plasma levels of PHI may lead to metastatic events such as cytokinetic vibration and dislodgement of the cancerous cell from its neighbouring environment and consequent embolism via lymph or blood flow to distant sites[68].

American Metabolic Laboratories (www.caprofile.net) include a test for PHI in their Cancer Profile. It can also be ordered from them as an individual test.

TM2-PK or Tumour Marker 2

Pyruvate Kinase (PK) is, as its name suggests, an enzyme related to the activity of pyruvic acid. In fact it is the enzyme that catalyses the final stage of the production of pyruvic acid, the precursor to the acetyl groups, prior to the start of the mitochondrial aerobic activity. Magnesium is essential for the function of this enzyme, but its activity is hindered by calcium.

The normal form of pyruvate kinase has four protein subunits. An altered and abnormal form of this enzyme is known as tumour marker 2-pyruvate kinase or TM2-PK. It is similar to pyruvate kinase (PK) but has only two protein subunits instead of the normal four. It is produced in increased amounts by un-differentiated or proliferating tissues, including a number of cancer cell types. Its production is thought to be due to the different metabolic requirements of cancer cells. It enables the cells to use a metabolic shortcut that saves energy which is then used for cellular replication[69].

An increase of the amount of TM2-PK in the blood can indicate a variation in the activity of the normal E-M pathway. Raised levels of TM2-PK have been found in the blood of people with solid tumours and this test has, for instance, been used with considerable success to distinguish between benign and malignant cervical tumours[70]. The level of TM2-PK has been shown to increase with disease progression and tumour stage in lung cancer[71]. It has been suggested as a better marker than CA19-9 and CEA in gastrointestinal cancer[72].

However, like PHI, TM2-PK is not raised only in cancer cells[73]. The amount present can also be increased in other conditions where there are problems with normal cellular glucose metabolism. So although this test is helpful, it is even more useful if the results are viewed in conjunction with the results of all the other tests you have done, and for this interpretation you will need professional advice. This test is offered at Neuro-Lab (www.neuro-lab.com).

There will be more references to these tests later, in other appropriate chapters. As we go through the material ahead you will come across a number of other tests. While each one, individually, is important, the most secure information is obtained by taking them all together and obtaining a more complete indication of your overall metabolism and any possible problems.

Solutions

Fatty acids break down to acetyl groups directly, and not via pyruvic acid, and so they do not produce lactic acid with its attendant risks. Thus, if there are problems with any of the above tests it is a good reason to reduce your intake of carbohydrates and obtain a large amount of your energy input from high fat foods. These should not, of course, contain the very long chain saturated animal fats, nor should they be overheated fats such as occur in fried foods or crisps, or the processed vegetable oils derived from hard seeds. Nor should they include dairy fats unless these come from organically-reared and grass-fed animals. Good sources of dietary lipids (oils or fats) are raw nuts, avocados, olives, coconut oil and flaxseed oil. These, plus large quantities of vegetables and some lean fish or similar protein, form the basis of some of the most commonly recommended diets.

An important aim should be to restore mitochondrial function. Many substances and activities offer such possibilities:

- increase your intake of the coenzymes needed for the Pivotal Point. These include lipoic acid, magnesium and vitamins B1, B2, B3;

- increase your intake of vitamin B5, it is needed for the step after the Pivotal Point;

- increase your intake of the B group vitamins in general, as almost all of them are needed for the Krebs Cycle in the mitochondria. This includes biotin which is needed to get the Krebs Cycle started;

- make good any other nutrient deficiencies involved in glucose metabolism, such as chromium, vanadium, zinc, magnesium and manganese;

- a number of phytonutrients, from a range of vegetables and dark-coloured fruits, can assist in this process so increase your intake of these foods;

- exercise: this increases the flow of oxygen to the cells;

- make a habit of deep breathing rather than shallow breathing, this also increases the flow of oxygen to the cells. In addition it can have a beneficial effect on your mood;

- reduce stress to improve oxygenation;

- increase your intake of the essential fatty acids, generally in the form of flaxseed oil combined with appropriate protein [Chapter 17].

CHAPTER 10

DEFICIENT MITOCHONDRIA

Since the time of Otto Warburg, other researchers have followed the concept of oxygen deprivation as the cause of cancer. Goldblatt and Cameron[74] were able to show that fibroblasts (cells) from the heart became cancer cells when they were deprived of oxygen, but not otherwise.

The experimental work of cancer scientist and researcher Dr. Paul Gerhardt Seeger, as early as 1938, showed that most cancers start in the mitochondria and the cytosol[75]. Part of the mitochondrial breakdown of the acetyl groups as they are passed along the Krebs Cycle discussed above, [Chapter 8] involves a side sequence of reactions called the 'respiratory chain'. One of the enzymes involved in this respiratory chain is called cytochrome oxidase. Like all enzymes it is a protein, in this case a trans-membrane protein. In other words, it sits in and penetrates right through the membrane of each mitochondrion. Seeger showed that in cancer cells this enzyme is largely missing. He also showed that when he took healthy cells and artificially destroyed their cytochrome oxidase they turned into cancer cells.

You now know that this means that these mitochondria are then blocked or not functioning, that the cell has to rely totally on anaerobic energy production in the cytosol, and that this in turn leads to the production of large amounts of lactic acid. The more lactic acid produced by a tumour, or the cancer cells within it, the more aggressive the cancer becomes. Aggressive cancers that produce large amounts of l-lactic acid can generally evade the actions of your immune system. Less aggressive cancers, that produce less l-lactic acid, are more likely to be detected and dealt with by your immune system when it is appropriately stimulated. This lactic acid is a major contributor to the acidity of the tissues.

Others have stated that the ultimate cause of cancer is mitochondrial malfunction, not oxygen deprivation[76], though ultimately it may be a case of 'the chicken or the egg' since the mitochondria cannot function without oxygen and, without functioning mitochondria, the oxygen delivered to the cell is of little use. However, we now know that there are many important differences between the structure and function of mitochondria in healthy cells and those in cancer cells[77], and this topic and the various mechanisms by which mitochondrial dysfunction can lead to cancer have been reviewed in some detail[78].

A considerable body of research puts mitochondrial dysfunction as the cause of cancer and an increased risk of metastasis[79]. Mitochondrial problems have been related to specific types of cancer, such as breast cancer[80] and prostate cancer. In fact, the level of mitochondrial dysfunction has been suggested as a prognostic tool to determine the probable progression of prostate cancer with higher levels of mitochondrial dysfunction being found to be associated with increased malignancy[81]. Mitochondrial dysfunction can be viewed as an age-related disease following on from damage caused to the mitochondria by reactive oxygen species (ROS)[82] and a wide range of other causes, and leading to metastatic cancer.

Mitochondrial damage and overall health

In a broader context, there are now suggestions that mitochondrial dysfunction may be a contributing factor to a large number of degenerative diseases, as well as cancer[83, 84]. Mitochondrial damage has been shown to contribute to, or aggravate, atherosclerosis[85], heart disease[86], strokes[87], type 2 diabetes[88], brain and nervous system disorders, and neurological degeneration[89], including Alzheimer's disease[90] and Parkinson's disease[91]. It has been postulated to play a role in rheumatoid arthritis[92], fibromyalgia[93], allergic asthma[94] and many other health problems, too numerous to list. Finally, mitochondrial damage in stem cells can lead to unhealthy stem cells[95] and you will read about these and their importance in relation to cancer in Chapters 14 and 15.

This adds weight to the view that whether or not you have cancer you should make all the sensible lifestyle changes suggested here. These will, in all probability, reduce your risk of developing many, if not all, of the most feared diseases of aging, including cancer, heart disease, strokes and senility. When there are so many positive outcomes to a suggested programme for the restoration of good health, it adds great weight to the probable correctness and benefit of that programme.

Consequences of mitochondrial dysfunction

Much more could be said about mitochondrial dysfunction, but we will return to our original discussion and expand on the cellular metabolism of glucose and specifically how it relates to cancer. As we have discovered, as a result of the failure of mitochondrial function, cancer cells convert the pyruvic acid derived via glycolysis from glucose into l-lactic acid. This lactic acid can be rebuilt into glucose, mainly in the liver. However, very little energy is released during glycolysis in the E-M pathway and greater energy input is required to rebuild the lactic acid back into glucose. This means that cancer cells get no benefit from this recycling and they rely heavily on new intakes of sugar, in the form of glucose, for their energy.

In the healthy state, whenever there is spare glucose available to the cells it is taken up by the liver and built up into glycogen. Glycogen is the large carbohydrate molecule made up of hundreds or thousands of glucose units that was referred to earlier as 'animal starch'. Under normal circumstances this glycogen is then available for breakdown to energy when a sudden burst of activity is required. In fact your energy reserves can be thought of as becoming available to cells in the following sequence:

1. Firstly, there is the glucose circulating in your blood. This is available for immediate energy production, but the supply is limited and if the level were to fall too low you would pass out. So this is a short-term energy source, designed to smooth out sudden short-term needs.
2. Secondly, the glycogen stored in the liver is then called into play. It is broken down by glycogenolysis, into glucose which then leaves the liver and enters the blood where it replaces the glucose that has been drawn from the bloodstream by cells elsewhere. This glucose too is delivered to the cells that need it.
3. Thirdly, fat is drawn from your adipose tissue storage deposits. Unless you are very underweight there is an even greater amount of energy available from this source. However, it takes longer to

mobilise than the previous two sources. The triglycerides are released from the adipose tissues and broken down into fatty acids which are then taken up by individual cells and broken down to acetyl groups which, in turn, go through the Krebs Cycle, as we have seen.

Glycogen is found in muscle cells as well as in liver cells. The amount (per unit of muscle) is less than the amount in the liver but the total amount in your body, in this form, is greater as your body contains a large amount of muscle. However, not all of this glycogen is available for energy production. Much of it is part of your muscle structure.

As you will learn later [Chapter 11], Dr. Fryda believed that cancer, or the specific activity of cancer cells, is the cells' way of dealing with an excess of this glycogen (or animal starch) should it accumulate in the cells. She suggests that the cells actually turn cancerous as a way of dealing with excessive amounts of stored glycogen that, for whatever reason or malfunction, cannot be released. Why the excess glycogen is there in the first place you will learn about in the next chapter.

The reactions that occur in the mitochondria require large amounts of oxygen. Four atoms of oxygen are needed for each round of the Krebs Cycle as the two carbon atoms of the acetyl group are converted, by the end of the cycle, into two molecules of carbon dioxide. In the process a number of toxic free radicals are produced, and this is one of the reasons you need antioxidants, to protect you from these toxic oxygen species. You need oxygen, but it can also damage you. It has to be handled and processed carefully.

Oxygen is essential for the conversion of food into energy, the process known as oxidation, or, more accurately, oxidative metabolism. Food is made of similar material to the cells and tissues of your body, fats, proteins and carbohydrates. To prevent your own cells, and the mitochondria and other organelles in them, being oxidised, while you metabolise the food you have taken in, you have a number of antioxidant enzymes and they need their attendant coenzymes or helpers.

Because mitochondria contain such large amounts of oxygen they need particularly large amounts of antioxidant enzymes for self-protection from a variety of oxidising agents including oxygen, oxygen radicals and toxic superoxide radicals.

One of the most important of these antioxidant enzymes is superoxide dismutase, and to function correctly it needs adequate amounts of copper, manganese and zinc. It has been found that the mitochondria of cancer cells have unusually low levels of this protective superoxide dismutase and so are not protected from superoxides and other free radicals that are normally produced while the Krebs Cycle is operating[96, 97, 98, 99].

One possible scenario as to a cause or contributing factor of cancer is anti-oxidant deficiency which could lead to oxidative damage of the mitochondria. As a defence mechanism aimed at preventing this, the mitochondria shut down their high-level of oxygen-related activity and divert the cell to relying on the anaerobic E-M pathway for energy. In other words, according to this scenario, cancer can be considered to be a short-term solution to a cellular problem, a lack of protective anti-oxidant nutrients. The strategy works in the short term, but in the long term it may kill the host. This is one of the reasons that anti-oxidants are thought to be so important in the prevention and management of cancer.

The mitochondria of cancer cells have been found to be vulnerable to free-radical damage, both to their genes and DNA (mitochondrial DNA – mDNA), which are different to the genes of the rest of the cell that are housed mainly in the nucleus, and to the proteins for which the mitochondrial genes code[100].

Thus, oxidative damage can reduce the function and efficiency of the mitochondria. It can also block the entry of the acetyl groups into the mitochondria and so divert the pyruvic acid into the production of increased amounts of lactic acid.

One way to test the efficiency of the Krebs Cycle is to add one of its components to the mitochondria. This should trigger increased activity of the cycle, rather like using your hand to speed up a slowly spinning wheel. When, for instance, succinate was added to various cancer cell lines, there were almost none of the responses that would have been expected from healthy cells, indicating a pathological lack of mitochondrial activity. Supplementation with sodium succinate has also been shown to increase exercise performance[101, 102].

Proteins and fats in the mitochondria

So far we have focused on the breakdown of carbohydrates. What about fats and proteins? You now know that these both depend on the functioning of the Krebs Cycle for their complete breakdown [Chapter 8].

You will recall that proteins are made of amino acids. When their life is over, these amino acids are stripped of their nitrogen (as amino groups) which is excreted from the body, mainly as urea or ammonia. The rest of the molecule finds its way into a mitochondrion. Here it enters the Krebs Cycle at a point appropriate to its own structure.

Fats break down into the two-carbon acetyl groups, similar to those obtained from glucose. If they cannot enter the Krebs Cycle they move backwards and rebuild or form a variety of ketone bodies that are then excreted intact in the urine. These ketones are commonly present in the urine of people who are on a very high protein and low carbohydrate diet and the person does not consume sufficient carbohydrate to keep priming the Krebs Cycle. Ketones are found in the urine of people who are losing weight rapidly and burning body fat for energy, and are thus on, essentially, a high fat regime, and they are found in the urine of uncontrolled diabetics who are burning fat rather than taking glucose into the cells from the bloodstream.

This means that if the mitochondria of cancer cells are not functioning correctly they cannot fully burn fat or protein to produce significant amounts of energy. This further adds to the fatigue experienced by people with cancer.

However, there is a further consequence of this build up of ketones that can be helpful. The ketones can inhibit the controlling enzyme of the E-M pathway called phosphofructo kinase[103]. Far from inducing fatigue, this can have a beneficial outcome if cancer cells are present, as it can help to starve the cancer cells.

Studies on experimental animals have shown that reducing the caloric content of the diet can reduce both the incidence of cancer and can lead to tumour regression[104, 105, 106]. As this means that body fat is being oxidised for energy there will be a consequent rise in ketones and an induced reduction in the activity of the E-M pathway.

Cancer cells and energy

This mitochondrial failure leads us to a possible quandary. Cancer cells grow and replicate more rapidly than healthy cells. This is clear from the rapid growth of tumours compared to the surrounding healthy tissues. To achieve this rapid growth-rate cancer cells need a huge supply of energy. However, since cells normally derive 90 per cent or more of their energy from mitochondrial function and we now know that cancer cells have very little mitochondrial activity, possibly none, we have to wonder how they get the energy for their daily activity and this rapid growth-rate. You will not now be surprised at the phrases, 'cancer cells loves sugar' and 'sugar feeds cancer'. Cancer cells require very much larger amounts of glucose, by many orders of magnitude, than is required by health cells. How is this accomplished? Let's look at an overview.

Cancer cells have developed powerful strategies to steal far more than their fair share of the available glucose. There are several key players in this scenario and it is worth introducing them.

Cells normally take in glucose as a result of the action of the insulin produced by your pancreas. This insulin reacts with insulin receptor sites on the membrane of target cells and together they facilitate the entry of glucose into the cells. The amount of pancreas-derived insulin in the blood is the same for all cells, cancerous or healthy, so cancer cells have to find a way of obtaining more than their fair share.

Insulin is a protein hormone produced by the pancreas in response to a raised blood glucose level. It facilitates cellular uptake of glucose. For insulin to achieve this it has to find insulin receptor proteins on the membrane of the target cell[107]. In addition, there is another protein hormone that facilitates cellular uptake of glucose. It is called insulin-like growth factor-1 (IGF-1) and is produced by the liver. For IGF-1 to achieve its goal it has to find IGF-1 receptors (IGF-1R) on the membrane of the target cell[108].

IGF-1 is a powerful stimulator of cellular growth and reproduction and potent inhibitor of apoptosis (or cell death). These functions are beneficial in growth and development, and indeed IGF-1 is stimulated by growth hormone, but they are harmful in cancer[109,110]. (This is one reason to avoid processed foods to which growth hormone has been added in the production chain.)

Back to cancer cells and their voracious demand for glucose. Firstly, they have developed the ability to increase their number of insulin receptor sites. The average healthy cell has from 100-100,000 insulin receptor sites on its surface. Breast cancer cells, for instance, have more than six times as many insulin receptor sites, up to 600,000[111], thus benefiting disproportionately from the pancreas-produced insulin that is flowing past in the bloodstream[112].

Secondly, and to further increase their glucose uptake, cancer cells have learnt how to produce their own insulin and this obviously gives them a huge competitive advantage over your healthy cells when it comes to glucose uptake.

Thirdly, cancer cells are able to produce their own IGF-1 which not only increases their glucose uptake but is a known mitogen[113] and stimulates cellular replication and growth. Breast cancer cells, for instance, have as many as ten times as many IGF-1 receptors as do healthy cells[114, 115].

Arguably, and put simplistically, this gives breast cancer cells at least a sixteen-fold advantage over healthy breast cells when it comes to obtaining the glucose they need. In fact, the greater proximity of the receptor sites further increases the glucose uptake efficiency when compared to receptor sites located further apart, as on the walls of healthy cells.

Examples could be given for many different types of cancer. The final summary has to be that cancer cells have powerful ways of obtaining their required energy, in spite of the lack of functioning mitochondria. They obtain this energy at the expense of that available for the rest of the body's healthy cells. They remain unable to obtain a significant amount of energy from fats or proteins.

All this helps to explain and underscore the benefits of some of the dietary advice that has been given to cancer patients, for many decades, by CAM therapists. Eat a low calorie diet, and one that is low in starches and sugars but high in fibre-rich foods such as above-ground vegetables, and with moderate amounts of proteins and fats. In particular, if you have cancer or want to avoid a recurrence, and if you fear there could be a few cancer cells left, avoid all sugars, limit your intake of fruits to the berries, and avoid refined carbohydrates such as white flour or white rice.

Other cellular consequences of mitochondrial dysfunction

Here we have focused on the problems of mitochondrial dysfunction in relation to cancer, glucose metabolism, and the harm done to you by sugar in your diet. There are many other serious consequences of mitochondrial damage. One of these includes its role in apoptosis. Apoptosis is the process by which damaged or faulty cells are persuaded to commit voluntary suicide, as it is often called. If this mechanism is operating correctly, any cancer cell should self destruct. However, cancer cells have clearly found a way around this and refuse to do so. Their mechanism comes back to the role of the mitochondria. Mitochondria, via a number of complex mechanisms that we will not go into here, orchestrate this process of apoptosis. Clearly, if the cancer cells have managed to achieve a largely mitochondrial-free state, they have also managed to avoid mitochondrial-induced apoptosis. This adds to the importance of protecting and nourishing your existing mitochondria and endeavouring to regenerate new ones.

Regenerating your mitochondria

One way to do this is by participating in energetic aerobic exercise[116], another is by reducing your intake of calories[117], though if you are unwell this may not be advisable. Many natural compounds are helpful[118], among the most important of these are alpha-lipoic acid[119] (though current research suggests that r-lipoic acid may be even better), coenzyme Q-10[120] and acetyl-L-carnitine[121]. All the B group vitamins and the trace minerals that are required for the Krebs Cycle are also of vital importance.

Most of the organelles (organs) within one of your cells were made at the time the cell was formed. However, mitochondria are somewhat different. They are relatively independent. You will recall that there are some suggestions that they were once independent organisms that got caught up in our type of cells early in evolution. They certainly have their own DNA (mDNA). As such, they can reproduce even after the cell in which they live is formed. So if they have been damaged there is the possibility of replacement. A natural compound that plays a role in cellular function called pyrroloquinoline quinone (PQQ)[122] has been found to stimulate the formation of new and healthy mitochondria[123], and able to replace old and damaged ones.

There is even more to be said later about the importance of mitochondria and the consequences of mitochondrial dysfunction, so read on.

CHAPTER 11

ADRENAL EXHAUSTION AND DR WALTRAUT FRYDA

When I met Dr. Fryda in Bavaria in 2007 she was 82 years old and, by her own admission, almost as proud of her ability to produce a PowerPoint presentation as of her theory of cancer. This latter she had formulated within a year of graduating from medical schools in Jena, Berlin and Innsbruck. She spent the following two days expounding it to a small group of us in a beautiful village nestled in amongst the Bavarian mountains.

According to Dr. Fryda, cancer is caused by adrenal exhaustion[124, 125]. She has continued to work with this concept throughout her professional life and has found it to be confirmed repeatedly by her clinical experience.

In brief, her hypothesis is this. Stress leads to exhausted adrenal glands which lead to a state of adrenal exhaustion whereby there is a lack of adrenalin and diminished oxygen circulation. This is accompanied by decreased glycogen mobilisation from the cells in the form of glucose into the bloodstream and so to excess cellular glycogen storage. In an effort to reduce these glycogen stores the cells turn anaerobic, focus on the inefficient E-M pathway and increase their l-lactic acid production. This further inhibits mitochondrial function and the action of the Krebs Cycle and stimulates the development of more cancer cells. We have again, in effect, a short-term solution to a problem, excessive glycogen accumulation in the cells, but one that can eventually be fatal to the organism as a whole, to you.

Here is a more detailed description of her ideas.

Your first response to stress is to produce the alarm signal in the brain. As a result, a hormone called ACTH is sent out throughout your body. This alerts your adrenal glands to the need for the production of increased amounts of the adrenal hormones, adrenalin and noradrenalin. If the stress continues, if you have repeated stressful incidents, if your glands are not provided with all the nutrients they need, especially a range of the B group vitamins and vitamin C, your adrenal glands eventually become overworked and exhausted. Their hormone output slows or comes nearly to a halt as a result. Both adrenalin and noradrenalin are produced in the medulla or centre of your adrenal glands and their output diminishes, significantly.

However, there is an important distinction between these two hormones, and one that concerns us here. Noradrenalin, but not adrenalin, is also produced in other parts of your body. It is produced in cells called chromaffin cells (due to the colour or chroma they stain when chromium salts are applied to them). These chromaffin cells occur in your adrenal glands but also in other parts of your body. They occur in the ganglia (nerve structures) along the trunk or spine of your sympathetic nerves, in the synapses at the end of each of your nerve cells, in your brain, in the mucous membranes that line your intestinal tract, and in a few other internal organs. This means that if your adrenal glands become exhausted, the production of adrenalin falls but noradrenalin is still produced at these other locations. This leads to an increased ratio of noradrenalin to adrenalin and causes an imbalance of the two hormones.

To understand the consequences of this it is necessary to consider some of the actions of adrenalin and noradrenalin. Firstly, you will recall that adrenalin is an important hormone in the maintenance of your normal blood glucose level. In this, it works in opposition partnership with the hormone insulin. Insulin works to lower your blood glucose level when it is too high, adrenalin raises it when it becomes too low. Between the two of them your blood glucose level is, in health, maintained within a narrow normal range. We touched on this in earlier chapters.

The maintenance of a normal blood glucose level is important for many reasons. Most of your body's cells can utilise fat for energy if a supply of glucose is not available, but your brain, at least in the short term (less than three days) cannot. It has, in the short term, an absolute need for glucose. Adrenalin, but not noradrenalin, achieves this steady supply of glucose by stimulating the breakdown of glycogen (or animal starch) by the process of glycogenolysis. Without an appropriate supply of adrenalin, your blood glucose level will fall, your brain cells will starve and you will feel awful: tense, irritable, weak, jittery, and more, the common symptoms experienced if you are suffering from hypoglycaemia. Noradrenalin does not stimulate glycogenolysis.

Worse is to come. When your adrenal glands become exhausted and cannot produce adrenalin, not only does glycogenolysis not occur to refresh your blood glucose level, but there remains a build up of unused glycogen inside your cells. This occurs, and worsens, because insulin continues to pump glucose into your cells whenever your blood sugar level rises, such as after a meal, even when it is not needed by the cells concerned for the production of energy or glycogen. The main cells that accumulate glycogen are those of your liver and muscles. In adrenal deficiency these cells become engorged with glycogen. If the situation is prolonged this is then followed by the engorgement of all your other cells that are capable of storing glycogen.

Fryda states that cells saturated with glycogen cannot continue to function normally and that this is an important early factor in their metamorphosis into cancer cells.

A second action of adrenalin dictates where the oxygenated blood flows in your body. To understand this we first have to consider your autonomic (think automatic) nervous system. This is divided into two parts, your Sympathetic Nervous System (SNS) and your Parasympathetic Nervous System (PSNS). Your SNS activates your flight-or-fight mechanism and deals with all types of stress. This requires increased flow of blood to your limbs, heart, eyes and lungs and away from around your digestive and waste disposal systems and your trunk in general, so you can deal with the sudden emergency or stressful situation. Your PSNS manages your internal housekeeping, your digestion, waste removal and so on. This system can only operate when your SNS is turned off. The blood can then flow back from your extremities to your trunk around your digestive system for digestion and your kidneys for waste removal.

During stress, shock or trauma your SNS is turned on and your PSNS is turned off. Adrenalin ensures that your blood flows to where it is most needed and that the areas affected by an emergency get a generous supply of blood, nutrients and oxygen, at the expense of the areas within your trunk that have slowed down. Noradrenalin does not do this. Noradrenalin only restricts blood flow to the less important areas, it does not stimulate increased blood flow to where it is needed and thus does not create the same increased supply of oxygen to cells that are called on to deal with the stress.

Combined with our first consideration, this means that the cells that, due to adrenalin deficiency, have become engorged with glycogen and that have come under pressure or are facing stress, are now, again because of a lack of adrenalin, also deprived of much-needed blood flow and hence of a supply of oxygen which they need if they are to deal with this glycogen. These cells will thus either die, leading to tissue damage and organ death, or they will endeavour to find alternative methods of dealing with the situation, of getting rid of the unwanted glycogen. Fryda believes that the organism will choose the latter option rather than death and will revert to a more primitive type of metabolism to achieve this. This inevitably leads to an increase in the process of anaerobic breakdown of the glycogen, to unhealthy fermentation and the E-M pathway, instead of to healthy glycogenolysis, as the cells try to flush out, or use up, the glycogen in the quickest way possible. As a result the cells turn cancerous.

Remember that during times of adequate adrenal function, the glycogen stored (healthily) in the muscles and liver is broken down to release energy when it is needed. If heavy activity is demanded and if a bottleneck does occur at that Pivotal Point in carbohydrate metabolism between pyruvic acid and acetyl coenzyme A, it leads to the production of d-lactic acid. This d-lactic acid cannot be catabolised in the muscle cells and so travels through the bloodstream to the liver where it is rebuilt into glucose.

When there is insufficient adrenalin and oxygen, and when the excess glycogen ferments, l-lactic acid is produced instead of d-lactic acid, **this l-lactic acid is toxic. It increases the rate of cellular division or mitosis.** In other words, this l-lactic acid stimulates mitosis which leads to an accumulation of unwanted cells that build into a tumour, a body of cancerous cells. These tumour cells, unlike healthy cells, require and are able to use large amounts of glycogen for their energy as they only metabolise glucose as far as the Pivotal Point. So, in effect, they become glycogen-sucking pumps, taking glycogen out of the system and providing a way for cells to get rid of the excess.

At first glance this might seem to be a useful adaptation, but it is yet another short-term solution that can have disastrous long-term consequences. It is only beneficial in the short term, as an immediate answer to the lack of adrenalin and the resulting build up of excessive glycogen. In the long term this adaptation can, of course, be fatal. Unrestricted and inappropriate cellular division and multiplication, as a means of storing unwanted glycogen, are obvious precursors to the development of tumours.

You will discover later [Chapter 14] that in Beard's theory, wayward trophoblasts represent yet another short-term solution to a problem (i.e. the healing of damaged tissues) that has failed to recognise when its job is done. In this consideration of adrenal stress the tumour cells are a short-term solution to another problem (that of glycogen accumulation due to adrenal exhaustion). Unfortunately, the mitosis, once started, fails to stop, even when the stress is reduced and healthy adrenal function is restored. This is a major point to remember and adds emphasis to the statement that prevention is much easier than cure. If you have cancer and if you now realise that it was preceded by a period of damaging stress, and that this was possibly the trigger for the start of Phase Two, it is not enough to simply remove or get over the stress. You still have to deal with the cancer cells that are present and steadily producing new cancer cells. Nonetheless, reducing stress is an essential part of restoring your health and of preventing future cancer cell development.

This stress-related scenario is why an essential part of dealing with or treating cancer, as well as preventing it, is to reduce your stress level, to make changes in the way you think, feel and respond to situations, to learn to relax, have fun, fill your heart with joy, and to let go of anger, hate, jealousy, fear or any other such negative emotions. A course of psychotherapy, periods of meditation, the use of techniques such as EFT (the Emotional Freedom Technique), autogenic therapy, tai chi, or any other de-stressing programme that appeals to you and works for you at the deepest level, is vitally important. Change your lifestyle if you can. Reduce some of the expectations and demands placed on you by yourself or other people, if you can. If you cannot change your outer world, change your inner world. Change your attitude and responses to situations, people and events. Give your adrenal glands a chance[126]. Put less demands on them. Allow the balance of adrenalin and noradrenalin to return to normal. In this way you will increase the flow of oxygen to all your tissues, allow your cellular glycogen levels to return to normal and reduce the risk of developing cancer or encouraging new tumours.

However, even this is not the full story as to what can happen during adrenal exhaustion. Adrenalin plays an important role in the function of your immune system. When foreign objects or organisms enter your body adrenalin stimulates the production of granulocytes and macrophages, cells that are part of your immune defence arsenal. These protective cells engulf and then destroy the invaders. This process also leads to shivering, glycogenolysis, the formation of d-lactic acid, the production of more adrenalin and the rise in temperature characteristic of an acute infection. This is healthy. This rise in temperature is an important part of the way your body deals with foreign substances. It is only at these raised temperatures that the enzymes that catalyse many of your defensive reactions are effective. Lack of temperature leads to reduced defence against pathogens. Lack of adrenalin hinders this rise in temperature.

People who develop cancer commonly report that they rarely get an acute infection with a rise in temperature. They may get a cold but their temperature rarely rises. They may even feel proud of this, thinking that it indicates their healthy nature. Unfortunately this is not so, it means that this healthy mechanism, this evidence of effective immune function, is missing or inadequate. Helping your body to raise such an inflammatory response and achieve an increase in body temperature is an important part of several proposed cancer recovery strategies including mistletoe therapy. The aim is to raise the normal resting temperature of your body and to encourage an additional increase in body temperature, as and when appropriate, such as when foreign or unwanted cells have to be dealt with. This is distinct from hyperthermia when external heat is applied to the body, though this has at least partially similar aims. Mistletoe and related therapies encourage the body to raise its temperature for itself.

Fryda insists that raising your temperature (with mistletoe) or improving immune function (with a variety of supplements and herbs) is only part of an overall recovery plan and the total plan absolutely must include or be accompanied by efforts to improve the function of the adrenal glands and overall health. It is important to give these glands a rest by reducing the stress load.

Fryda considers the decreased action of the immune cells to be of secondary importance, in relation to the development of cancer, to the process of glycogenolysis that should have been stimulated by adrenalin. Immune cells, such as the B and T lymphocytes, can encapsulate foreign invaders, be they chemicals, viruses, bacteria or other organisms, thus rendering them harmless, but they are still *in situ*, still present. This engulfing is a viable strategy when the foreign organism is tiny and the surface area to volume ratio is large. Its effectiveness when dealing with a large tumour mass, with a relatively small surface area, is vanishingly small. Thus, she claims, the lymphocytes were useful as a backup when adrenalin was doing most of the work, but when there is limited output of adrenalin, the immune cells are nearly on their own and they just can't cope. As a result the tumour grows.

Thus, without adequate adrenalin the immune system becomes less effective. There is a body of cells that is growing as a result of the excessive glycogen and mitosis and the lack of oxygen, but this cellular mass, this tumour, is not recognised as something foreign and so it is not, and cannot be, attacked or broken down. As a result it can continue to grow unrestricted. At a certain size it will need its own blood supply to nourish its internal cells, but this is usually managed successfully, and it then puts up a protective wall to further ensure its survival.

So, let's summarise this. Fryda postulates that a long-term state of less than optimal health, consisting of excessive stress, leading to reduced adrenal output, a build up of cellular glycogen, increased cellular mitosis, plus compromised immune function, is a systemic state and precedes tumour formation. The stressors, she suggests, could be mental (lifestyle), physical (radiation, electro-magnetic fields, local friction), chemical (carcinogens), pathogens (*candida albicans*, *helicobacter pylori* or other parasites) prolonged infections (particularly due to slow viruses, such as HPV) and, in fact, any of the known causes of cancer.

When subjected to these stressors the body first finds short-term alternative ways of coping, a variety of quick fixes. It pays less attention to the fact that in the long term these coping mechanisms can be fatal to the total organism – to you.

TESTS

Adrenal stress test

An adrenal stress test is offered by Genova Diagnostics and several other laboratories, so ask around if you want to find a local laboratory. The results of the test will provide you with important information as to the state of your adrenal glands.

The test involves the analysis of saliva samples collected at four times in the day: on waking, at noon, late afternoon and last thing at night.

The most obvious goal is to reduce your stress level in any way you can. This may not be easy if you have just been diagnosed with cancer, nonetheless it is vital.

The next step is to repair and nourish your adrenal glands so that normal adrenalin output is restored and the adrenalin is available when required for the minor stresses of normal body physiology. Many nutrients can help to achieve this, particularly the B group vitamins and vitamin C. Liquorice is a useful herb. It should be taken at the times in the day (when samples were collected) when your results were below normal.

Lactic acid

Cancer cells can produce forty times more lactic acid than normal cells.

(a) Measuring l-lactic acid in your blood will provide information as to whether or not your cells are reverting, or have reverted, to more primitive cells and there is a danger of Phase Two of the Cancer Process being in operation. This test is offered by Neuro-Lab [www.neurolab.com], as is the test for d-lactic acid. The latter is also a component of the ONE test offered by Genova Diagnostics. Other laboratories also offer these tests, so you can shop around.

(b) The presence of l-lactic acid. If it is present, the harmful l-lactic acid (do not confuse this with L-lactic acid which is different) must be dealt with. This can be done by taking some of the positive, d-lactic acid. The protocol Dr. Fryda suggests is described in Part 3 [Chapter31].

This use of d-lactic acid should, in her view, balance out the l-lactic acid and encourage or enable your body to deal with and destroy the tumour. It should also discourage or inhibit the formation of new cancer cells. This should be helpful even if the primary tumour has been removed, and even if the surgeon thinks he or she has 'got it all'. It is important to keep this in mind as cancer is a systemic problem. Even when the tumour has been removed there is a major question that has not been answered during, and subsequent to, surgery: Why did cancer start in the first place and what has been done to change that fundamental situation?

If the tumour has not been removed surgically its breakdown will lead to the production of large protein molecules. These are difficult to eliminate and can lead to what Fryda calls a toxic fever. Unfortunately, this fever is rarely sufficient to destroy the tumour but may be sufficient to weaken the host. To aid in the process of eliminating these proteins she recommends an enzyme supplement such as Wobenzyme N, a synergistic combination of plant-based enzymes, pancreatic enzymes and antioxidants. Other pancreatic enzyme supplements can also be helpful and there will be a discussion of them later [Chapters14 and 16].

From this scenario you will realise that if you ever do get a temperature you should not do anything to suppress it. Leave it alone, be happy, encourage it. It could be a sign that you are improving, that your immune function is increasing, that your body is fighting the toxins.

Dr. Fryda also uses a product called Regeneresen, a live cell RNA therapy made from gland and organ extracts that has been specifically designed to stimulate the adrenal glands back into life.

Finally, Fryda makes some specific comment on the benefits or otherwise of surgery, chemotherapy and radiation and their relation to her theory. On all three so-called therapies she has this to say:

- In general: *"It would be best in most cases to apply this (lactic acid) treatment to the adrenal glands first and to achieve cross-over status **before** starting any of these conventional (MDS) therapies, if indeed the latter are to be used at all."* (Cross-over is the point where the d-lactic acid has started to become effective and is discussed in Chapter 31.)

- On surgery: *"...this can either be such a trauma that it damages the immune system irrevocably, or it can be such a stress that it stimulates the adrenal glands to mobilise their final remaining reserves. In the latter case you will need to support your adrenals in every way you can or their exhaustion will only increase or become absolute. On the other hand (if the tumour is not removed surgically), the breakdown of large tumours could overwhelm the detoxification capacity of the body and in this case and on this basis surgery could be justified."*

- On chemotherapy and radiation: *"...these are both immune suppressants. They may reduce the body to such a vegetable state that again the chromaffin system (mentioned above) is restimulated, and again, if the tumour is large and surgery is not applied the treatment, especially when combined with these procedures, could overwhelm the system."*

- Overall: Many people feel that there 'is not time' to start on her programme without any of the conventional remedies and, although Dr. Fryda would not agree, that is a decision that must be up to the individual.

Fryda has used this theory and the resultant therapeutic approach for many years and claims considerable success, she also offers a number of comments:

- her treatment is based on sound theory, on sound biochemistry and physiology;

- the treatment provides no strain to the organism, as is experienced by surgery, radiation or chemotherapy;

- the treatment leads to no pain or distress, other than during the three cross-over days, during which time they are generally mild, and to no unwanted, unpleasant or damaging side-effects;

- even in the case of patients that she has not been able to save she has been able to improve their quality of life enormously, to prolong it, and to keep pain to a minimum until the last few days.

It is interesting and helpful to note, in view of Fryda's hypothesis, that researchers have found that when they artificially stimulated the production of adrenalin in rats, by treating them with imipramine or its precursors serotonin and dopamine, two things happened. Firstly, tumours injected into the rats failed to implant or take hold. Secondly, existing malignant changes disappeared without trace[127].

It is very common to find that people who develop a tumour have experienced a period of major or significant stress in the two or three years prior to the diagnosis. It is commonly a stress of the 'hopeless and helpless' kind. This is the type of stress where you appear to have no viable option that will lessen your stress or lead to a less stressful state. You can't follow action A because B would result and this would be just as bad or worse. Alternatively, it is the type of stress where, for some other reason, you feel you are powerless to take positive action of any sort, where someone else can 'pull the strings' or where you cannot force a resolution.

The work of Dr. Fryda suggests that adrenal exhaustion is behind almost all cancers. If this applies to you, you need to know about it. Two things have to be accomplished, you must deal with the past issues and you must treat the present damage to your adrenal system.

At the emotional level you will need to work on resolving the issues. If the situation is ongoing you should find appropriate help in order that you can deal with it and resolve the emotional issues within yourself. No matter how hopeless the situation may seem to you there is almost certain to be some professional who can help you to resolve it. This may mean changing practical aspects of the situation, or it may mean changing your emotional response or reactions to it. Anything you can do to lessen the stress as you experience it will help you to reduce your risk of getting cancer, avoid a recurrence if you are in remission or, if you currently have cancer, will help you in your recovery.

You may well need, or benefit from, professional psychotherapy to help you to accomplish this. There are also many books on the subject[128, 129, 130]. If the stressful situation is fully in the past, behind you, it is still important to release any negative energy associated with it to ensure there is no further strain on your adrenal glands as you think back over it. In this way you can minimise the likelihood of any further damage. Leaving it buried but unresolved in your past is like ignoring a boil.

At the physical-chemical level you will need to work on correcting and rebalancing your adrenal function and feeding the glands the nutrients and phytoceuticals that will support them.

To accomplish these outcomes it is useful to have measurable markers, and this is where the **adrenal stress test** comes in again. Arrange it via your practitioner and do it at intervals until all the readings are within the normal range. Remember, the test is simple and merely involves spitting into small collecting tubes at stated times throughout one 24-hour period and then sending the four samples off for analysis, and it provides useful information as to the progress (or not) that you are making.

More on lactic acid

In closing this chapter it is worth adding one more comment on lactic acid. Lactic acid as produced by your cells is not good. However, the story is different in relation to lactic acid producing bacteria.

A type of lactic acid bacteria, *Lactobacillus casei* strain Shirota, has been shown to have antitumour activity in experimental animals. One clinical trial using *L. casei* showed a significant decrease in the recurrence of superficial bladder cancer and the authors suggested that the habitual intake of lactic acid bacteria could reduce the risk of bladder cancer[131]. A similar result has been obtained in relation to colon cancer. *Bifidobacterium longum,* a lactic acid-producing intestinal bacterium has been shown to inhibit colon cancer and modulate the intermediate biomarkers of colon carcinogenesis[132]. The authors studied *Bifidobacterium longum,* a lactic acid-producing enterobacterium, and concluded that taking this probiotic (*B. longum*) orally can produce strong antitumour activity. Similar chemistry occurs in almost all cells and thus it is possible to suppose that the same benefit could be achieved in relation to the prevention of other possible cancers.

According to the National Cancer Institute, *"...a probiotic containing live, cultivated, freeze-dried lactic acid bacteria with gastrointestinal (GI) protective, anti-inflammatory, immunomodulating and potential antitumour properties"* is beneficial. Oral administration of probiotic bacteria helps to maintain adequate colonization of the GI tract and modulate the composition of the normal micro flora. Upon colonization of the GI tract, the probiotic bacteria form a protective barrier, interfere with the attachment of pathogenic bacteria and other harmful substances, and may bind to and degrade carcinogens. This may prevent inflammation and possibly cancer. In addition, these bacteria produce lactic acid, thereby creating an acidic environment within the G.I. tract that is unfavourable for pathogens[133].

CHAPTER 12

STRESS, THE IMMUNE SYSTEM AND DR. ABO

Stress can do more than damage your adrenal glands and lead to all the problems that this can cause. Stress can also have a powerfully negative effect on your immune system, and this too, it is claimed, can cause or contribute to cancer. In fact, Dr. Toru Abo, the famous Japanese immunologist renowned for his discovery of extrathymic T cells and of the fact that the autonomic nervous system is responsible for the equilibrium of leukocytes (white blood cells), and professor of immunology at Nigata University School of Medicine in Japan, gives this greater emphasis than does Dr. Fryda. He claims that stress-induced immune dysfunction is the cause of cancer[134]. In a sense, this can be considered a parallel hypothesis to that of Dr. Fryda. Both theories claim stress to be the cause of cancer, Dr. Fryda focusing on the result of stress-induced lack of adrenalin on cellular metabolism, and Dr. Abo on the impact of stress-induced output of cortisol on the immune system.

Stress can be physical, such as excessive demands on your time and energies, or physical pain. It can be chemical, such as is caused by a wide range of toxins including carcinogens. It can be emotional, a topic touched on in Chapter 19. Negative stressors can be chronic, long term and persistent, eating away at your natural resources.

Strictly speaking, stress can also result from positive causes, since stress is defined as anything that significantly changes you and your body from the resting relaxed state. However, positive stressors rarely cause a long-term negative perturbation of the status quo and often have the opposite effect and produces positive benefits. Humour, for instance, produces psychological and physiological effects on your body that are similar to the health benefits of aerobic exercise[135], and is beneficial to general wellbeing[136]. Humour and laughter are said to increase the level of salivary Immunoglobulin A, and increase spontaneous lymphocyte blastogenesis, a natural killer cell activity[137]. Laughing certainly helped Norman Cousins[138]. He suffered from extreme inflammatory pain due to either reactive arthritis or ankylosing spondylitis, both of which involve aberrant immune function. The pain was such that his doctors prescribed morphine. Cousins found that ten minutes of belly-laughter could provide him with two hours of freedom from pain, and without the side effects of morphine.

Stress can also either boost or suppress the immune system and its activity depending on the time duration of the stress. Acute stress stimulates the activity of your sympathetic nervous system and triggers the activities that will enable you to deal with the consequences of the stress, such as infections, wounds and other physical damage. Chronic stress can have the opposite effect and can inhibit the activity of the immune system.

Stress can impact on the immune system in other ways, one of which is via its action on your hormonal system. Put simply, this is how it works. Stress triggers your sympathetic nervous system (SNS) and produces a neurological response. This nerve message acts on a small sub section of your brain known as the hypothalamus. Your hypothalamus then releases a hormone called corticotropin-releasing hormone which acts on a gland, your pituitary gland, situated just below the hypothalamus and at the base of your brain. The pituitary gland, often called the 'master gland', is the link between your brain and your endocrine or hormonal system. When your pituitary gland receives corticotrophin-releasing hormone it releases a compound called adrenocorticotropic hormone (ACTH), also known as corticotropin, though this term is rarely used nowadays. ACTH travels, via your blood, throughout your circulation system. It triggers your adrenal glands, situated on top of your kidneys (ad-renal), to produce both adrenalin and noradrenalin from the medulla (middle) of the glands, as described by Dr. Fryda above, but also cortisol from the cortex (outer layer).

In general, acute stress triggers adrenalin output, chronic stress triggers cortisol output. All chronic stress increases the output of cortisol. This cortisol plays many roles, but our interest here is on the immune system. Cortisol acts on white blood cells to inhibit several immune pathways[139]. This reduces the inflammatory response and may be one of the reasons why, as stated earlier, it is common to find among many people with cancer that they say, *"But I've always been so well, even if I get the flu I rarely get a temperature."* Instead of being proud of this it should alert them to a failure of their immune system.

Instead of the normal inflammatory response, this long-term stress and cortisol release leads to a mild, low-grade inflammation, produced by white cells called monocytes that have become resistant to cortisol. It is this that is thought to lead to the stress-induced degenerative diseases including cancer[140].

As you saw in Chapter 11, stress induces adrenal exhaustion which leads to reduced circulation. This reduced circulation leads to increased activity of granulocytes[141] (a sub-set of immune system cells within the white blood cells which contain granules), which then release superoxide that damages the cells of the endothelial (blood vessel) walls. This superoxide-induced damage can lead to mutations and so to cancer. The increased level of granulocytes also leads to increased destruction of red blood cells and anaemia.

Immune deficiency leads to reduced production of lymphocytes, cells of the immune system that recognise foreign substances and cells. Without their vigilance cancer cells can go unnoticed and be allowed to reproduce. It is Dr. Abo's contention that this reduced production and activity of lymphocytes is one of the main causes of cancer (if not the main cause), and that this reduction is stress-induced.

Cancer cells are not healthy cells, they do not function as well as healthy cells and they are not strong. Remember, they have great difficulty in getting energy since they can only utilise glucose and can only do so very inefficiently and to a very limited extent. This should already tell you that cancer cells are not strong. Researchers find that they have to inject a million or more cancer cells into an experimental animal before the animal develops cancer. The majority of the injected cancer cells are destroyed by the animal's lymphocytes. It is recognised that we all develop many cancer cells, probably daily, but that our immune system deals with and destroys them. They do this very efficiently, the pass mark for that function is not 50%, as it is for many of the exams we humans face, it is 100%. One mistake, one cancer cell that is allowed to escape, signals failure, and the development of cancer in the host. Those lymphocytes work hard and successfully – unless you damage or hinder them.

In the face of this hypothesis, the use of surgery, chemotherapy and radiation therapy, all of which damage the immune system, is clearly not the answer. Surgery stimulates the sympathetic nervous system and this is undesirable. If lymph nodes are removed this reduces lymphocyte production, and these are the cells you need, to recognise and fight cancer cells. If you must have surgery, keep it to a minimum, as is now being increasingly recommended, at least for both breast and prostate surgery. Chemotherapy is generally aimed at reducing cell division and reproduction. This applies to healthy cells as well as to cancer cells, especially to rapidly dividing cells. This includes the cells of your immune system and so there is reduced production and activity of your immune cells, just at the time when you need them most. Radiation can nowadays be very accurately targeted, at least at the tissue level. It cannot be targeted at individual cells. Identifying individual cancer cells and irradiating each one individually might work, but is not currently feasible, particularly since there are generally millions (1cu mm) or billions (1cu cm) of cancer cells to deal with in any tumour. Thus, radiation damages the healthy cells that are intermingled with cancer cells plus those that surround the tumour. Inevitably, this means that many lymphocytes are killed. As the radiation kills cancer cells many toxins are released into the bloodstream, thus there is an increased need for more, not less, lymphocytes and this aggravates the problem, further reducing immune efficiency.

Management strategies

Dr. Abo's suggestions for both the prevention and the management of cancer are discussed in more detail in Chapter 33. He focuses on the ultimate goal of optimising your immune function in general and your lymphocyte count and efficiency in particular. In brief, his protocol involves the following:

- Reduce stress and the stimulation to your SNS. If you cannot change the outer stressors you can at least change your reaction to them [See Chapter 11].

- Do whatever you can to stimulate your parasympathetic nervous system. It is common to find that people who develop cancer are generally SNS dominant rather than parasympathetic nervous system dominant (PSNS dominant). Here is one of the possible reasons as to why that is so. People who are PSNS dominant are generally much more laid back than those who are SNS dominant; they react less strongly to stress and so have a stronger immune system.

Note that his focus is on reducing stress and a fundamental balancing of the autonomic nervous system, the ratio of SNS to PSNS function, and not on the use of either herbal remedies or nutrients that help fight infections, or on antibiotics. Either of these approaches would be band-aid approaches. Reducing the stress in your life allows your body to rebuild its own immune function.

CHAPTER 13

ANAEROBIC VERSUS AEROBIC ACTIVITY

In Chapters 9 and 11 we spoke of the anaerobic E-M pathway and the aerobic activity that occurs within the mitochondria of the cell. There are further aspects to consider in relation to the change from aerobic cellular metabolism to anaerobic metabolism. In summary, we now know that cells turn to anaerobic cytoplasmic fermentation due to adrenalin deficiency, which leads to both a lack of available oxygen and an excessive store of glycogen. With mitochondrial function compromised there is excessive dependency on the E-M pathway to 'use up' their excessive stores of glycogen, and the consequent production of l-lactic acid which further stimulates mitosis and (cancer) cellular reproduction.

In fact, Warburg suggested that tumours are effectively segregated waste dumps for toxic material held inside the body and that they derive their energy from the fermentation of sugar.

Cancer does not cause cells to turn to anaerobic fermentation. It is oxygen deprivation and the need for cells to turn to anaerobic fermentation that turns healthy cells into cancer cells. Once formed, however, there are benefits to the cancer cells to be derived from this focus on anaerobic fermentation.

Whereas the end-product of E-M pathway fermentation is l-lactic acid, the end product of the full mitochondrial oxidation of a glucose molecule is carbon dioxide. In healthy tissue this carbon dioxide is expelled from the cells and attaches to the haemoglobin in the red blood cells. When this happens, oxygen is 'pushed off' the haemoglobin molecule and so is available for uptake by the cells. This is obviously desirable but is a function that is missing from cancerous tissues which produce l-lactic acid instead of carbon dioxide. Cancer cells thrive in an oxygen-poor environment and by refraining from producing carbon dioxide they fail to trigger the release of oxygen from haemoglobin and thus help to maintain low tissue levels of oxygen in the location of the tumour.

Once cells have changed from aerobic to anaerobic respiration the system is self-perpetuating. The lack of carbon dioxide leads to a lack of oxygen which leads to increased fermentation and production of more l-lactic acid, etc., and to increased cellular replication. This is another reason why prevention is much easier than cure and why simply backtracking out of cancer is not sufficient. As well as removing the causes, strong correctional strategies are also required.

It has been suggested that this cellular replication is caused by a faulty gene called p53 gene but at best this may be a contributing factor. You will remember from Chapter 7 that cancer cells get their energy by producing and secreting their own insulin, and that they stimulate their own growth by producing their own insulin-like growth factor-1 (IGF-1). This causes them to self-stimulate and induces the production of a compound called hypoxia-inducible factor 1 (HIF-1) which controls oxygen delivery via its effect on angiogenesis[142, 143]. HIF-1 also controls the cells' adaptation to the lack of oxygen by stimulating fermentation[144].

Other causes of oxygen deprivation include:

- clumping up of red blood cells which slows the flow of blood and reduces blood flow through many of the fine capillaries;
- a deficiency of essential fatty acids [Chapter17].

CHAPTER 14

TROPHOBLASTS AND DR. JOHN BEARD

In the preceding chapters we have considered possible causes of cancer and the ways in which healthy cells can be converted into cancer cells. The focus was on the lack of oxygen to the cells and compromised mitochondrial function. Predisposing factors to this include adrenal exhaustion and lack of mitochondrial nutrients and available oxygen.

It is now time to turn our attention to what happens once cancer starts to develop and how a tumour starts to form and grow. It is generally believed that we produce cancer cells in our bodies most days, and certainly very frequently. This raises the question: How do we normally handle them and either destroy or eliminate them? How does the body itself treat these mini but frequent occurrences of cancer? Could this same process be called in to help when tumours have formed? This is where the work and insights of Dr. John Beard come in[145].

Adult stem cells and cancer

One of the major foundation stones of most successful CAM suggestions for cancer recovery was first suggested over a hundred and fifty years ago when it became known as the embryonal rest theory of cancer[146, 147]. However, little seems to have evolved from this start.

This early work was followed by the independent research of John Beard D.Sc., an English developmental biologist who also worked in Germany and Edinburgh. He was a distinguished scientist, honoured by the French Academy of Sciences in 1890, nominated for the Nobel prize for Medicine in 1906 and published more than 100 scientific papers. He was the first to describe apoptosis, which you will recall is the programmed cell death by which old, damaged, faulty or worn out cells commit voluntary suicide; the first to recognise the importance of the thymus gland, an essential component of your immune system; and the first to recognise the similarity of trophoblastic cells (see below) and cancer cells. By 1904 he was generally thought of as one of the leading embryologists in the world.

By then his research had led him to a study of the developing foetus and a recognition that placental tissue looked remarkably similar to cancerous tissue. He developed the theory that we will explore in the following pages, that cancer develops from *"...displaced trophoblast or activated germ (stem) cells."* He published this work in 1904. It raised a storm of debate and gradually increasing condemnation and ridicule. In 1911 he published his book, *'The Enzyme Theory of Cancer'*, but his ideas were too far ahead of his time and of the understanding of most of his colleagues. Although these ideas were followed up by a few doctors, they were largely ignored and buried, and Beard died embittered and in obscurity in 1924. In more recent times it has been suggested by some that his work on this topic should have earned him a Nobel prize rather than condemnation, yet it is still a long way from being properly or fully recognised. His book has recently been republished with a foreword by Dr. Nicholas Gonzalez[148].

In the intervening hundred years a small number of people have worked with his theory, though mostly within the CAM rather than in the MDS system. Now these ideas are being rediscovered by modern medicine and thought of as the 'stem cell theory of cancer'[149]. It is disturbing to recognise how much distress could have been avoided if Beard's work had been incorporated into cancer therapy a hundred years ago. Indeed, much suffering could be avoided today if more attention was paid to this theory by the medical profession that is actively involved in cancer treatment.

To understand his work we need to explore some of the characteristics of cells and their development. To do this we will first consider, by way of an analogy, the development of a human being. Individual human beings start out undeveloped and then mature into adults with unique life-paths, skills and aptitudes based on irreversible decisions made during their development. A baby has the potential to develop into a wide range of possibilities and choose a nearly limitless number of life choices. Then decisions are made, this school is chosen over that; one subject is chosen instead of another. The individual may choose the arts or the sciences. By the time they have done their final school exams it is almost impossible, if they want to go on and do a degree, to swap from an arts-based schooling to a science degree. If you decide to be a tennis player it is almost certainly too late, by the time you are an adult, to opt for a training as a ballet dancer. The options decrease even further, when you make such decisions as accepting this job instead of that, to marry or not to marry, to have children or not to have children. The non-specialised baby has the maximum potential, but is the least specialised, trained or competent. The more specialised and experienced you become, the fewer possibilities you have for changing your direction in life.

It is similar with cells. Cells start out in life as immature undifferentiated cells with the possibility of becoming any type of cell in your body, but with no specialised skills. They then mature into differentiated cells, very clever at what they do but with, eventually, no potential to change into another cell type.

This is an important concept to grasp in relation to cancer. Undifferentiated cells are cells that can develop into a wide range of types of cells with specialised structures and functions appropriate for their chosen 'career' or future path in life. These undifferentiated cells are totipotent, they have the potential to develop into any type of cell, but until they do they all look alike.

Once a cell 'decides' or is stimulated to become a nerve cell, a liver cell, a colon cell or a skin cell it matures along this chosen path becoming more and more clearly, both microscopically and in its physical and chemical structure and function, a cell of its particular chosen tissue. Just as a human who has chosen to be a childless bachelor of forty cannot suddenly change his mind and decide to be an entrenched family man with three children while he is young enough to play games with them, a cell that has differentiated into a nerve cell cannot suddenly decide it would be more interesting to be a liver cell.

When I did my medical training I was taught, by the medical doctors that covered the subjects, that, when new cells of a particular tissue type were required, an existing cell of that type divided into two daughter cells, and hey presto, you had the additional cell(s) you wanted. I was also taught that cancer came about when fully formed, mature differentiated cells suddenly 'went off the rails' and started to behave abnormally, deteriorate and multiply endlessly. This had to be so, the doctors who taught the course argued, because the cancer cells of a particular tissue had recognisable, if damaged and altered, characteristics reminiscent of the tissue in which they were situated.

We now know that new tissue cells do not come from the division of one old mature tissue cell into two new daughter cells. The recognition of this fact, as we shall see, has a huge impact on the approach to detecting and treating cancer. In fact, it is probably fortunate that we do not rely on elderly mature cells for the production of new ones as old cells have worked hard and been metabolically active throughout their lives, and have probably developed faults.

So where do new cells come from? Unbeknown to my teachers, and to the teachers in virtually all medical schools, even to this day, our English biologist, Dr. John Beard, had published his entirely different concept of the development of new healthy tissue cells, and hence of cancer, back at the start of the last century.

In 2005, during a Christmas visit to Australia, I was amused to see a headline in the Sydney Morning Herald trumpeting what they claimed to be a new theory as to the cause of cancer. It was hardly new. It was closely aligned to the work that Beard had published a hundred years earlier.

This 'new' theory of cancer, particularly of epithelial cancers (those that start at or are in the lining of organs or ducts, which includes the majority of solid tumours), has been growing, slowly, over the last decade or so. This is now accepted by some of the cancer specialists who are prepared to think 'outside the box', be they CAM therapists or medical doctors who are prepared to take a wider view than most of their colleagues.

In brief, this theory states that cancer does not develop from mature cells, but from residual undifferentiated adult stem cells (as opposed to embryonic stem cells) that have lain dormant in your body since birth. It is time to explore this further.

Adult stem cells, also called somatic (or body) cells, are distinct from embryonic stem cells. Adult stem cells are found in a large number of organs and tissue throughout the body, in amongst the fully differentiated cells of that organ or tissue in 'stem cell niches'. They may eventually be found in all tissues. They are known to occur particularly in rapidly dividing or dying tissues such as peripheral blood and blood vessels, in the epithelium and the skin, in muscles and the heart, in the liver and digestive tract, and more. They can, when appropriately stimulated, differentiate into all the various cell types of the organ or tissue in which they are located. Their job is to replace old or damaged differentiated cells and repair the tissue, when this is required. To do this they rapidly develop up into fully differentiated cells of the appropriate type.

For instance, hematopoietic (from *haima* – blood; and *poiesis* – to make) stem cells, found in the bone marrow, can form all the various types of blood cells. Bone marrow stromal (connective tissue) stem cells can differentiate into bone cartilage and fat cells. It used to be said that damaged or destroyed nerve cells in the brain could not be replaced; we now know that there are brain stem cells and that they can differentiate into astrocytes, neurons and oligodendrocytes, three important types of brain cells.

Stem cells can divide and replace themselves so there is no need for there to be a large number of them in any specific tissue. They can divide in three ways to produce (1) two replacement stem cells, (2) one replacement stem cell and one cell of the local tissue type or (3) two cells of the local tissue type. Once removed from the body, unlike embryonic stem cells, their capacity to multiply is reduced, thus limiting their use in medicine.

It is noteworthy that there is a major problem with the concept of cancer being due to mature differentiated cells, suddenly multiplying out of control. The more mature and differentiated cells become, the more they actually lose their ability to subdivide and reproduce. By the time they are fully mature, fully differentiated and fully committed to being a cell of whatever tissue they have chosen to become, most of them have essentially lost their ability to multiply, a skill much needed, and demonstrated, by cancer cells. From this we might start to suspect that cancer does not come about, for instance, as a result of mature liver cells suddenly multiplying and becoming a liver tumour.

We have to look elsewhere for the origins of cancer. A useful place to start, when learning to understand this new-old theory of cancer, is with an understanding of the development of the human embryo. Put simply, at conception sperm and ovum come together and the fertilised ovum is formed. This partnership of sperm and ovum creates a product that is foreign to the mother. Even though it is her ovum, the complex (which includes the man's sperm) and the cells produced by it, as it multiplies, constitute a foreign body. Foreign bodies are usually attacked or repulsed by the immune system of the host. One would expect, therefore, that the mother's body would attack and eliminate this foreign organism.

In this case the foreign organism has entered an environment that is essentially hostile to it but at the same time this seemingly helpless foreign organism is totally dependent upon this environment, the adult female, for survival, nourishment and growth. It needs a home, a place to rest and to grow, and a supply of blood, oxygen, macro nutrients, vitamins, minerals, trace elements, and many other factors essential for its life and development. Somehow, this little complex of two, three or four cells has to persuade this vast maternal organism of several trillion cells to provide for its needs and not to attack or eliminate it.

The cells in this embryonic cluster are totipotent, meaning they are fully undifferentiated and have the potential to differentiate into any type of cell. They subdivide symmetrically, producing two identical daughter cells, and they do this slowly as they descend down a fallopian tube until there is a total of about a dozen cells, clustered together. Under the microscope they look something like a small blackberry, with some of the cells on the outside surrounding a few in the centre. Technically this is called a morula (after mulberry).

Somehow this morula has to find a safe haven, a place to shelter so it is not swept away, and where it can locate the appropriate source of the nourishment it needs for its continued growth into a full embryo and then a foetus and finally a baby. This is no small task.

The epithelial lining of the female's uterus is essentially an impenetrable wall with no 'holds' to latch onto. Yet somehow the morula has to attach to the uterus so that it is not swept away. Keep in mind that this epithelial lining of the uterus is so cohesive that it withstands the repeated periods of endometrial building and dispersing that occurs each month and also, when pregnancy occurs, the huge pressure that this pregnancy inevitably puts on it. It is a very strong wall that the tiny little morula has to penetrate.

Even if it can gain a 'foothold', the morula's job is not done, it then has to force its way through this epithelial layer to the very tough and even stronger basal layer underneath. This accomplished, it cannot rest on its laurels, it next has to penetrate through this basal layer to the underlying stroma or connective tissue that is sufficiently strong to hold the uterus together, for this is where there is a supply of blood and a source of the nutrients it needs. Yet even now it is not safe.

In the very early stages the individual cells can still each acquire their own nourishment from their surroundings, but if the cluster simply continued to grow, by subdivision, the central cells would soon be cut off from access to their surroundings and they would soon starve for lack of nourishment. They would die, and the pregnancy would terminate.

So the growing morula, having penetrated this far, has to force branches of the maternal blood supply system to grow and extend capillary channels for its own use, so that they divert nutrients from the mother to the morula. When, and only when, this is accomplished has the morula found a secure home and embryo development is possible. That's the story in brief. We need to go into this in more detail as what you will learn will help to explain to you the possible benefits of some of the tests you can do to learn more about (your) cancer itself.

Once the morula's cells start to differentiate it turns into a blastocyst. The cells divide into two groups with two distinct tasks. The outer cells become trophoblastic cells. It is these cells that have the job of invading the uterine wall. Once implantation has occurred these trophoblasts will form the placenta that protects the embryo and ensures a supply of nourishment for it. When they are eventually nourished by this activity the inner cells of the blastocyst start to multiply further and they then gradually differentiate into the individual organs and tissues of the developing embryo. Once these embryonic cells have a secure supply line they can act on the basis of the fact that they will continue to be fed and protected by the actions of the surrounding trophoblast cells of the placenta throughout the pregnancy.

One activity of the trophoblasts is to produce a hormone called human chorionic gonadotropin or HCG [see Chapters 3 and 6]. This is essentially only produced by these trophoblastic cells of the placenta. Its presence indicates that a pregnancy is occurring, and it is the substance that is tested for in the common pregnancy test that you can purchase from any chemist. We will have more to say of this shortly when we consider doing the tests for cancer.

For the moment we will return to the embryo and follow, in more detail, the first challenge of the trophoblastic cells, namely to break through the epithelium of the maternal uterus. This layer of cells is strongly welded together by a variety of different adhesion proteins. To enable them to penetrate this layer the trophoblast cells start to produce specific projectiles or receptors on their outer cell membranes. On their own they might be ineffective, but help is at hand, and if the pregnancy is successful it is because the epithelial cells of the uterus have detected the presence of the trophoblastic cells and are willing to cooperate with them. The uterine epithelial cells produce projections that are attracted to and bond with those of the trophoblasts in very firm bonds or 'handshakes'. This achieves a starting anchorage. At least now the risk of the blastocyst being swept away and out of the uterus is reduced.

However, the blastocyst, now an embryo, needs, as we have seen, a more secure resting place than this. The next step occurs when the trophoblast cells start to secrete a range of enzymes known as matrix metalloproteinases or MMP enzymes. (Nearly all enzyme names end in –ase and most compounds with names that end in –ase are enzymes.) About 24 of these MMP enzymes are known, all of which contain, as their name implies, a metal atom in their structure.

To provide a brief and conceptual understanding of the tissues of your body, I offer this comparison. Think of the wall of a building. There are the bricks that make up the wall, but they do not necessarily touch each other; they are embedded in a matrix of cement. In a somewhat similar way many of the cells of your body, and in this case those of the uterine wall, are embedded in a chemical matrix, made up of a significant amount of specialised proteins. These metallo matrix protein enzymes are able to act on the metallo link of the matrix proteins (the link binding the metal to the protein) and so are able to weaken and break down the cement between the cells. As a result, the localised part of the uterine wall starts to weaken. Once these MMP enzymes have weakened the structure of the uterine wall, the trophoblast can burrow more deeply into it. Finally, when the trophoblasts reach the underlying stroma and its connective tissue, they secrete more MMP enzymes that weaken this structure too, in a somewhat similar manner. It's somewhat like weakening the cement in a cavity wall in a building, and doing it layer by layer, first the outer wall, then on the inner wall.

In addition to the cells (bricks) and ground substance (cement) of your tissues there are fibres that hold the overall tissues together, rather like the steel rods that strengthen a concrete building. In the connective tissue of the underlying stroma, which the trophoblast has now reached, there are cells called fibroblasts. These are the cells that build or produce the fibres of the connective tissue in which the cells are embedded. As the MMPs break down the local proteins, various peptides (very small protein fragments) are produced. These peptides stimulate the fibroblasts into activity that will make life easier for the invading trophoblast. In addition, the MMPs from the trophoblastic cells combine with receptor proteins on the outer membrane of the fibroblasts and these, in their turn, start to produce more MMPs. Thus, the trophoblasts (from the embryo) and the fibroblasts (of the mother's uterus) are now working together to break down the stroma. At this point the developing tiny embryo is nearly home and housed. It has managed to implant itself in the uterus.

Testing for MMPases and the use of this in detecting and monitoring cancer and assessing the risk of metastatic activity will be discussed in the next book in this series. At this point it is worth mentioning that they are similar to other protein-digesting or protein-splitting enzymes, namely the protein-digesting enzymes, trypsin, chymotrypsin and carboxypeptidase produced by the pancreas for the digestion of food proteins. We will have more to say about these later [Chapter 16, Kelley].

Back to the embryo. It is now implanted, it has a home, it has escaped the danger of being flushed out of the system. The next step in this developing pregnancy is for the embryo to acquire a supply of blood, oxygen and nutrients. Without these it still cannot grow and survive. The process whereby it achieves this is called angiogenesis and this occurs when the embryo diverts some of the mother's blood to itself and stimulates the growth of arterioles, venules and capillaries to form and penetrate within itself, bringing in the needed supply of nutrients and providing an excretory route for waste products.

To achieve this angiogenesis the trophoblastic cells initiate another activity. They secrete a type of growth hormone called vascular endothelial growth factor or VEGF, and another one called platelet derived growth factor or PDGF. (These will also be discussed in more detail in the next book when we consider some of the tests you can do to help you plan a recovery programme that is specific to your unique needs.) VEGF and PDGF cause the local blood vessels, within the stroma of the uterus, to grow and send out new branches that can penetrate through the surrounding trophoblasts of the placenta and feed the embryo inside its protective wall. Growth of the embryo within the protective trophoblastic outer layer has been very slow until this point. Its whole aim has been focused on invading, anchoring, penetrating and ensuring a supply route.

The embryo does this to the uterine wall. But as we shall see, these same processes are also initiated by cancer cells. Cancer cells do the same thing when they grow into the first tumour and when they metastasise and find a new home. Cancer cells need to invade tissue, anchor, penetrate and secure a blood supply. Then, and only then, can they feed the cells in their centre and so only then are they able to grow more rapidly into a mass or tumour of a significant size.

Cancer cells behave in a way that is similar to that of the trophoblastic cells of pregnancy. In fact, Dr. Beard put it more strongly. He stated that cancer cells behave in *exactly* the same way as trophoblastic cells. He goes even further and states that trophoblast cells *are* cancer cells. It is for this reason that this discussion of embryo development is relevant when we consider how cancer starts and how we can block or reverse the process.

Back, again, to the embryo. The stage is set for a dramatic change. The embryo complex is securely anchored and has its own dedicated blood supply. It can now afford to grow at a very much accelerated rate. This is all well and good for the embryo, but such growth can be exponential and if it were allowed to continue indefinitely the embryo could rapidly outgrow the uterus. In other words, if penetration of the uterine wall and cellular growth were allowed to continue at the initial rate, unchecked, and the cells could continue to derive nourishment and multiply as rapidly as they do at the start, the viability of the mother, her life, would be threatened. Occasionally this does happen. If this accelerated growth doesn't stop at the appointed time then a type of cancer, specific to pregnancy and called choriocarcinoma, occurs and threatens the life of both the mother and, as a result, the developing embryo.

John Beard, around 1900, noted, and was able to demonstrate, even with the relatively limited tools at his disposal, that this enormously fast growth of the embryo, this doubling and redoubling of the number of cells, always slows dramatically around day 55 of the pregnancy. He also noted that this is the exact time at which the pancreas of the embryo becomes active.

The first thing to ponder here is why the pancreas of the embryo has to become active at all at this time. After all, the pancreas has, essentially, two main jobs to do. Firstly, the exocrine (external activity) pancreas is involved in digestion. This activity is taking place before any food crosses the intestinal wall and enters fully into the body and into the bloodstream. But the embryo gets its food supply from its mother, via the blood supply, not from an oral food source, and so digestive activity by the embryo will not be required until after birth, some seven months later. Secondly, the endocrine pancreas (involved in internal activities) has the job of normalising the level of glucose in the blood. But the blood comes from the mother, and her pancreas is doing this job. Control of its blood glucose level will only be demanded of the embryo's pancreas after the baby's birth, seven months later. So why does the embryo's pancreas become active at day 55?

Beard noted that choriocarcinoma, if it occurred, started around day 55 and only if the embryo's pancreas did not start to work. He wondered if it was the activity of the embryo's pancreas and the enzymes it produces that halted the rapid invasive action of the trophoblasts and the wayward development of overly rapid cellular division and growth, and thus prevented the choriocarcinoma of pregnancy. From there it was a small step for him to take to speculate that if the embryo's pancreatic enzymes could be used to attack or stop choriocarcinoma, then perhaps pancreatic enzymes could be effective against other types of cancer cells and tumours.

Although most of the trophoblastic cells form the placenta, Beard noted that some of them, in fact millions of them, are not used in this way. Most of these other trophoblastic cells make their way to the foetal gonads, the testes if it is going to be male and the ovaries if it is going to be female, ready for conception some years ahead, when the individual matures and reproduces in his or her turn.

Beard came to the conclusion that cancer evolves from the presence and transformation of aberrant germ cells that have lost their way en route to the foetal gonads, during embryogenesis, and become what he called 'irresponsible' or 'wayward' trophoblasts. He also noted that they dispersed throughout the developing foetus and formed reserve pools in all the tissues of its body. These wayward trophoblasts are what we now call stem cells, adult stem cells, to distinguish them from placental stem cells.

These adult stem cells, like all stem cells, are undifferentiated cells, and remember what this means. They are totipotent and have the potential to differentiate into any tissue that is needed, and they can divide and multiply rapidly, especially at the start, once they receive the appropriate triggers. After that, as they become more differentiated and specialised, their ability to reproduce slows down until, once they have become fully differentiated, it stops altogether.

We now know that these cells are called upon whenever new cells are needed, anywhere in the body. The lining of your digestive tract, for instance, is replaced approximately every five days. This is not accomplished by the old and mature intestinal cells dividing to produce new younger and (in some magic way) healthier daughter cells. Remember, these mature cells are highly differentiated cells and we now know that fully differentiated cells do not replicate readily. It is the locally situated undifferentiated adult stem cells that are called upon when replacements are needed.

You will recall that these adult stem cells can multiply in at least two different ways. They can multiply symmetrically by subdividing into two identical daughter stem cells. They can do this when more stem cells are needed at a particular location. They can also multiply asymmetrically. When this happens one of the daughter cells is a stem cell and replaces the original one, the other daughter cell differentiates and develops into a new cell with the character of, and ready to replace, the old cells lining your digestive tract (or in any other tissue). As this daughter cell matures and develops, its ability to reproduce slows until it stops entirely.

A similar activity takes place when any other cell types, anywhere else in your body, become old and need to be replaced, or when wound healing is required. The process is carefully controlled. Excess conversion of stem cells into skin cells would produce a growth above the skin. Too few new cells would lead to incomplete healing of the wound. The process is well controlled and is usually exact.

Remember, the reason for discussing this topic is that this starting phase of a pregnancy is, according to Beard, exactly the same as the process that occurs in the development of cancer. He states very clearly that the process is not similar to it, it is not analogous to it, but that it is exactly the same as, cancer. Beard further stated that these stem cells (his wayward trophoblasts) *are* cancer but that we are safe from their potentially negative activity as long as they are controlled or do not get the trigger to continue their activity beyond what is required for local repair and replacement.

Think of the developing embryo as being analogous to a group of cancer cells set on breaking down the structure of the local tissue. In the case of cancer this could be breast, prostate, lung, colon or other tissues where cancer is known to occur, invading it, layer by layer, and calling upon it for a blood supply that it can use for its own nourishment, then growing at an exponential rate and, in the process, destroying its host. The difference between a pregnancy and cancer is that, at some point during a pregnancy (day 55) the rapid embryonic growth is brought under control, whereas in the case of cancer the growth of a tumour is not brought under control by the host. Beard attributed this to a failure on the part of the individual's pancreas and its enzyme output.

When some of the undifferentiated, or partially differentiated, tumour cells move off through the bloodstream, and invade other tissues (metastasise) they do so by the same mechanism as is used by the developing embryo. They produce and use MMPases, they develop VEGF, they do all the things that the trophoblast cells did to and within the uterine wall. They even persuade the local tissue to co-operate with them, just as the cells of the uterine wall recognised and co-operated with the trophoblastic cells.

The original cancer cells will have begun to differentiate into the tissue in which they are situated, and will have started to develop some of the characteristics of this tissue, though possibly imperfectly so. Back in Beard's day it was easy to make two assumptions. Firstly, it was easy to assume that, in the primary tumour, they were once-healthy breast cells that had turned into breast cancer cells. Secondly, it was easy to assume that the new metastatic growth, which consisted of cells with similar characteristics, also derived from once-healthy breast cells and were secondary cancers. These assumptions are now thought to be wrong. It is now thought possible that the cells of a breast tumour have some of the characteristics of breast cells because they *started* to become breast cells, *not* because the are *broken down* breast cells.

Once a faulty stem cell begins to multiply and is not controlled, we have the amazing situation that, just as occurs in pregnancy, the host tissue actually works co-operatively with the developing cancer cells, to enable the establishment of the tumour. If a tumour cannot behave in this way and cannot invade the local tissue it is labelled a benign tumour. It can grow to a considerable size but it cannot invade the host's tissue, it cannot break through the various layers and so it cannot spread and is not generally life-threatening, not, at least, unless it damages surrounding organs by the sheer pressure of its size.

It used to be thought that all the cancerous cells in a tumour were capable of metastasising. Now it has been shown that only about one per cent of the cells in breast tumours are capable of doing this and that these are the highly malignant stem cells[150].

Beard was convinced that a fully adequate production of pancreatic protease enzymes, enzymes such as trypsin and chymotrypsin, plus amylase, was essential for the prevention of cancer[151]. Others came to be of the same opinion[152, 153, 154, 155]. It follows from this that the use of supplements of pancreatic enzymes should be helpful in the management of cancer. We will have more to say about this in later chapters.

TESTS

HCG

In view of the above discussion, the presence of HCG in the blood or urine is thought to be the best early warning sign of the start of Phase Two of the Cancer Process. It can generally be detected within about six weeks of the start of the development of permanent cancer cells.

As far back as 1994 it was shown that cancer cells express HCG in all its forms[156], that HCG was consistently found in at least 85 different cancer cell lines and that, *"...synthetic HCG... is a common biochemical denominator in cancer."*[157]

Not only is HCG a useful indicator of the presence of cancer cells, it is a harbinger of worse to come. HCG and HCGLS (see below) inhibit immune activity, increase angiogenesis and stimulate metabolic, regulatory, growth and cell proliferation in target cells and organs, thus increasing the possible development of any type of cancer[158]. These may seem to be inappropriate actions for the host (you), but remember, this activity is designed primarily to support and help the developing embryo. If it is happening in tumour formation this is a fault of the host in not controlling it.

In other words, the level of HCG indicates how metastatically aggressive a tumour may be. *"Neither non-embryonic cells nor benign tumour cells express HCG, but HCG-beta is a defining phenotype statement of malignant transformation."* [159]

HCG is an oligosaccharide glycoprotein hormone, meaning that it is composed of groups (probably up to about eleven) of saccharide molecules (glucose or related sugar or carbohydrate compounds) or units attached to amino acid sequences (peptides or proteins). It consists of 244 amino acids and is made up of two subunits, alpha and beta. The alpha subunit consists of 92 amino acids and is the same as the subunit found in luteinizing hormone (LH), follicle stimulating hormone (FSH) and thyroid stimulating hormone (TSH). The beta subunit is unique to HCG.

In the 1950s, through the work of Dr. Manuel Navarro and Dr. Howard Beard, a Yale trained biologist and chemistry professor, the Anthrone Colour Test, done on urine, was used to detect HCG[160]. However, this did not discriminate between the alpha and beta subunits and only indicated total HCG-like components.

In 1977, Dr. Robert Williams, working with the Framington study and using frozen serum samples collected prior to the diagnosis of cancer for nine patients with pancreatic cancer and eight with gastric carcinoma, was able to report the detection of HCG in the blood two years before a tumour was detected[161]. However, there were also a number of false positives, presumably due to the presence of alpha subunits unconnected to the presence of cancer.

In combination, the alpha and beta subunits sit at the core of the molecule and are hydrophobic (repel water). This core is then surrounded by a layer of hydrophilic amino acids. In either blood or urine, HCG exists in a number of forms. Some of it is present as free HCG, some as free alpha subunits, some as free beta subunits and the rest as fragments such as nicked HCG and nicked free beta HCG.

An excellent test for HCG levels in blood and urine is offered by American Metabolic Laboratories (www.caprofile.net). This laboratory has developed its CA Profile since 1980. At that time the panel consisted of three tests, for HCG-beta, PHI and CEA. Using that test the results showed that, *"94% of patients (n = 133) with proven cancers displayed at least one abnormal result... and ...26% of patients without proven cancer (n = 197) displayed one or more elevated tumour markers. A number of these 'false positive' results were in individuals with signs or symptoms of cancer (e.g., enlarged lymph nodes, breast lumps, etc.), but without pathologic diagnoses. Some were later diagnosed with cancer."*[162] Thus, even false positives can have their uses and provide possible triggers to encourage the individual to take better care of their health.

The panel now consists of a number of components. Among other results it gives three results for HCG, two blood forms: IRMA HCG and IMM HCG and a urinary level called urinary HCG or HCG-U. This grouping of three HCG tests offers a much more secure test with very much less likelihood of producing false positives or false negatives.

- The IRMA HCG result comes from a test done by an ImmunoRadioMetric Assay (hence its name) and detects only the intact HCG molecules, not any of the fragments or separate subunits.

- The IMM HCG result is obtained by chemiluminescence and detects not only the intact HCG molecules, but the subunits and fragments and the HCGLSs (HCG-like substances). For this reason the IMM result is usually higher than the IRMA result.

- The HCG-U detects all HCG except for the HCGLS and so, if this reading is positive, it increases the probability that you do not have a false positive reading.

For many years the laboratory only offered the two blood tests and they were generally found to be giving accurate information. However, there was always a small possibility of false positives caused by non-specific heterophilic-immune binding HCG fragments or HCGLSs. These, if present, can be found in blood samples, but they do not enter the urine. Thus, the addition of the urine result has increased the certainty of the interpretation of the results. In other words, by doing the urine test for HCG you can, if it is found, rule out the possibility of basing your interpretation on false positives, while still getting the useful information from the two blood tests.

Some laboratories rely only on urine HCG but this too is open to errors if it is used as the only test for HCG. The reason is as follows. With increasing age there is the possibility of developing gonadal insufficiency. This means that there is a decrease in the output of oestrogen or testosterone. In response to this there is an increased output of two hormones from the pituitary gland, luteinizing hormone and follicle stimulating hormone as the body tries to whip the tired gonads into increased output. As a result of this increased pituitary output there will be a small output of HCG-like substances that are common to luteinizing hormone, follicle stimulating hormone and thyroid stimulating hormone.

Clearly this is not related to trophoblastic cells, but it does show up in the urine. By assessing the levels of IRMA-HCG, IMM-HCG and HCG-U it is possible to make a more secure assessment of the results and to avoid chasing after false positives.

If you are either male, or are female but could not be pregnant, you should not have any of this hormone in your blood. If you do, it suggests the probability that you have transformed trophoblastic cells, cells that have the potential to turn into, are turning into, or have turned into cancer cells. If this is the case, then now is the time to take action to correct the situation. It is most unwise to ignore this early warning sign – and there is a *lot* you can do.

The level of HCG can rise within days of cancer cells developing, within days of you entering Phase Two of the Cancer Process. This is long before a tumour is large enough to be detected, it may even be many years before this is possible. There is considerable evidence that an abnormal level of HCG, even if it is only small, generally leads on to a tumour in the future, possibly months or sometimes years in the future.

If you have had cancer and had surgery and been told that, *"They got it all, and you do not need further treatment"*, you can use this test to determine the truth, or not, of this statement. According to Dr. Schandl at American Metabolic Laboratories, *"After successful surgery, provided all of the tumour has been removed and there are no metastatic foci, the markers should be negative in three to six weeks, depending on the extent of the surgery."* If you do the test six or more weeks after your surgery and your results are not within normal limits, it suggests that they did not 'get it all', that there are trophoblastic cells there, ready at any time to grow into a tumour, and that you have more work to do to get out of the danger zone.

If you have not yet had surgery, but are going to have it, and you have been advised that they 'hope to get it all', you would be wise to do this test before surgery, to get a starting bench mark, and then afterwards to make sure that the level has returned to zero. This before and after test will give you useful information as you monitor the situation in the future. If there is a recurrence it will be helpful to know how the level of HCG relates to the pre-surgery or pre-treatment level.

An abnormal level of HCG can also indicate the likelihood of metastasis occurring. It can be thought of as a time bomb, waiting for a trigger.

If you have cancer and embark on recovery programmes, be they CAM or MDS programmes, you can use repeated HCG tests to monitor the progress you are making. If all is well, the levels of the various forms of HCG will eventually return to normal and none will be detected.

However, it is worth keeping in mind that few tests, including the various tests done by your doctor, are perfect. The laboratory advises that they like to have at least two out of three of the HCG results positive before feeling confident of the existence of cancer. Conversely, there have been a few relatively rare occasions when someone with diagnosed cancer has been found to have had normal HCG levels or only one slightly raised level. This test should serve as a guide, rather than as an absolute on its own, and, if there is concern, be assessed in combination with a total clinical picture.

HCG (IRMA and IMM) can be measured on a blood sample, specifically on a sample of the serum, the part of the blood that does not include the blood cells. This serum is separated off by centrifuging the sample before it is sent to the laboratory.

If you choose to discuss the subject of HCG with your doctor you may be told that HCG is only present in choriocarcinoma, the type of cancer which can occur during pregnancy, and is of no relevance in any other type of cancer. This seems to be the generally held MDS wisdom, at least at the clinical level. However, using 85 different cancer cell lines, intact HCG has been found in cell membranes in association with metastatic aggressive tumours of many different histological types and origins, and in the blood and urine of patients with bladder, gastrointestinal tract, lung, and skin (melanoma) cancers as well as in embryonal carcinomas[163, 164], and cancer of the lung, pancreas and liver[165, 166, 167] but not found in benign cells. It therefore seems likely that raised levels of HCG may be associated with all types of cancer, in line with the trophoblastic origin of cancer postulated by Beard (above). Certainly, any indication of a raised level of HCG should be taken very seriously and responded to accordingly.

It is worth pointing out here that the usual (urine) pregnancy test, alluded to above, is inadequate for detecting the presence of HCG that is found if cancer is present. The level rises very much higher in pregnancy than in cancer and the pregnancy test is far too insensitive to detect the very small amounts that indicate cancer.

There is a very important difference between this test and the medical tests for tumour markers. This test will tell you if there is cancer anywhere in your body. Thus, one test gives you great coverage. It will not tell you where the cancer is, if it is detected; however, this is not important as we are not focused on locating and eradicating a tumour, but rather we are focused on correcting the cellular errors that constitute Phase Two of the Cancer Process, wherever they are occurring in the body. The MDS system does need to know the location of a tumour as that is the focus of its treatment. The HCG tests in the CA Profile are thought to be better than 93% reliable, compared to the medical tests for tumour markers where the correlation can be significantly less. Further, they are usually location specific. For instance, a clear result when you do a PSA test (commonly done to test for prostate cancer) will tell you nothing about the possibility of cancer anywhere else in the body. Similarly, if you have your CA 15.3 (commonly done to test for breast cancer) and it is clear, you may feel you can relax, thinking you don't have breast cancer, but that too tells you nothing about the possibility of cancer anywhere else in your body.

CHAPTER 15

STEM CELLS AND DR. BIAVA

Dr. Pier Biava, an eminent Italian cancer researcher, author of many papers and several books, has written an interesting book entitled *'Cancer and the search for lost meaning'*, subtitle, *'The discovery of a revolutionary new cancer treatment'* [168]. Based on an autobiography of his career it takes the reader step by step through his development of the concept of cancer as a complex disease related to the activity of aberrant stem cell replication. It is a complex read but essentially an endorsement of Beard's hypothesis of the importance of damaged stem cells (aberrant germ cells). This comes, inevitably, with a lot more of the technical information, cellular and epidemiological evidence and physiological chemistry that has emerged in the hundred years since Beard wrote his work.

In the foreword to Beard's book, Ervin Laszlo points to an interesting parallel that will help us here with our understanding of the nature of cancer from a non-reductionist perspective. Laszlo likens cancer cells to individual terrorists or criminals and points out that you can no more 'cure' cancer by killing individual cells or cell clusters (tumours) than you can stop criminal or terrorist behaviour by killing or imprisoning individuals or small groups of troublemakers. The answer, in both situations, is to focus on the health of the overall organism, be it society or the total human being, and that when endeavouring to reach your goal it is essential to be aware of the effect of the treatment you apply (social or medical) on the total organism (society or the human body). This will only come about, in health care, when we remember, and take seriously, the concept that the whole (human being) is more than the sum of its parts (from tissues, down to organs, cells, molecules, and atoms).

While Biava is not opposed to destroying the tumour, he suggests, like others before him, that cancer cells can be reprogrammed back into healthy cells. In suggesting that cancer is the result of a loss of meaning to the purpose of life in our modern society, Biava is echoing Dr. Fryda's hypothesis that cancer is the result of stress, and particularly, as others have suggested, stress of the helpless and hopeless variety.

Biava's research led him to focus on the shift that occurs with stem cells as they move from unlimited multiplication to controlled differentiation. Think back to the unlimited multiplication phase of the first 55 days of pregnancy that Beard recognised, and the controlled differentiation phase of the remainder of the pregnancy, the switch, as Beard pointed out, occurring when the embryo becomes a foetus and its pancreas comes into play. Biava looks for the communication that occurs from the mother's uterus to the embryo that leads to this change and to the start of organogenesis. When searching for a cure for cancer he therefore looks for a way to communicate and instruct this change from (unhealthy if excessive) multiplication to (controlled and healthy) differentiation, from out-of-control cancer cells to controlled healthy cells.

Based on his research and its results Biava insists, as do most of the scientists or doctors discussed in this book, that it is essential to stop taking the (MDS) reductionist view and change to a more comprehensive and complex view of cancer and the related inter-cellular communications.

Biava recognised that carcinogens, when administered to a pregnant adult female, can cause either malformations and miscarriages on the one hand, or tumours on the other. His research led him to the idea that the nature of the outcome, whether it was a malformation or a miscarriage, or a tumour, depended on the phase of the pregnancy during which the exposure to the carcinogens occurred. In studies on experimental animals, he found that if the carcinogen was administered early in the pregnancy, during differentiation and organogenesis (the period in which the organs and systems were being formed), the number of miscarriages or of malformations in the offspring increased, but not the incidence of tumours. He ascribed this to the fact that during this phase there is a tight control on cell differentiation. If the carcinogen was administered later in the pregnancy, after organogenesis, there was an increase in the number of tumours in the offspring and a concomitant decrease in the number of malformations. Of this he says, *"...once organogenesis is complete... the system of correction and control of cell differentiation becomes less efficient."*

Biava suggested that certain factors, that are present during the time when cells are differentiating into the different organs, are able to slow down or inhibit tumour growth, and that these factors are only present at the moment in which the stem cells start to differentiate and not when they are fully and actively multiplying. From this he suggested that it could be possible to obtain at this time 'from the uterus' factors that are able to inhibit or slow down tumour growth. For the best results these have to be extracted at the point when embryos start to differentiate. He was eventually able to isolate a low molecular-weight fraction that he called the 'Life-Protecting Factor' and found that it stimulated apoptosis.

In further studies, working with zebra fish (*danio rerio*), he found that when the embryo is made up solely of totipotent undifferentiated embryonic stem cells there is increased chance of tumour proliferation rather than slowing it down. This is in line with the experimental fact that when totipotent embryonic stem cells are used in the experimental treatment of certain pathologies there is an increased risk of the subsequent development of cancer. From this he concluded that **tumour growth is arrested during cellular differentiation**. This arrest happens in different ways, but these all depend on the fact that stem cell differentiation factors regulate proteins such as Protein 53 (p53) and another protein called retinoblastoma protein (pRb). These proteins control cell cycling (the process of one cell differentiating into two daughter cells). *"As a result, cancer multiplication is arrested, and... genetic damage at the origin of the disease is repaired and the cells differentiate or, if the mutations cannot be repaired, genes prompting programmed cell death (apoptosis) are activated and the cells die."* [See his book.]

Cadherins are calcium-dependent adhesion proteins. Put simply, their presence enables cells to stick firmly together. A reduction in the level of certain cadherins indicates a weakening of the connections between cells and, in cancer, an increased risk of metastasis occurring[169]. Biava points out that cancer cell apoptosis and re-differentiation increases when differentiation factors are added to tumour cells. Put another way, when cells are induced to differentiate (specialise) there is increased apoptosis of cancer cells. This is shown by the rise in E-cadherin, and that, *"...differentiation factors have the same function and role in regard to cancer cells as in embryos."*

De-differentiation (the reverse of specialisation) factors play the same role in the embryo and in cancer cells. The activity of p53 suppressor gene and the output of p53 protein are increased every time the embryo genome experiences a mutation or a cell develops cancer. Thus, p53 protects against mutations. If the genetic insult is overwhelming, then p53 fails to repair the DNA damage and apoptosis is triggered. In other words, either the cancerous cell is persuaded to revert to being a healthy cell or it is destroyed.

DNA and the Epigenetic code

DNA is the substance of which our genes are made, it is our biological inheritance from our parents. Epigenetics is the study of how these genes are expressed as a result of modifying factors that occur *outside* (epi-) the genes. When we talk of genes 'expressing themselves' in this way we mean that the genes are being active and showing their presence by the results that occur. We have talked, for instance, about protein 53 that encourages apoptosis or the death of damaged cells. If outside (epigenetic) factors inhibit the activity or the 'expression' of the gene that codes for this protein you are more likely to have a lowered level of p53 and to develop a tumour.

The human body contains approximately 100,000 different proteins. It used to be thought that there was a specific gene that coded for each of these proteins. It seemed to be a simple, and therefore, to the way of Newtonian thinking, logical arrangement. However, as work has advanced on the human genome it has became clear that less than 21,000 genes, or a mere 2% of the total human genetic code, is used to code for proteins. So the question then became, *"How do the cells know which protein to make in response to a gene that codes for several of them?"* In fact, the production of the individual proteins is accomplished by a variety of different regulatory processes that control the action of single genes. Higher regulatory capacity enables greater complexity of the number and type of proteins produced. A medium-sized gene can codify more than 3,000 different proteins.

Much of the DNA, in combination with a network of other molecules, constitutes the epigenetic code and controls this regulatory function. The epigenetic code regulates gene expression during embryonic development and leads to appropriate differentiation into specific cell and tissue types. The genetic code in each cell is the same, the epigenetic code is tissue and cell specific. So the differences between cells are epigenetic rather than genetic. The genetic code can be thought of as the computer's hard disk, and the epigenetic code the use that is made of this by the operator. The information that is stored in the cell's DNA is communicated, via various forms of RNA, to the ribosomes (cell organelles), where the various proteins are synthesised.

MicroRNA is tiny, with only 21-23 nucleotides (or individual segments or 'letters' of the code), but it is essential for life. It can regulate codifying genes, regulate gene expression by a number of mechanisms and influence cell differentiation. By intruding into the cell's RNA it can selectively deactivate any gene, with enormous beneficial possibilities for the cell.

Think back to Chapter 14 and the developing morula, blastocyst, embryo and foetus. The early totipotent cells of the blastocyst start to differentiate and form three layers, the ectoderm, mesoderm and endoderm. The ectoderm (outer layer) will develop into the skin, mammary tissue and nerves of the baby that is to be. The mesoderm (middle layer) will develop into the bones, connective tissues, muscles and blood vessels. The endoderm (centre) will develop into the digestive system and the glands feeding into it and the lungs and bronchial tubes. This development is done by asymmetric reproduction of the stem cells which produce one replacement stem cell and one daughter cell of the resulting tissue. The resulting daughter cells will have different levels of differentiation and of reproductive potential. They may be:

- pluripotent cells, able to differentiate into cells of all three layers;
- multipotent cells, able to differentiate into many cell lines, but of a limited number of them;
- oligopotent cells, able to differentiate into only a few cell lines;
- unipotent cells, able to differentiate into only one type of cell line;
- definitively differentiating cells;
- terminally differentiated cells.

As you progress down the list they become more and more differentiated, more and more specialised and less and less able to reproduce or multiply.

Nature versus nurture

Biava is of the opinion that more than ninety per cent of cancers are caused by epigenetic factors, by diet and the environment, and that less than ten per cent are due to viruses or inherited faults. He points out that tumours inherited at birth are rare, whereas there are more frequent cases where heredity causes a greater tendency for the individual to develop cancer during life. With regard to environmental toxins he points out that the smallest dose of a carcinogen, even if it is fully metabolised and eliminated, leaves irreversible effects that, when they all come together, can lead to cancer.

Radiation can cause long-delayed damage and is probably a component, along with other carcinogens, in the final trigger that starts Phase Two of the Cancer Process. Radiation-induced cancers leave a particular and detectable pattern in the tissues and this is still showing up in Japanese women with breast cancer many decades after the Second World War. It seems that radiation-induced cancers can occur many decades after the original radiation exposure, and that its occurrence is commonly delayed until the age at which that particular type of tumour is most likely to develop[170].

Cause of cancer

Biava considers that there is no single clear-cut mechanism by which a healthy cell turns into a cancer cell. Instead, he sees the process as the result of a complex network of signals between cells or the actions of soluble extracellular factors. He notes a number of facts to support this view:

- fibroblasts adjacent to tumour cells are able to direct tumour progression;
- cells near connective tissues can promote the transformation of immortalized cells by releasing a proliferating stimulus;

- cells connected to inflammatory processes can withstand, instead of fight, tumour growth.

Thus, the development of cancer cells is a micro-evolutionary process as a result of which cancer cells acquire the ability to:

- be self-sufficient in growth signals;
- be insensitive to signals that block growth;
- survive and avoid apoptosis;
- potentially replicate without limit;
- maintain continued angiogenesis;
- invade tissues and create metastasis.

His research has shown that the development of all types of human tumours is governed by a single final process. He focuses on the accumulation of genetic mutations up to an 'early crisis' point. Prior to this point, what he calls a check-point, p53 protein can block the cellular cycle and induce the transcription of p21, another protective protein, one which then repairs the damaged DNA. If this is unsuccessful then attempts are made to induce apoptosis.

If apoptosis fails and the cell continues to live, the cell can mutate further and reproduce chaotically, leading to rampant genetic instability and genetic catastrophe, at which point the cell is fully a cancer cell capable of leading to an invasive and progressive tumour. His studies have shown that this chaotic process is stabilized in time by an 'attractor' that leads the genome of the cancer cell to a new configuration, somewhat similar to that in the placental or trophoblastic part of the embryo process. Thus, he comes to Beard's hypothesis, proposed a hundred years earlier, that cancer cells are mutated stem cells.

Tumour cells and stem cells have a number of similarities

It is time to consider some of the similarities between stem cells and cancer cells.

- Both have proto-oncogenes. Proto-oncogenes are genes that can be converted into or turn into oncogenes (genes that encourage cancer), either when they have mutated or been allowed to over-express themselves. They are active embryonic genes that are responsible for cellular replication. These proto-oncogenes are clearly important at the start of embryonic growth. They are progressively inhibited as differentiation progresses, until they are turned off completely. This can be thought of as gradually putting on the brakes until further growth is halted once the tissues have been fully formed. In cancer cells, these proto-oncogenes may be mutated to oncogenes and so may not 'turn off', thus growth continues, unchecked. Oncogenes produce embryonic growth factors that are responsible for continued cellular replication.

- Both have onco-suppressor genes that are responsible for turning off cellular reproduction. An example of one of these is the p53 gene which, in healthy cells, produces normal p53 protein. In cancer cells these onco-suppressor genes are often mutated and produce a mutated, and ineffective p53 protein. Tests are available to determine your level of normal p53 gene expression, the amount of protein it produces, and the possible and unwanted presence of mutated p53 gene and its faulty protein. The presence of the latter, of course, means that normal p53 activity and defences do not occur. As soon as a cell has activated certain oncogenes and deactivated certain onco-suppressor genes, it goes into uncontrollable multiplication.

- Both stem cells and cancer cells contain growth factors. Several of the cancer cell growth factors are also embryonic growth factors, including those that lead to angiogenesis (the formation of new blood vessels). Cancer cells deactivate signals that stop cell growth and activate growth factors.

- Both have oncofetal antigens (proteins) on their membranes. It is thought to be these that are the receptors for differentiation factors that send growth signals into the cell.

Examples of these (oncofetal antigens) include:

(a) carcinoembryonic antigen (CEA), which is readily tested for and often associated with colon cancer;
(b) alpha-fetoprotein, which has been found in a number of types of cancer, including liver cancer;
(c) trophoblast glycoprotein precursor; and
(d) immature laminin receptor protein or oncofetal antigen protein.

These proteins can often be detected in the blood of people with cancer. A test for CEA is included in the CA profile offered by American Metabolic Laboratories. A test for alpha fetoprotein gene expression is offered by Neuro-Lab. They are useful in both the detection of the presence of cancer cells and the monitoring of recovery programmes.

- Both embryonic and stem cells rely on anaerobic metabolism.
- Both types of cells share a number of common metabolic or signalling paths, such as ones called the APC/beta catenin/TCF/WNT path and the Hedgehog/Smoothened/Patched path, and their molecular effectors. These pathways lead to different outcomes in embryo and stem cells. In embryo cells they lead to health and to normal embryonic development and cell differentiation. In cancer cells they are mutated and result in unstoppable replications since the mutations inhibit the cells' path to full differentiation.

So now we are clearly at a stage when we can say that cancer cells are mutated stem cells in which (a) there is an imbalance of the epigenetic code in an embryonic sense and (b) there are mutations that have split the differentiation and multiplications programmes. That is, both the genetic and epigenetic codes have been altered.

Current MDS thinking, in practice, is generally based on genetic mutations, but these on their own are not sufficient to cause cancer. It is the alterations to the epigenetic code that are critical. This means that, in Biava's view, it is the epigenetic factors, the dietary, environmental and other such external insults, that are the necessary triggers that alter the expression of the genetic code (genes) and convert healthy adult stem cells into mutated stem cells and hence into cancer cells. Thus, Biava claims that approximately 93 per cent of cancers are caused by diet and lifestyle (epigenetic factors) and only seven per cent by genetic factors.

In this scenario:

- a healthy stem cell mutates and either dies or survives as a cell with damaged DNA;
- this cell with damaged DNA either dies or becomes a cell with rampant genetic instability;
- this potentially rampantly unstable cell either dies or becomes one of several types of mutated stem cells, being multipotent, oligopotent, a differentiating stem cell or a differentiated cell.

This scenario points to a logical programme of cancer management and recovery. Such a programme should involve working on the epigenetic aspects of the disease (diet and lifestyle in the very broadest sense) and developing a programme that aims to repair the cellular damage and reprogramme the cells so that normal cellular development is resumed. This means correcting all the Predisposing Factors of Phase One of the Cancer Process and correcting any errors shown up by the tests described here in relation to Phase Two of this Process.

Not only has Biava's work led to a greater understanding and elucidation of the mechanism of cancer and tumour development and to the production of his 'Life Protecting Factors', it has since led to the development of natural remedies, incorporating extracts from the zebra fish, that have similar cancer-inhibiting effects. These are thought to be due, at least in part, to their positive effect on the p53 gene. However, there are additional mechanisms by which the zebra fish extracts act. For instance, *"Previous studies have shown that proteins extracted from zebra fish embryo share some cytostatic characteristics in cancer cells... our study shows that zebra fish embryo proteins significantly inhibit Caco2 growth and induce programmed cell death by activation of p53-independent mechanisms, acting mainly through the pRb/E2F1 apoptotic pathway."* [171].

TESTS

P53 protein will be discussed in much greater detail in the third book in this series. For the moment it is sufficient to note that the p53 gene is arguably our best defence against getting cancer, and in the fight against cancer once it has started. Healthy, 'wild' p53 acts in many different ways to protect against cancer. If cancer has started, you would hope to find that the level of p53 has risen in response. If you have insufficient activity of this gene, or if the gene is mutated, then corrective action is required.

Neuro-Lab offers tests for wild and mutated p53 gene and for the amount of p53 protein that is produced. The detailed interpretation of the results is complex and you should discuss this with your practitioner.

CHAPTER 16

THE PANCREAS AND WILLIAM KELLEY

The next part of the story involves William Kelley[172, 173, 174, 175], an American dentist with a long-standing interest in cancer. In brief, he developed metastatic cancer of the pancreas, was given weeks to live, advised that he was too ill for surgery and told to go home and put his affairs in order. Instead, he took control of his own health and recovery programme, cured himself and lived another forty years. During this time he helped thousands of people who were suffering from cancer. Here is his story.

Kelley's first early warning signs of ill health were spread over three years and included burping and flatulence, worsening eyesight (for which he was given glasses), then fatigue, followed by muscle cramps in the back (for which he was given a muscle relaxant) and chest pains (for which he had several ECGs that were all normal), plus depression and confusion.

By the end of this three-year period he had seen his doctor so often the doctor was getting impatient with him and of all his various complaints. The doctor then gave Kelley a thorough examination and told him he was fine and that he should stop worrying as his problems were all in his mind. Kelley tried to put this advice into practice and get on with his life, but he gradually grew weaker and lost interest in most things, including his profession – which he loved. He noted changes in hair colour (going grey) and texture (becoming dry) and that it was falling out, and also some developing varicose hernias, which he subsequently attributed to protein wasting.

When he finally returned to his doctor he was at last sent to an internist who did a range of tests, including x-rays, which showed a liver that was swollen to three times its normal size, lesions in his lungs and a large tumour on his right hip. He was advised to have biopsies done of his pancreas, liver and intestines, as cancer was strongly suspected at all three sites. His wife was told that he had tumours in all three organs. He declined the biopsies, knowing the dangers of biopsy-induced metastasis.

You will recall that [Chapter14 and HCG] in the 1950s, Dr. Manuel Navarro had announced that he could detect HCG produced by only a few million trophoblast cells[176] using the Beard-Anthrone Colour urine test (BAT) for HCG (not related to Dr. John Beard of the earlier chapter). This test measures the level of HCG in the urine and is a forerunner of the current urinary test done by American Metabolic Laboratories (above). The blood tests for HCG were either not available or Kelley did not know about them. When Kelley did this urine test his result was 'extremely positive' for cancer.

After examining Kelley, his surgeon refused to operate, thinking that Kelley was too ill to survive the operation. Instead, he advised Kelley that he did not have long to live and that he should go home and put his affairs in order. In spite of the various health problems he had had, the diagnosis surprised Kelley and made him stop and think about a lot of the things he was doing. His pancreas was so damaged his blood sugar level was out of control, swinging widely between hyper- and hypo- glycaemia and he would go into insulin shock several times a day. His heartbeat was rapid and erratic. His liver was so enlarged that he could easily feel the distension below his ribcage and cup it in the palm of his hand. In fact, he used it to determine when he was eating right or wrong foods as it varied in size accordingly. The state of his intestines caused him to be in constant pain.

In spite of his diagnosis and what he had been told, he decided not to give in or give up but to take his health into his own hands. Firstly, he took control of his diet. He knew, soon after eating a particular food, whether it made him feel better or worse, partly by his symptoms in general and partly by the size of the liver tumour that he could feel with his hands. As a consequence of these inputs he evolved his diet plan.

He then turned his attention to his tumours. His first thought was to destroy the cancer as fast as possible. Building on the work of Beard he recognised that the best way to do this would be to use pancreatic enzymes and he used these in large quantities. That was when he learnt about the dangers of tumour lysis toxicity. He found that if he took too many enzymes and did not do sufficient detoxing to get rid of the detritus, he broke the tumours down too fast and the toxic symptoms of nausea, vomiting, headaches, and general 'unwellness' became unbearable. His aim had to be to adjust the speed of tumour lysis or breakdown so that the toxicity symptoms were present (indicating that tumour breakdown was occurring) but mild (so they did not overwhelm his tissues with the released toxins).

Over time he developed his five-step plan which consisted of:

1. the correct diet for the individual – this will depend on your metabolic type [Chapter 25];
2. a fully adequate enzyme and supplement programme;
3. an extensive detox programme to reduce or prevent tumour lysis toxicity and to remove existing toxins. He did this using castor oil wraps, heavy doses of Epsom salts, daily enemas, which he learnt about from the medical Merck manual of the time, and monthly liver flushes;
4. neurological stimulation - for which he used chiropractic and related procedures;
5. resolving emotional issues.

Using these methods Kelley cured his own cancers. They were diagnosed in 1964 when Kelley was 39 but they had clearly been developing for several years. Not only did Kelley not die as rapidly as his doctors had predicted, he lived another forty years, until 2005 when he was aged 79, and died, not of cancer, but, it is thought, of congestive heart failure.

Throughout that time he treated and helped thousands of people with cancer. He helped as many people as were prepared to wholeheartedly and unreservedly follow his programme, using the same methods he had applied to himself, all the time convinced that the trophoblastic or stem cell theory of cancer, as elucidated by Dr. John Beard, was correct. The large doses of pancreatic enzymes were a key component of his protocol and, he believed, they were a large part of the reason for his total recovery and the recovery of those who followed his protocol to its fullest extent[177, 178].

If Kelley was able to do this for himself with his extensive problems and using the information he had in the last century, you can surely do the same in this century. We have learnt more since Kelley's time. There are many more tests available that help to guide and direct a recovery programme and there is more new equipment that is readily available. Some of this equipment can be used in the home, such as Far Infra Red Saunas, foot baths, and appliances for preparing interesting raw and dehydrated meals. We also have equipment for targeted hyperthermia and other clinical procedures. There is more knowledge now about specific therapeutic agents and there are more supplements containing these agents readily available than were available to Kelley.

Kelley's methods have also been tested since that time[179, 180] including by Dr. Nick Gonzalez, some years after Kelley's recovery. At the time, Dr. Gonzalez was a medical student, working under the auspices of Dr. Robert Good of the Sloane-Kettering Cancer Center of New York City. Dr. Gonzalez went through Kelley's records and identified 22 cases of biopsy-confirmed pancreatic cancer diagnosed at major medical institutions.

Of these 22 patients with pancreatic cancer who had consulted Kelley:

Ten did not follow his protocol; thought to be because they considered it to be too difficult or too demanding. They lived an average of 67 days.

Seven partially followed his protocol and survived for an average of 233 days.

Five followed the full protocol. One had Alzheimer's disease and died eleven and a half years after starting his protocol. The other four were all alive when the study was written up. The average survival time, at that stage, was nine years[181].

The five-year survival of pancreatic cancer by the MDS system is essentially zero with average survival being very much less than this, as indicated by the first ten patients. The results achieved by those who followed the Kelley regime are impressive. It is shameful that the MDS system has not been willing to take more notice of these results.

Dr. Gonzalez is now in practice in New York and focuses his practice on helping people with cancer using diet, supplements, pancreatic enzymes and other lifestyle changes[182].

How pancreatic enzymes work

Immune cells such as Natural Killer Cells normally destroy foreign cells or pathogens such as bacteria. However, they do not kill cancer cells as readily. There are many reasons for this. The membrane or wall of cancer cells is about fifteen times thicker and stronger than the membrane or wall of healthy cells. Furthermore, it often has a protective coating that resists breakdown.

Kelley stated that, as tumours grow they produce an enzyme called malignin. This breaks down what he calls the 'left-handed proteins' of healthy body tissue. These are proteins made up of the normal L-amino acids. Malignin increases the production of cancer cells which in turn increases the output of malignin and thus the growth rate of the tumour is increased in a self-perpetuating manner. Malignin is the mirror image of trypsin (one of the major pancreatic protease enzymes) which he says is capable of breaking down the right-handed proteins (containing D-amino acids), found in the tumour. According to Kelley, *"Large quantities of trypsin in the bloodstream stop malignin's acceleration of tumour growth. Also, the non-growing tumour can now be recognized by the body's defensive warriors, white blood cells and antibodies. These defensive warriors engulf the liquefied, dead non-growing tumour debris from the digestive activity of the enzyme trypsin."* He further states that amylase, a carbohydrate-splitting enzyme, is needed to work with trypsin.

A study of the effect of pancreatic enzymes on glycolysis in cancer cells[183] leads to the conclusions that:

1. the aerobic and anaerobic glycolysis of cancer tissue is inhibited by pancreatic extract;
2. other amylase-containing extracts made from malt diastase, takadiastase and salivary gland also inhibit glycolysis in cancer tissue;
3. cancer tissue is unable to form lactic acid from hexose diphosphate or hexose monophosphate;

4. in the soluble muscle enzyme system, the production of lactic acid from hexose diphosphate is inhibited by pancreatic extract, while the production of lactic acid from hexose monophosphate is not inhibited by pancreatic extract[184].

The study is worth quoting. The full abstract is given here:

"Historically, large doses of proteolytic enzymes, along with diet, nutritional supplements, and 'detoxification' procedures, have been used in alternative therapies to treat all forms of cancer, without formal clinical studies to support their use. A 2-year, unblinded, 1-treatment arm, 10-patient, pilot prospective case study was used to assess survival in patients suffering inoperable stage II-IV pancreatic adenocarcinoma treated with large doses of orally ingested pancreatic enzymes, nutritional supplements, 'detoxification' procedures, and an organic diet.

"From January 1993 to April 1996 in the authors' private practice, 10 patients with inoperable, biopsy-proven pancreatic adenocarcinoma were entered into the trial. After one patient dropped out, an 11th patient was added to the study (however, all 11 are considered in the data tabulation). Patients followed the treatment at home, under the supervision of the authors. As of 12 January 1999, of 11 patients entered into the study, 9 (81%) survived one year, 5 (45%) survived two years, and at this time, 4 have survived three years. Two patients are alive and doing well: One at three years and the other at four years. These results are far above the 25% survival at one year and 10% survival at two years for all stages of pancreatic adenocarcinoma reported in the National Cancer Data Base from 1995.

"This pilot study suggests that an aggressive nutritional therapy with large doses of pancreatic enzymes led to significantly increased survival over what would normally be expected for patients with inoperable pancreatic adenocarcinoma." [185]

TESTS

Kelley's test for cancer

Symptoms

Kelley listed a number of cancer early warning signs, based on the assumption that a weak pancreas was one of the major factors that allowed cancer to develop. Poor pancreatic function leads to poor digestion, disordered blood sugar levels and subsequent fatigue and energy slumps. Inadequate protein digestion leads to gradual protein starvation of the individual and so to muscle wasting. His warning signs include:

- digestive upsets such as burping, flatulence or passing wind;

- increased and constant tiredness and lethargy;

- sudden weakness or deterioration in eyesight, due to weakened (protein) focusing muscles;

- muscle weakness and cramps, also due to reduced muscle (protein) mass and strength;

- sudden changes in hair colour (going grey) and texture (becoming dry and/or falling out);

- mental changes, depression, confusion.

Clearly these are non-specific symptoms and need not indicate cancer. However, if they apply to you and are persistent, you might well choose to do the CA profile described above and determine your HCG levels.

Pancreatic enzyme challenge test

Kelley recognised the trophoblastic or stem-cell theory of cancer causation (as described by John Beard), the implication that pancreatic weakness was a major contributing factor to the development of cancer, and the importance of pancreatic enzymes in breaking down the tumour. He thus used these enzymes for a self-administered test for cancer.

As part of this test people were advised, for a period of six weeks, to take five grams (5,000mg) of good quality pancreatic extract with each meal and at bedtime, a total of twenty grams (20,000mg) a day. Most supplements contain around 400mg so this can mean taking a large number of capsules (12 or more) on each occasion. The quality is important as enzymes are fragile and can easily be denatured if inappropriate methods are used to extract and encapsulate them. The regular digestive enzyme supplements that are commonly available are generally inadequate as they are designed primarily for digestion rather than for absorption and systemic circulation. Beef, lamb and pork pancreas supplements are commonly available. Pork protein is the closest to human protein, which is why pork insulin is used for diabetics, and so it is thought that pork pancreatic extract and enzymes may be the best, but some people prefer not to eat pork and so may prefer to use lamb-derived pancreatic extract.

Kelley identified three possible outcomes to this challenge test, and recognised their implications:

Resultant Symptoms	Probable Diagnosis/Conclusion
Nausea, vomiting, headaches, lethargy.	A tumour mass is probably present that should be palpable. The symptoms are due to the toxicity caused by it being broken down by the enzymes.
Feeling better, digestion improves, more energy.	Probably pre-cancerous. Likely to develop cancer within 2-4 years. The pancreas is under-functioning and in no state to either prevent cancer or deal with it if it starts. It is being helped by the supplements.
Health is good and the enzymes lead to no change in state of health.	Cancer is unlikely at this time and the pancreas is probably functioning pretty well.

Kelley found it took him eighteen months to restore his health and he remained on a maintenance programme for the rest of his life. This obviously required discipline, but it did mean he lived for approximately forty years longer than the doctors had said he could! A considerable amount of effort is required if you embark on his programme, but based on Kelley's results and those of his patients it could mean adding many healthy years to your life, as it did for Kelley. Kelley's suggestions are incorporated into the final Fundamental Regime [Chapter 35]

TATI

Trypsin is one of the important pancreatic enzymes, one that acts on tumour cells. We now know that many tumour cells, including those of the ovaries, bladder and kidneys, develop a compound called tumour-associated trypsin inhibitor or TATI[186]. 'Trypsin positive' tumours of the colon[187] and liver[188] also lead to a poor outcome.

High levels of TATI are associated with a number of types of cancer and indicate a poor outcome. TATI has been compared with CA125 as a marker and prognosticator for ovarian cancer. In one study of 66 patients it was found that the five-year survival of 27 with raised levels of TATI was 8%, whereas the five-year survival of the 39 patients with normal TATI levels was 45%. TATI was found to be a better predictor of outcome than CA125 [189].

This is in line with the work of both Beard and Kelley in recognising the efforts that need to be made to increase the pancreatic enzyme attack on tumour cells and the experienced benefit of endeavouring to break tumours down with high doses of pancreatic enzymes.

In short, and if you do not want to explore further into the biochemistry, this means that not only do we know, experimentally and experientially, that the pancreatic enzymes can break down tumour cells, but we are also developing an understanding of why this is both beneficial and needed and how this is done.

CHAPTER 17

CELL MEMBRANES
AND DR. JOHANNA BUDWIG

Cell membranes were described in Chapter 7 and it was clear that the membranes are critically important in relation to cellular function. They are not merely the skin that holds the cell together, far from it. They are probably the brains of the cell, they are certainly a very active part of the cell's metabolism with serious responsibilities. You will recall that their activity controls what messages are received from the blood flowing past, or from adjacent cells, and whether or not these are passed through and on to the inside of the cell. The nature of the membrane affects what substances can enter or leave the cell. In these and other ways, it can be said, in effect, that the nature of the cell membrane controls the way the cell will behave. It's as if the cell membranes filter the mail, deciding what correspondence (information) and parcels (goods, nutrients, waste materials) can enter or leave the cell. To this extent they have ultimate control. Healthy cell membranes lead to healthy cells. Unhealthy or sluggish cell membranes lead to unhealthy or sluggish cells.

In Chapter 7 I described the membranes as being made up of a lipid-on-lipid bilayer with lots of parallel fatty acid chains, with protein receptor sites and channels on and through the membranes. You also learnt that the main lipids are not, in fact triglycerides, but phospholipids, more correctly called phosphatides, commonly referred to as lecithins, and that these are triglycerides where one of the fatty acids is replaced by what we called a phosphate complex. It is time to look at this phosphate complex in more detail.

The basic unit of the phosphatides is phosphatidic acid. This is made up of glycerol with two fatty acids and one phosphate group attached, respectively, to each of the three carbon atoms. In the phosphatides a further group is attached to the free 'end' of the phosphate group on the end carbon atom. There are four possible attachments and these give rise to the four types of phosphatides or lecithins:

- when the compound attached to the phosphate group is choline, the phospholipid is phosphatidyl choline;
- when the compound attached to the phosphate group is inositol, the phospholipid is phosphatidyl inositol;
- when the compound attached to the phosphate group is ethanolamine, the phospholipid is phosphatidyl ethanolamine;
- when the compound attached to the phosphate group is serine, the phospholipid is phosphatidyl serine.

However, there is one more variation we need to consider. Remember the two fatty acids attached to the other two carbon atoms of glycerol. There are six possible fatty acids that can fill the two places on the glycerol carbon atoms of each phosphatide. These are linoleic acid (an omega-6 fatty acid), alpha-linolenic acid (an omega-3 fatty acid) and arachidonic acid, palmitic acid, oleic acid and stearic acid. The last four can be made in your body from other fats that you eat. The first two cannot, and they have to be obtained from your diet. They are the 'essential' fatty acids. The richest source of these is flaxseed oil with over 55% alpha-linolenic acid, in which people are most commonly deficient. It is worth commenting that arachidonic acid, an omega-6 fatty acid, was, in the past, considered to be 'essential', but we now know that it can be made from linoleic acid, another omega-6 fatty acid. Both the type of phosphate complex and the nature of these fatty acids will determine the nature of the phospholipid, and hence of the cell membrane.

This detail is given here to stress the importance in your diet of both lecithin and the essential fatty acids. Remember, the correct structure of your cell membranes is critically important, and for this you need significant amounts of the two essential fatty acids in the diet, and in the correct proportions. Without them your cell membranes will be substandard and your cells will function with diminished efficiency. When this happens ill health is a high probability.

You now know [Chapter 9 and Chapter 11] how important it is for there to be sufficient oxygen inside your cells for correct mitochondrial function. For this to happen there has to be free entry of oxygen across the cell's membrane and then across the mitochondrion's membrane. You may do a lot of aerobic exercise and practise a range of deep-breathing techniques; this may get oxygen into your lungs and into your red blood cells, attached to haemoglobin. These oxygen-charged red blood cells will then circulate round all your body, passing every single cell, but if the cell cannot take the oxygen in, across its cell membrane, then much of your effort will be wasted. The same is true of all the other nutrients, including those needed by your mitochondria to keep the Krebs Cycle functioning correctly.

We have established that oxygen deprivation and poor mitochondrial function are the final mechanism by which carcinogenic damage to the cells converts them into cancer cells, so our focus now is on how to get more oxygen into your cells and then into your mitochondria to prevent this mitochondrial malfunction.

The work of Dr. Johanna Budwig, a renowned German biochemist, is relevant here. She was an expert on fats and oils; it is commonly thought that she was nominated several times for a Nobel Prize. She lived to be nearly 96 years old. In 1951 she proposed a diet that she claimed could help to prevent and treat a range of health problems including heart disease, arthritis and many other chronic degenerative diseases up to and including cancer. This Oil and Protein Diet was recently (1990) re-examined by Dr. Dan C. Roehm M.D., FACP, an oncologist and former cardiologist. Dr. Roehm claims that, *"...this diet is far and away the most successful anti-cancer diet I have found in the world."*[190]

The background to her diet includes a recognition that generous amounts of the essential fatty acids should be consumed each day. Budwig's theory is firstly, that the average diet is very deficient in these fatty acids and secondly, that they are used most efficiently when they are combined with the sulphur-rich amino acids of proteins, and particularly with dairy proteins, and that the oil and protein should be intimately mixed together before they are eaten. The important amino acids are found in beneficial quantities in the organic cottage cheese, yoghurt or quark that she recommends and, in her words, translated from the German, *"...the resultant fatty-acid-sulphur-rich-amino-acid complex is an 'enlivened' fatty acid complex that stimulates the proper use of oxygen by your body's cells."* This is clearly a crucially important statement.

Remember, your red blood cells carry oxygen to just outside your cells where it is released. This released oxygen is drawn from the plasma into the cells by, again to use Dr. Budwig's words, *"...the effect of the 'pi-electron' oxidation-enhancing, or enlivened, fatty acids."* These electron-rich fatty acids play a decisive role in the function of the respiratory enzymes in your mitochondria, which are essential for proper cellular oxidation. Without them, oxygen entry into the cells is compromised and there is limited energy production. Healthy cells need oxygen, plenty of it. Cancer cells do not need oxygen and, in fact, thrive in an oxygen-impoverished environment.

In the absence of sufficient alpha-linolenic acid (found in flaxseed oil), an oxidase enzyme is produced and this encourages cancer and the anaerobic fermentation type of metabolism that is characteristic of cancer cells.

Her theory is that:

- the use of oxygen by the organism can be stimulated by protein compounds or foods with a high sulphur content when these foods are intimately combined with foods rich in alpha-linolenic acid;

- the sulphur-rich compounds make the oils water-soluble;

- ferments of cell respiration closely connected with the highly unsaturated fatty acids are needed for proper oxidation;

- appropriate sulphur-rich foods include quark, nuts, sesame seeds and tahini, onions, leeks, chives, garlic and black pepper, but especially cottage cheese, quark and natural yoghurt. Whey protein isolate (not whey powder which also contains lactose, a sugar) can also be used; it is not as rich in the sulphur-amino acids as are the other dairy products but it offers additional benefits to the immune system. The cysteine content, a sulphur amino acid, can be boosted by adding cysteine powder or a cysteine-rich whey protein powder to the Budwig mix;

- the sulphur-rich foods that most easily combine with the oils are the various denatured dairy products.

The two components, cottage cheese, quark or yoghurt plus the flaxseed oil, should be very thoroughly combined before eating to allow them to interact. If this is not done, the high intake of poly-unsaturated fatty acids can do more harm than good as they are so readily oxidized. Use a blender or electrical mixing wand. Dr. Budwig's protocol and diet are discussed in Part 3 when we consider solutions.

The Budwig diet, and particularly the use of the yoghurt and flaxseed oil combination, is important. Dr. Budwig recommended a combination of two parts of natural, organic yoghurt or quark, intimately combined with one part of flaxseed oil by sixty seconds of electrical mixing and then allowing the mixture to stand for ten minutes before it is consumed.

Some people express concern at the use of dairy products at all, and this point merits attention. It is generally recognised among CAM therapists that there is little need for dairy products in your diet, once you have been weaned, and that for many people the consumption of dairy products can lead to health problems. There are many reasons for this:

1. The intestinal production of lactase, the enzyme that breaks down lactose, the milk sugar, decreases after weaning. For some people, so little lactase is produced that the consumption of milk and whey powder, both of which contain lactose, can cause diarrhoea and other problems.
2. If you were weaned onto cows' milk products too early, before your intestinal mucosa and immune system were fully formed, you may have developed an allergy to cows' milk, but possibly not to goat or sheep milk.
3. In many people, the consumption of dairy products in general is acidic and mucous-forming and can lead to glue-ear in children, and to the excess production of nasal and bronchial mucous.

In relation to cancer, there is a further problem. There are two groups of proteins in milk, the fat-soluble proteins, the major one of which is casein, a phosphoprotein, and the water-soluble proteins, such as whey protein and lactoglobulins. Casein has been shown to be a risk factor in cancer. In experimental rats it has been shown that there is a dose-response curve between some carcinogens (aflatoxin produced by moulds and associated with liver cancer[191]) and cancer on a high (20%) casein diet, but that this relationship is not detected on a low (5%) casein diet[192]. Rats given aflatoxin and fed a diet with 20% casein were all dead, or nearly dead, within 100 weeks from liver tumours. Those given the same dose of aflatoxin and fed a 5% casein diet were alive and healthy. Campbell suggests that the effect is specific to casein, and did not exist in relation to soy, wheat or other plant proteins. He also reported that by adjusting the casein intake of the same rats he could turn cancer on and off as if with a switch[193].

E.J. Hawrylewicz, research director at Merry Hospital and Medical Center in Chicago, found that to produce significant tumour growth in laboratory rats he had to feed them a diet consisting of 20% casein. Both scientists agree that they could not increase cancer occurrence on a diet below 5% casein but that vegetable protein sources should be favoured over animal proteins, especially dairy proteins[194].

IGF-1 is a natural growth hormone found in human blood. However, increased levels have been associated with increased risk of cancer[195]. For instance, one study showed a 7-fold increased risk of breast cancer among pre-menopausal women with the highest blood levels of IGF-1[196]. If dairy cows are treated with a genetically engineered bovine growth hormone (rBGH) they produce up to 15% more milk, but this milk contains increased levels of IGF-1. The IGF-1 is protected from breakdown in the human stomach by the casein of the milk[197].

Other researchers have reported similar concerns about a high casein diet. They have shown that increasing the dietary level of casein increased the incidence of breast cancer in rats, by the same oestrogen system as is operative in humans[198]. Thermolysed (heated) casein has been shown to cause colon cancer[199], suggesting that melted cheese, such as found on pizzas and baked dishes with melted cheese, could be particularly dangerous, followed by dishes on which cheese is allowed to melt prior to serving.

Why is casein such a problem? Casein affects the way that carcinogens react with cells and with DNA, and the way that cancer cells develop and multiply. It also, as we saw above, protects the IGF-1 in milk from breakdown and thus increases its absorption into the bloodstream.

This brings us back to the diet as suggested by Budwig, and the question as to what dairy proteins, if any, are advisable.

1. Sweet (non sour) milk contains casein and should be avoided.

2. Many commercial cheeses contain casein and should also be avoided.

3. Whey protein isolate contains the water-soluble milk proteins, not casein, and so is considered to be safe.

4. Remember whey protein isolate is not the same as whey powder. The latter contains lactose which is problematical for people with a lactase deficiency. More importantly it is a sugar, and sugars should be avoided entirely by people with cancer. Whey protein isolate is a useful and economical protein for people on a largely plant-based diet and it also helps to boost glutathione levels and immune function.

5. That leaves us with the question of the use of yoghurt, as promoted by Budwig and stated by her to be highly beneficial in any cancer recovery protocol.

When milk is fermented by lactic acid bacteria and changed into yoghurt many different chemical reactions occur. One result of the process is the changing of large complex proteins, such as casein, into smaller proteins and peptides of lower molecular weights[200]. These lower molecular weight proteins and peptides have been shown to be stronger antioxidants than the original proteins. Furthermore, the yoghurt has been shown to contain less oxygen than the starting milk. The antioxidant effect of yoghurt was measured against its ability to reduce the oxidation of polyunsaturated omega-3 fatty acids[201], such as those found in fish and those in the flaxseed oil used in the Budwig mixes, and found to be protective. Thus, this 2010 research is endorsing at least part of Budwig's claim of many decades ago that the yoghurt protected (and she said energised) the flaxseed oil.

It has proved difficult to find exact figures for the amount of casein in yoghurt as opposed to the amount in milk and cheese. However, since milk protein is broken down during the fermentation stage of yoghurt production, and since the antioxidant protective effect, ascribed to the presence of smaller protein fragments and peptides is marked, it is reasonable to assume that there is significantly less casein in yoghurt than in milk or cheese. If this is indeed the case it makes yoghurt a safer food than cheese or milk.

In addition, the relatively small amount of yoghurt used in the Budwig mixes (2 parts of natural yoghurt to 1 part of flaxseed oil) if it is the only yoghurt or other dairy product consumed in the day, will generally lead to a protein content of considerably less than 5% of the diet.

With regard to IGF-1, this is another reason for choosing organic products, ones in which the cows' production of milk will not have been artificially stimulated with hormones.

There is a further benefit to the use of fermented dairy products such as naturally fermented yoghurt or quark. They contain lactic acid, in the form of d-lactic acid. We have already seen [Chapter 11] from Dr. Fryda's work that d-lactic acid is the form that is produced in your cells when muscles are exercised faster than the available supply of oxygen and that it can neutralise or counter balance the harmful l-lactic acid produced by cancer cells and that encourages mitosis, the duplication of the cancer cells.

Dr. Budwig also recommends the consumption of a glass of sauerkraut juice every morning before breakfast, another rich source of d-lactic acid. This is consistent with Dr. Fryda's explanation and her practice of recommending patients to take 3 x 30 ml of d-lactic acid daily.

CHAPTER 18

CANCER AND YOUR GENES

Like many health problems, cancer often seems to run in families and so people are inclined to believe that whether or not they develop cancer is already determined by the genes they inherited from their parents. This is partly true, but only partly so. In fact there are very few cancers that are predetermined by the genes you inherited and which greatly or inevitably increase the likelihood that you will develop cancer, such that there is little or nothing you can do to avoid it. Even for people who have a cancer-disposing gene, or genetic mutation, the risk of developing cancer is not constant, as the following example shows.

BRCA1 and BRCA2 are a proteins whose job is to repair DNA damage on your chromosomes or destroy the cell if the repair cannot be effected. As such, the genes that code for their synthesis are tumour suppressor genes. However, when these genes are mutated the proteins cannot perform that function and they become, in effect oncogenes. If your risk of determining cancer was dominated by these genes you could expect the risk of developing cancer for people with the mutated genes to remain relatively constant, but this is not the case.

An obvious example of the latter situation relates to the BRCA1 and BRCA2 genes that increase your risk of developing breast and ovarian cancer if you are a woman, or prostate cancer if you are a male. Yet even if you inherit these genes and have an increased risk of developing one of these cancers, this outcome is not a certainty. There is a very good chance that by applying all the recognised prevention strategies, you will help to reduce the risk.

In a 1997 study of 120 carriers of a BRCA1 or BRCA2 mutation it was found that by the age of 70 the average estimated risk of breast cancer was 56 per cent; of ovarian cancer, 16 per cent; and of prostate cancer, 16 per cent. There were no significant differences in the risk of breast cancer between carriers of BRCA1 mutations and carriers of BRCA2 mutations[202].

In the more recent New York Breast Cancer Study, the lifetime risk of breast cancer for women with inherited mutations BRCA1 and BRCA2 was found to have risen to 82%, and the lifetime risk of ovarian cancer to 54%. In addition, it was found that the risk for breast cancer by age 50 among mutation carriers born before 1940 was 24%, but among those born after 1940 it was 67%[203]. Clearly there is more operating than genetics. Lifestyle and environment have evidently led to a huge increase in the risk, over and above that that can be attributed to the mutated genes. Conversely, this almost certainly means that by improving your diet and lifestyle you can reduce your risk. In other words, no matter what your genetic make-up you can greatly reduce your risk of developing cancer by improving your diet and lifestyle, factors over which you can have significant control. For instance, the more recent study found that physical exercise and lack of obesity in adolescence were associated with significantly delayed onset of breast cancer.

In truth, many of the health problems that seem to run in families, including cancer, may be related to your genes, but even more so they are related to your environment and lifestyle. I once had to deal with a family who wanted to lose weight. Both parents were verging on obese as were their three daughters. The daughters took the view that there was little they could do to control their weight as they had inherited 'obesity genes' from their parents. In fact, what they had inherited was their parents' lifestyle, in particular, their eating patterns. When I probed them, individually, for details of their diet I found they each had a three course breakfast of cereal with milk and sugar, followed by bacon, eggs and fried bread, finished off with toast and marmalade. They all went to school with a sandwich or similar to see them through the morning, then they came home from school for lunch and were presented with three courses, soup, meat and vegetables, followed by a generous helping of sweet dessert such as apple pie and ice cream. After school there was a similarly generous afternoon tea of bread and jam, followed by cake and biscuits, and again, of course, a three course dinner. None of them thought this was an unusual eating pattern, it was what their (obese) mother thought was appropriate.

In other situations you may have inherited genes that increase the likelihood, but not the inevitability, of developing a certain health problem. For instance, there are genes that control the amount of enzymes you make in certain metabolic pathways. An example would be the desaturases and elongases which control how effectively you use omega-3 fatty acids. Without the EPA and DHA produced by these reactions you are more prone to heart problems, but you can greatly change this disadvantage by increasing your intake of the cofactors that go with these genes, in this case vitamins C, B3 and B6 together with the minerals zinc and magnesium. You may have genes that produce relatively little of the enzymes that catalyse the production of thyroxin in your thyroid gland, but if you increase your intake of iodine and trace elements such as selenium, copper and zinc, you can compensate for this.

The story is, arguably, similar in relation to cancer. You may have a genetic make-up that leads to an inadequate production of some of the detox pathways, or that doesn't produce sufficient anti-oxidant activity. All this really means is that if your parents, grandparents, aunts, uncles or siblings have had cancer then you would be wise to be extra vigilant in avoiding the predisposing factors already discussed. In other words, do all you can to ensure maximum health, maximum nutritional benefit, the avoidance of toxins and so forth.

However, that aspect of your genes is not the main focus of this chapter. The genes that form the core of this chapter are those that operate after you have cancer. There are many of them, and, once you recognise which ones apply to you, you may well find that there is remedial action you can take.

A cancerous tumour starts with a single cancerous cell, and it is the progeny of this cell that form both the initial tumour and the body of cells that move off from the original site, travel through the bloodstream and lymphatic channels, and form metastatic colonies. Most of the cells that travel from the original tumour fail to survive, but if even one does, and is able to penetrate other tissues, as discussed in Chapter 14, then a metastatic tumour is formed. When the rate of reproduction is high the cancer is said to be aggressive.

Cancerous tumours are distinguished from benign tumours, such as moles or uterine fibroids, in that, in the latter case, the tumour growth eventually stops, and no cells are able to escape from the tumour and set up metastatic tumours elsewhere in the body. It is rarely the tumour itself that kills, but much more commonly it is the metastatic activity.

In health, when cells multiply they do so in a controlled way, and this multiplication stops when the initial goal, such as tissue repair, has been accomplished. In cancer, there is uncontrolled cellular reproduction that continues indefinitely. Proteins are enzymes, the biological catalysts that facilitate the majority of the reactions that occur within the body. Without these enzyme catalysts most of the reactions that occur within the body would happen at an indescribable and uselessly slow rate. When certain genes are damaged they are known as mutated genes and they in turn, by their catalytic activity, lead to the production of mutated enzymes or mutated proteins. Cleary this reproduction has side-stepped or avoided the normal control mechanisms that should have kept the process in check.

One of the ways that cancer cells manage to survive is by changing many of the normal genes. Most genes initiate the production of proteins within the cells and most of these mutated genes include:

- Mutations of the genes that control the cell cycle and hence mitosis or cellular reproduction.
- Oncogenes. These either lead to the production of mutated protein enzymes or an excessive production of normal enzymes. For a cell to grow and divide, certain growth signals need to be present. In cancer cells, these oncogenes can stimulate cellular growth and reproduction even in the absence of such growth signals. One example of such an oncogene is the gene called EGFR, or HER1, that codes for the receptor site for epidermal growth factor. Closely related to this is the gene SIS which codes for the production of PDGF or platelet derived growth factor. Oncogenes are dominant, so if even one of the pair that sits in your DNA is damaged, cancer will develop.
- Mutated tumour suppressor genes. Suppressor genes code for such proteins as p21 and p53. In their normal healthy state these are helpful proteins. P53, for instance, stimulates apoptosis or the death of faulty or damaged cells whenever it detects damage to the cell's

DNA. When this gene is mutated it produces mutated p53 which does not induce apoptosis and so the damaged cell can continue to reproduce. P21 regulates steps in cellular reproduction and is at least partially controlled by p53[204]. It encourages the self-destruction of transformed cells and the level generally rises if cancer is present, indicating a positive response. A low level of p21, when cancer is present, suggests that there is inadequate apoptosis[205, 206]. The MAD gene (mitotic arrest defective) codes for a protein that monitors a particular stage in the cellular division sequence. In health, if a fault is found the cell's reproduction is stopped[207]. If the MAD gene is mutated this policing action does not occur. Tumour suppressor genes are recessive and so both of them must be defective for the damage to occur.

- Telomerase. Each time one of your strands of DNA reproduces, a small piece at the end is lost. It is a bit like applying glue to a strip of wallpaper. Because you are holding the very end you cannot put the glue on it so when the strip is put up this bottom piece is cut off. Each time your DNA is copied a tiny end piece is cut off. This end piece is a telomere. Each strand of DNA has a string of telomeres at the end, one is lost after each reproduction, and when they have all been used up, the DNA can no longer divide and the life of that cell is over. An enzyme called telomerase can side-step this dead end. It does so by catalysing the addition of telomeres back onto the strand of DNA. Healthy cells do not contain telomerase, most cancer cells do, and you can test for this enzyme in your blood.

- Apoptosis. A number of genes are involved in initiating apoptosis if that is appropriate. Any of these genes can be mutated and, if they are, then this element of control is lost.

- Angiogenesis. As we saw in Chapter 14, when a few cells get together they can survive by utilising the blood flowing past them; but when a tumour grows beyond a relatively small number it needs its own blood supply. This process of angiogenesis is required for normal tissue growth and repair, it is stimulated by VEGF (vascular endothelial growth factor) and the activity of this factor is needed for normal tissue growth and repair. But if any of the genes that affect it are mutated, such as mutated oncogenes or mutated tumour suppressor genes, then increased activity of VEGF can lead to increased angiogenesis, to the benefit of the growing tumour.

- For a tumour to become dangerous, as we have seen, it has to metastasise. To achieve this, the travelling cancer cell (again see Chapter 14) has to be able to invade the target tissue. This, in general, is no mean feat. Cadherins are proteins that cross cell membranes and help to bond cells together[208]. If the gene that codes for one of these, for E-cadherin for example, is mutated or down-regulated this adhesion is weakened and metastatic invasion is made easier for the travelling cancer cells[209]. Most cancers are carcinomas or cancers that involve the epithelial cells. Then there are genes that code for compounds that enable cells to stick to their surroundings. An example of this is the integrin gene, which, if mutated, fails in its task and so allows for the invasion of the cancer cell. There are also specific proteases (protein-splitting enzymes) that intentionally do break down the tissues. They have a role to play in health, but if mutated they can then 'run amok' and facilitate the breakdown of healthy tissue, enabling metastatic invasion.

- There are also genes that code for metallo matrix proteins, MMPs. These were mentioned in Chapter 14 and they too can be mutated.

You may ask how this focus on your genetic make-up and genetic changes sits with the claim in Chapters 9 and 11 that cancer is due to a lack of oxygen to the cells and the induced fermentation replacing the healthy aerobic biochemistry of the mitochondria. After all, the popular concept is that carcinogens damage the DNA in the cell's nucleus and it is this that is the cause of cancer. But, as with most diseases, there are primary and secondary causes of cancer.

The primary cause of influenza might be the specific influenza virus, but not everyone that is exposed to the virus will get influenza. The secondary causes have also to be present, such as poor health, weakened immune response, excessive exposure to cold and wet conditions or nutrient deficiencies. Even if these secondary causes are present, if the virus can be avoided influenza will not result.

The primary cause of most cases of diabetes might be thought of as a lack of insulin, but the secondary causes include an excessive intake of sugar, deficiencies of chromium, vanadium, a number of B group vitamins, and more. Similarly, the prime cause of hepatitis may be thought of as the appropriate virus, yet without the secondary causes, such as other damages to the liver, the disease can generally be avoided.

In the same way, the prime cause of cancer can still be thought of as a lack of oxygen. Secondary causes include all the diet and lifestyle insults, physical, chemical and emotional, that the body sustains. These insults include the toxins and carcinogens – these interfere with normal healthy cellular chemistry and inhibit the ready availability and easy uptake and utilisation of oxygen by the cells. We saw, for instance, in Chapter 8 how the presence of toxic elements such as antimony, arsenic and mercury can inhibit some of the enzymes of the Krebs Cycle and hence of the mitochondrial usage of oxygen and the full aerobic activity of the breakdown of the acetyl groups. Your red blood cells carry oxygen through your bloodstream, from your lungs to the various target tissues. When these red blood cells clump together, as a result, for instance, of an excessive intake of long-chain saturated fatty acids and their toxic counterparts, produced by over-heated fats, trans fatty acids and other degraded products of food processing, they cannot carry this oxygenation to your individual cells.

Lack of oxygen is the primary or ultimate cause of cancer and this can be triggered or produced by the secondary causes of environmental problems, including viruses, moulds and radiation, lifestyle in general, diet and emotions. These secondary causes can also lead to the genetic changes that aggravate the situation. Once the primary lack of oxygen has triggered a cell into a precancerous state, the various oncogenes or mutated versions of helpful genes can then permit or facilitate the development of more cancer cells by increased mitosis, thus enabling the tumour to grow and become established.

So yes, there is a genetic component to Phase Two of the Cancer Process, but it is not a genetic profile that you were born with nor is it inevitable. The changes from healthy genes to mutated genes come about as a result of many of the lifestyle factors that we know cause or contribute to cancer. You may have a genetic profile that increases your risk of or vulnerability to the secondary causes, but if you do all you can to increase oxygenation to your cells you will reduce your risk, in spite of your genes.

How you can deal with these mutations will be discussed in book three of this quartet. In that book too, we will explore a much more detailed and extensive supplement programme than is considered here.

CHAPTER 19

MENTAL, EMOTIONAL AND SPIRITUAL CAUSES

THE ANTHROPOSOPHICAL VIEW OF CANCER

Anthroposophy is a philosophy of the individual as a spiritual being, temporarily occupying a physical body for the period of this lifetime. It was initiated and outlined by Rudolf Steiner, an Austrian philosopher and medium in the early twentieth century. His ideas have led on to many practical endeavours since that time. These endeavours include biodynamic gardening and farming as a more thoughtful and perceptive form than the more common organic gardening and farming. The Waldorf schools incorporate into education the concepts of children as spiritual beings, recently incarnated. The Camphill Movement caters for children and adults with special needs. There are more. His ideas have penetrated into art and dance, science, politics and economics and into many other fields. Of interest to us here are the concepts of anthroposophical medicine, and particularly their role in the understanding of cancer. A wide range of books, written by him, about him, or based on his lectures, often taken down verbatim, can be obtained by most anthroposophical or Rudolf Steiner bookshops, as can books about his approach to medicine and healing[210, 211, 212, 213].

Anthroposophical medicine was founded in the 1920s by Rudolf Steiner in conjunction with Dr. Ita Wegman as an extension to conventional medicine. It is practiced by fully qualified medical doctors who incorporate into their work their training in anthroposophy or spiritual science. It is based on a holistic approach, the understanding of the human being as a four-fold being, and focuses on maintaining or restoring health and well-being rather than on disease processes[214, 215].

Anthroposophy, in its simplest form, sees the human being as a four-fold being made up of physical body, etheric energy field, emotional soul or astral field and your individual spirit or ego, and we need to explore these here, albeit briefly.

Physical Body

You have a physical body in common with minerals and other inert objects. On its own your physical body obeys the normal chemical laws including the laws of chemistry and thermodynamics. One of the latter laws states that, without an outside force, disorder (or entropy) will always tend to increase. This means that purely physical objects will tend to break down, disintegrate and become more disordered. They will not, of themselves, form into a more organised object. For instance, if a tin can is left alone it may rust and gradually breakdown, it will not become a cleaner (or newer) or better shaped tin can. A lump of clay may break down into small particles, it won't build itself into a sculpture. We see this state in the human being after death when all that is left is the purely physical body, when the other aspects, the etheric, soul and spirit have withdrawn. As a result of the absence of the latter three the physical body slowly disintegrates into a more and more unstructured state of smaller and smaller particles or entities as the body's structure gradually breaks down.

Etheric or energy field

In common with the plants, you have an energy field or etheric body. It is this energy field that works against the breakdown of order and the increase of entropy, and helps to maintain the structure and function of the living entity, be it plant, animal or human. The etheric body or energy field enables plants to grow from a disorganised seed into a highly organised plant. It does the same for the human body. You can think of your body as a physically-filled energy field or physically-filled etheric space. This can be visualised by imagining a magnet placed below a sheet of paper onto which powdered iron fillings are scattered. Each time you do this and then tap the paper the filings will line up along the same magnetic patterns.

This concept of an etheric energy field described by Rudolf Steiner at the start of the twentieth century is in line with the research of Dr. Harold Saxton Burr, author of over 93 scientific papers and E. K. Hunt, Professor Emeritus of Anatomy at Yale University School of Medicine where he was a faculty member for over forty-three years until the late 1950s.

Dr. Burr discovered and stated that all living things are formed and controlled by measurable electro-dynamic fields that could be measured. He called them L-fields, or the blueprints of life and believed that doctors should be able to use them to diagnose illness even before symptoms develop. He offered as an example, *"...malignancy in the ovary has been revealed by L-field measurements before any clinical sign could be observed."*

Dr. Louis Langman of New York University and Bellevue Hospital Gynaecological Service examined 102 women who had, *"...significant shift in the voltage gradient between the cervix and the ventral abdominal wall, suggesting malignancy. Surgical confirmation was found in 95 of the 102 cases."* This was confirmed by biopsy.

Dr. Burr found that when he induced cancer in cancer-susceptible mice he could detect changes in the L-field within 28 hours, leading to a maximum voltage shift after eleven days and stated that, *"It is clear from these findings that the crest of atypical growth in the host organism produced measurable and reproducible electro-metric correlates."* [216, 217]

Since then, and with the work of Fritz Albert Popp, a theoretical biophysicist from the University of Marburg in Germany, we have learnt a lot more about biophotons, very weak energy photon emissions of biological systems which can also be thought of as weak electromagnetic waves in the optical range of the spectrum[218].

Currently, the German-based International Institute of Biophysics is a focus for research into this area. Their stated mission is to, *"...explore the reasons of morphological and functional stability of living systems, investigate the role of electromagnetic fields in the functioning of living systems and expand the ... knowledge of intercellular communication."*

Various aspects of research and discovery in relation to this energy field are described in *'The Field'* by Lynn Taggart[219].

Current research by body workers is leading to the conclusion that, *"...the connective tissue matrix and its extensions reaching into every cell and nucleus in the body is a whole-person physical system that senses and absorbs the physical and emotional impact in any traumatic experience. The matrix is also the physical material that is influenced by virtually all hands-on, energetic and movement therapies. It is suggested that the living matrix is the physical substrate where traumatic memories are stored and resolved."* [220] Steiner also stated that memories reside in the etheric.

The physical and etheric state, in combination, are seen in the human being, in the purest form, when the individual is in a coma. To a lesser extent it is evident when they are in very deep sleep, when the brain is in its final brainwave state of delta. Here, the brainwaves are of the greatest amplitude and slowest frequency. They typically centre around a range of 1.5 to 4 cycles per second. During life they do not go fully down to zero, the point that indicates brain death, but in deep dreamless sleep they fall typically to between two and three cycles per second.

Emotional soul or astral field

In common with the animals, we have a soul or astral body, though the word 'body' here is not to be thought of so much as a physical substance but as a 'space' or field of energy. Consciousness resides in the astral. The concept of 'animals' here applies to all creatures, from single-celled bacteria, through microscopic 'animals', to birds, fish and the higher animals. A frightened ant does not stop and think whether or not to run away or stop and fight. It acts instinctively. In general, all ants will react pretty much the same way. Animals act out of instinct, out of their emotions, based on the activity of their astral forces. This state is seen in humans when they are 'behaving like an animal', when they are acting without thinking, when they are out of control. That control would come from their higher, fourth element.

Spirit, "I" or ego

As a human being you have a fourth element, your spirit, and it is unique to you. It is your spirit, your ego (using the term in a non pejorative way), that makes you unique. It is your spirit that decides just how you will respond to the events of life that can act on you and trigger different emotions. Your spirit allows you to control your emotions and not be ruled by them.

How does this relate to cancer? There are two things to consider.

Firstly, a characteristic of the etheric energy field is growth, unlimited and unbridled growth. That is best seen in plants that remain green, plants such as ivy and bindweed. Once flowering starts, growth stops.

Secondly, it is not uncommon for the soul and spirit to act together and for the physical and etheric bodies to act together. This is seen at night during sleep. During sleep the soul (along with consciousness) and spirit leave the body. While they are away the physical and etheric bodies can repair themselves and recover from the ravages brought about by the activity of soul and spirit during the day. The soul and spirit can have their own experience. However, since memory resides in the etheric, and the etheric is still in the bed along with the body, few of the soul experiences that occur during sleep are remembered when you wake up. Dream recall is the fleeting and distorted memory of events 'grabbed' by the etheric in the last few moments before the soul leaves the astral realm and returns to the body. This is true of the final awakening, it is also true of the near waking that happens several times through the night as you cycle in and out of REM sleep.

Back to cancer

The full anthroposophical concept of cancer is complex and profound, and if you wish to explore it I would recommend further reading in general[221, 222] and on the use of mistletoe[223, 224, 225, 226]. What follows is a very simplified version of a first approximation, yet it will help to understand what is being done for you in the planning and monitoring of cancer management if you choose this option.

When the soul and spirit are either out of the body or not fully engaged, etheric growth is active. If it is not properly controlled the growth can become excessive and out of control. In the anthroposophical view, this can lead to cancer. This control should be done by the soul and spirit. In other words, a deficiency of astral or soul activity can permit excessive etheric growth, and hence, if other contributing factors are also present, can lead to the formation of excessive tissue, or tumours.

This is one of the reasons that anthroposophical doctors will recommend specific soul activities as part of almost any healing protocol, and particularly in relation to cancer. They do this with the aim of engaging the astral or soul forces and harnessing or reducing any excessive etheric forces. For instance, I always ask a patient, *"What makes your heart sing? What do you truly enjoy doing, what do you revel in?"* Once that has been determined I encourage them to do it.

> When I first met him, with prostate cancer, client PD was working in a hectic and tense office in London, actively involved in detailed design and marketing. He had enjoyed running his company, but did not do so any longer. When I asked him what made his heart sing he had a ready answer. Many years ago he had inherited a derelict cottage on several acres of land in the Highlands of Scotland. His heart was there, but he felt it would be self-indulgent to retire early, sell his company, give up his business, and move north. I encouraged him to do so. He did, and I now get wonderful emails full of the stories of bees and red squirrels and photos of the restored cottage and poly tunnels of vegetables. As to his cancer, now, many years later, his PSA readings are comfortably low and he is in excellent health.

If you are uncomfortable with these spiritual ideas they can also be described in a more physical way. For instance, positive emotional activity can have a positive effect on the immune function, whereas depression can have a negative impact[227]. "Bereavement causes a fall in activity of the T-lymphocytes[228] and natural killer cells[229], cells that are very important in fighting infection."

TESTS

An active astral body is associated with a fully active thyroid gland, a fully active immune system and the ability to generate a fever whenever there is an infection. Someone with an actively engaged soul will generally have good body heat.

Cancer came as a huge surprise for one of my clients. WJ told me she had always been healthy. She almost never got the flu, and even if she did she didn't get a temperature and could readily continue to work. She was even proud of this. In fact, her body had been unable to mount a response to any virus or bacteria. Shortly before her fortieth birthday she suddenly found a breast lump. She was aghast. How could she, who had always taken good care of her health, and who had always seemed to be healthy, suddenly develop a tumour? When I asked her if she enjoyed her life, if her heart ever sang, she looked at me as if I needed my head read. *"How could I,"* she asked, *"have fun? I'm an accountant, a single mother and have three children to bring up on my own. There is no time or money for fun."* Clearly part of her recovery was going to depend on changes in this aspect of her life.

Appropriate tests include all those indicated for the thyroid gland. Take your body temperature three times a day. You can measure it under your tongue. Take it first thing in the morning, before you get up. Then take it in the early afternoon; you are looking for the highest reading you can get; for some people this is at 2.00 pm, for others it is later in the afternoon. Then measure it again last thing at night.

You should have the lowest reading last thing at night and early the next morning, with the highest reading being around two o'clock in the afternoon. Plot the results on a graph with the temperature up the side and the times and days along the bottom. A flat line is not good. A wide swing from morning to afternoon and back down at night is a good sign.

You will need a practitioner to organise tests in relation to your immune system, analyse the results and prescribe an appropriate response.

Management strategies

Anthroposophical doctors generally use mistletoe extracts at the heart of their therapy. There are several reasons for this. At the spiritual level mistletoe has certain similarities to a tumour. It does not have roots of its own, it is not an independent plant. Instead it grows from and on another plant, usually a tree, and depends on that plant for its nourishment, just as a tumour depends on its host's body for nourishment. At the physical level mistletoe contains a number of lignins and other compounds that challenge and stimulate the immune system, or, at the spiritual level, stimulate a closer astral involvement with the physical-etheric partnership. The anthroposophical treatment goes beyond this. Using eurythmy, a form of movement, and other artistic activities it further draws the soul into full expression. In addition, it incorporates a variety of other herbal and homoeopathic therapies.

If the treatment results in a fever this is seen as a good thing, a sign of improved astral and etheric balance. At the physical level a fever is often accompanied by, or due to, increased levels and activities of lymphocytes, of NK cells, T cells and B cells as happens when they start to attack cancer cells. Clearly such a fever, if it is experienced, should be encouraged and supported, not stopped or suppressed.

To learn more:

Books and advice can be obtained from Rudolf Steiner House, Tel: 020-7723-4400

There are many excellent residential clinics where this form of cancer care is practised such as the Lukas Clinic Arlesheim, near Basle, Switzerland[230], the original anthroposophical cancer centre and the Raphael Centre in the U.K (See Resources).

OTHER MIND BODY CONCEPTS

There is mounting evidence to show that cancer is often preceded by a period of extreme or unusual stress, particularly stress of the kind where you feel helpless and hopeless, unable to change the situation in which you find yourself. This will, of course, challenge your adrenal gland and, eventually lead to adrenal exhaustion and the progression of events described by Dr. Fryda [Chapter11].

As with all physical health problems there are almost certainly emotional issues involved. We know experientially that when you are stressed, unhappy, irritated, frustrated, jealous or frightened you are more likely to experience physical health problems than when you are relaxed and happy. We know that, following a bereavement, people often suffer from viral or bacterial health problems, the results of a weakened immune system. We know that worry can cause indigestion, ulcers or heart attacks. It goes further than that.

There is now a wealth of chemical and physiological evidence that mental and emotional issues change both the absolute and the relative levels of brain molecules called neurotransmitters. These, in turn, have a direct chemical impact on the cells of your immune system, your hormone or endocrine system and on various organs. This means that correcting, resolving or balancing all such mental and emotional issues can have a profound and beneficial effect on your health.

This entire topic is vast and requires a full book in itself at the very least. It will be discussed further in Book 4 of this series (of which this is Book 2). It is mentioned here to underline the fact that improving your health at the physical level, on its own, is not sufficient. When you are fighting something as major as cancer it is essential that you work on all fronts and that you understand that they are all important.

CHAPTER 20
THE ULTIMATE CAUSE OF CANCER
– A SYNTHESIS

Many researchers have claimed to know the ultimate cause of cancer. For Dr. Warburg it was lack of oxygen in the cells and poor mitochondrial function, possibly aggravated by a lack of what he called 'active groups', what we would now call vitamins, minerals and other active groups or coenzymes, needed by the mitochondria. For Dr. Fryda it was adrenal stress, though this, as we saw, can lead on to lack of oxygen. For others it is the build up of toxic and acidic waste. For Dr. Budwig it was a lack of the essential fatty acids. For Dr. Beard in 1910 it was the behaviour of wayward trophoblastic cells and lack of adequate production and activity of pancreatic enzymes. For dentist William Kelley in the 1970s it was the lack of pancreatic enzymes and a poor diet, combined with the presence of toxins. For Dr. Biava it was errors of adult stem cell function.

All of these ultimate causes originated in the extra-nuclear cellular domain rather than in the cell's nucleus, whereas it is frequently the nucleus and its possible or alleged mutations that have been the main focus of conventional (MDS) medical thinking. For Dr. Beard and Dr. Biava, cancer developed not from mature and fully differentiated cells that had turned cancerous but from undifferentiated totipotent stem cells. For a number of people more interested in psychotherapy, it is emotional issues, or from a spiritual perception it is an imbalance of soul and spirit on the one hand versus the physical body and its energy field on the other.

We can divide these ideas into two groups. One relates to the reasons why a cell turns cancerous in the first place. The other relates to the reasons why, once cancer cells have formed, the body does not destroy or eliminate them.

We should credit Dr. Warburg with an understanding of the reasons why a cell turns cancerous, the lack of oxygen and appropriate mitochondrial function. This can by caused by many factors including:

(1) a lack of adequate vitamins and minerals needed by the various enzymes in the Krebs Cycle;

(2) inadequate amounts of the hundreds of different phytonutrients found mainly in vegetables, that support mitochondrial function;

(3) toxic elements which interfere with the enzymes of the Krebs Cycle;

(4) a lack of cellular oxygen;

(5) a build up of damaging l-lactic acid.

We can credit Dr. Fryda with exploring one very important reason for the lack of available oxygen, stress, and the resultant adrenal exhaustion.

We can credit Dr. Biava with a clear understanding of the nature and development of stem cells and the reasons why epigenetic events have to be considered as vital initiating factors, affecting the cell's cytosol and its readiness, or not, to commit apoptosis.

Overall

You could argue that we have not yet found the ultimate cause of cancer, but rather the mechanism by which it develops. What, after all, causes the lack of oxygen, the shut down of the mitochondria and adrenal exhaustion, all of which can cause healthy cells to turn cancerous? What leads to the lack of proper pancreatic function, the deficiency of pancreatic enzymes, and the failure of the immune system's defence strategies? Does it all develop from stress?

Here are just a few of the many dozens of possibilities taken from what we have already considered:

- Stress → adrenal exhaustion → adrenalin deficiency → glycogen-saturated cells → l-lactic acid → increased mitosis → encourages cancer

- Stress → adrenal exhaustion → adrenalin deficiency → hypoxia → encourages cancer

- Stress → adrenal exhaustion → adrenalin insufficiency → compromised immune function → encourages cancer

- Lack of aerobic exercise → inadequate flow of oxygen to the tissues → hypoxia → increased reliance on E-M pathway → encourages cancer
- Toxins, such as lead, arsenic or antimony → compromised mitochondrial activity → reduced Krebs Cycle activity → increased reliance on E-M pathway → encourages cancer
- Lack of antioxidants → toxic free radicals → block entry of acetyl groups into the Krebs Cycle → compromised mitochondrial function → increased reliance on E-M pathway → encourages cancer
- Deficiency of B group vitamins, lipoic acid, biotin, magnesium, manganese and other nutrients → compromised mitochondrial function → increased reliance on E-M pathway → encourages cancer
- Inadequate intake of vitamin C → compromised collagen structure → compromised cellular matrix → increased likelihood of metastasis → encourages cancer
- Inadequate intake of vitamin C → adrenalin converted to noradrenalin (toxic) → increased toxic load plus the consequences of adrenalin deficiency as above → encourages cancer
- Sugar and high G.I foods → raised blood glucose level → over production of insulin → drop in blood glucose level → adrenal exhaustion → hypoglycaemia → diabetes → increased glucose availability to cancer cells → encourages cancer
- Deficiency of selenium, manganese, copper, zinc and other nutrients needed for antioxidant enzymes such as glutathione peroxidase and superoxide dismutase → toxic wastes, generally acidic → increased acidity → acids from blood into cells → decreased cellular uptake of oxygen → encourages cancer
- Deficiency of essential fatty acids → compromised cell membranes → reduced cellular uptake of oxygen → encourages cancer
- Antacids → increased stomach pH → decreased stimulus to the flow of pancreatic enzymes → decreased ability to destroy cancer cells → encourages cancer

There are, of course, many more scenarios, but this is a sample of some of the serious ones. For although what you are learning here may be complex it is but the tip of a vast iceberg of what is happening underneath. None the less, it is clear that 'all roads lead to Rome' and that there is a great degree of commonality in all of these scenarios.

We can then credit Dr. John Beard and William Kelley with the second half of the equation, the reason why cancer cells, once formed, are not immediately destroyed:

(1) poor pancreatic function; and
(2) lack of pancreatic enzymes, particularly trypsin, chymotrypsin and amylase;
(3) lack of the cofactors or coenzymes needed for the enzymes to function (poor diet);
(4) toxins, both in general and from a chemical-laden diet.

Although all this may seem somewhat complicated, and although you may have struggled to reach this point, this is, in fact, a very simplified version of what happens when cancer develops. Much more work has been done, by many remarkable people. However, we have considered some of the major pioneers in this subject and have, I hope, achieved a scenario and explanation that can, and does, underpin many CAM therapies.

You may already have been to a CAM therapist and been, possibly, overwhelmed by all the many instructions you have been given and the severe disciplines that are being expected of you. Perhaps now, based on what you have read so far, you will better understand the reasons for them. If you have not already been to a practitioner then I hope that your new understanding will help you to understand the reasons behind the various suggestions and instructions you receive when you do go to one. You will, for instance, now understand the reasons behind suggestions such as that you should:

- give up all sugars (they feed cancer cells);
- possibly give up all grains (they are all too high in starches and hence glucose and too low in phytonutrients);
- eat a diet composed almost entirely of vegetables (rich in phytonutrients), nuts and proteins appropriate for your metabolic type (to ensure good quality and 'safe' protein intake);

- increase your intake of omega-3 fatty acids (for your cell membranes);
- eliminate your exposure to and intake of toxins (interfere with cellular metabolism);
- go on a heavy detox programme (toxins interfere, either directly or indirectly with mitochondrial function, and toxins are produced or released when you break down cancerous tissue);
- do enemas and other procedures that support your liver (and increase detoxification);
- get plenty of sleep;
- do at least thirty minutes of exercise daily if your health permits. Otherwise do as much as you can (increases oxygen uptake);
- Take time out both to relax and do things that fill you with joy.

This knowledge can help to reassure you that the lifestyle changes you are making, though possibly inconvenient, are worthwhile and 'make sense'.

PART 3

MANAGEMENT OR RECOVERY STRATEGIES

INTRODUCTION TO PART 3

Big Pharma and the MDS system would have us believe that the only possible way to treat or manage cancer is their way. However, it is wise to keep in mind the possibility that any of the views held today, including those by 'the men of medicine' may seem absurd in the not too distant future, just as those of a century ago are held today.

The following discussion of therapeutic protocols is based on the rationales and reasons discussed in the preceding sections of this book. It is not intended to be a full discussion of all the supplements and remedies that can be used to fight cancer. These will come in Book 3 of this Cancer Quartet. The following discussion and suggestions lay down the basics, building on the concepts discussed as to the cause of Phase Two of the Cancer Process.

Managing cancer can be thought to be similar to managing diabetes, or managing a bad cardiovascular system. Improve your diet and lifestyle, remove toxins and eliminate all predisposing factors. Then build on the work of Dr. Warburg, Dr. Fryda, Dr. Beard, Dr. Budwig and William Kelley. To take it further, there are more tests you can do to learn about the individual characteristics of your particular cancer and the particular disturbances to your metabolism, and there is a vast number of therapeutic agents you may use to correct the errors you find. These will be discussed in the third book of this series.

Whether you choose to follow the MDS model and have surgery, chemotherapy or radiation, to follow the CAM model instead, or to combine the two it is your decision. No one, at this stage has the absolute solution to the problem of cancer. The people working within the MDS system are convinced that it is the way to go and that if you opt out of that system and follow the CAM therapies you are being, at best, foolish and irresponsible. Yet even some of these people operate on two levels. The medical drug therapists enthusiastically prescribe chemotherapy and related treatments for their patients. Yet when scientists at McGill Cancer Centre sent out a questionnaire to 118 oncologists they found that of the 79 who responded, 64, or 81 per cent, stated they would never undergo a therapy with Cisplatin, one of the commonly used anti-cancer drugs.

More alarming, 58 or 73 per cent, *"...said that they would never undergo chemotherapy because in the first place it is ineffective and secondly it is much too toxic."* [231]

Conversely, colleagues within the CAM system would almost certainly be willing to do the various therapies they prescribe, knowing that at worst they do no harm and at best they have a lot to offer. Some people who work within the CAM system would, if they had cancer, have absolutely nothing to do with the MDS system, certainly nothing to do with either radiation or chemotherapy, being convinced that this system had little to offer and would almost certainly cause harm.

If you absolutely cannot decide which of the two you feel will give you the best possible outcome, then there is merit in combining the two therapies. There are several reasons for this:

1. There are examples that show that combining one or more of the CAM therapies with a MDS therapy actually improves the results of the latter. Curcumin, for instance, has been shown to increase the sensitivity of tumour cells to radiation and thus increase the effectiveness of the radiation[232, 233, 234]. Resveratrol has been shown to increase the effectiveness of chemotherapy aimed at increasing apoptosis[235].

2. Almost everything that is recommended here, within the CAM system, can safely be combined with the MDS approach and will only add to the beneficial outcome when compared to following the MDS system alone. Improving your diet will improve your overall health and increase your ability to withstand the negative effects of the MDS treatments. The same is true of eliminating toxins and correcting all the Predisposing Factors of Phase One of the Cancer Process.

3. Doing the various tests indicated here will enable you to apply specific CAM remedies that will help to support whatever you do with chemotherapy or radiation.

A word of necessary advice and a warning: If you do combine the two systems you should tell the practitioners in both fields what you are doing. This way, if there is any possible conflict, you can be warned. However, you will often find that doctors and oncologists warn you against CAM therapies, often with no sound reason for doing so. If they advise against a specific combination of therapies ask them for the evidence for what they are saying. Frequently you will find that they cannot give you any, or that they prevaricate. If they do the latter, then continue to push them, if you are to follow their advice it is appropriate for you to know what they are basing it on. Similarly, your CAM therapist should be working from an evidence-based position. Only very rarely is there any conflict, and even then, it is rarely serious.

In general, if a CAM therapy is suitable for you, you can usually continue to use it. If, however, you use a MDS therapy, even if initially it seems to be effective, your body may soon become resistant to it. This presents a number of problems.

Cancer cells have a certain innate 'intelligence' and rapidly learn how to defend themselves from chemical attack or barrages of radiation. If, using chemical drugs, every last single cancer cell is killed, all may be well, for now, at any rate. But there are two problems with this. Firstly, if even one cancer cell is left alive then once the therapy is stopped this cell is free and able to multiply and will act even more aggressively than before. Secondly, you have done nothing to reverse the initial cause of the cancer and if this is still in operation then cancer is likely to start all over again. Remember too, the danger of MDR cells discussed in Chapter 3.

It has been said before, but it is important to stress here, at the start of the section on Therapies: Whatever treatment or combinations of management strategies you choose, your aim should be to eliminate the original cause, eliminate the tumour(s) and retrain your cells. This means:

1. Attending to all the Predisposing Factors of Phase One of the Cancer Process. In the widest possible sense this means correcting your diet and your total environment, physical, chemical, emotional and spiritual, and correcting any health problems, down to the smallest detail. It is vital that the external agents that constitute or initiate the epigenetic activity are removed.

2. Learning what you can about the unique characteristics of your own particular cancer, the factors that, for you, make up Phase Two of your Cancer Process, and acting to make the appropriate corrections.

3. Breaking down the tumour(s).

4. Resolving emotional issues.

Before considering which of the CAM therapies may be appropriate for you and the extent to which you are willing to rely on them, it is appropriate to comment briefly on specific aspects of the MDS options.

After that we will be focusing on the various beneficial strategies you can adopt in response to the various topics covered in the preceding chapters in combination with the results you have obtained from whatever tests you have done.

CHAPTER 21

WHAT ABOUT SURGERY?

If the focus is entirely on a tumour, surgery has an obvious appeal. It is easy to assume that, if cancer is limited to the tumour, and the tumour is isolated, then cutting it out, in its entirety, should solve the problem. Unfortunately, it is not this simple, and in fact surgery can worsen rather than help the problem. As you will know, from what has been written here, it is more correct to consider cancer as a process, and as a systemic problem than as an isolated tumour. Surgery therefore only addresses part of the problem, the end tumour.

Remember also [Chapter 9, PHI test] that recent research[236] suggests that cancer cells may spread around the body much earlier than was previously thought[237], and they probably left the tumour long before your diagnosis and spread to other sites where they may be lying dormant until such time as they are triggered into reproduction and growth[238]. Your aim, therefore, should be to avoid any trauma or trigger that could stimulate their mobilisation, and to do all you can to improve your overall health.

Removing the tumour may be successful in rare cases but it has not resolved or focused on the problem of why it developed in the first place, or on what is going on in your body that allows the Cancer Process to continue. Thus, a new tumour could well form some time in the future, for the same reasons as the first.

Long-term effects of surgery can be scars and chronic pain. Another problem post surgery is lymphoedema[239], a condition of localised fluid retention and tissue swelling caused by a compromised lymphatic system. The lymph system is a primary part of your immune function and tissues with lymphoedema are at risk of infection. This problem may be mild and simply involve local swelling and possibly restriction of movement. It can, however, be sufficiently severe that further surgery and possible amputation are required[240]. In fact, lymphoedema has been shown to be a lifelong problem following MDS treatment for breast cancer[241].

However, it can be worse than that and there can be several other late-onset effects. Surgery can actually encourage increased cancerous activity and can increase the risk of metastasis. It is rarely the initial tumour that proves to be fatal. Frequently it is the metastatic recurrence that develops and proves to be fatal. Unfortunately, for those that favour surgery, this can lead to a significantly increased risk of developing metastasis[242, 243] and hence to an increased risk of metastasis that can be fatal. In fact, the original tumour may actually be doing you a favour and preventing metastasis. It does this, at least in part, by producing angiostatin and sending it out through the blood circulation, as a result of which any smaller colonies of cancer cells are deprived of the ability to build their own needed blood vessels and so cannot grow[244]. There are other methods by which the original tumour can exert this effect, such as by selective COX inhibition. *"Primary tumour excision was associated with accelerated local and systemic tumour recurrence."*[245] Once the original tumour is removed, these brakes have gone and any of the metastatic colonies, which may have left the original tumour a long time previously, only to lie dormant waiting for their opportunity, can now grow and flourish.

There is another factor to consider. In brief, the initial tumour is walled off and it is difficult for individual cells to (a) leave the tumour; (b) force their way into the bloodstream or lymphatic vessels; (c) travel safely through the turbulent bloodstream full of white blood cells of the immune system; (d) break out of the blood vessels; and (e) invade a target tissue. These tasks are very much more difficult than you might imagine. Thus, an isolated tumour may well stay that way, isolated. Once the tumour has been cut into, such as for a biopsy, or surgically removed and the local tissues disturbed, it is much easier for rogue cancer cells to escape, travel and settle elsewhere.

Although there is considerable evidence that surgery increases the risk of metastases there is debate as to the ways this comes about. Metastases are more likely if a large number of cancer cells travel together. This is achieved, in part by the use of galectin-3, an adhesion molecule present on the surface of cancer cells[246].

Another way is thought to be as a result of increased ability of the travelling cancer cells to adhere to the target tissue. Surgical stress has been shown to lead to the release by neutrophils of soluble receptor for IL-6 and these in turn have been shown to increase the ability of colon cancer cells to stick to the target endothelium[247].

The process of metastasising is further assisted by angiogenesis[248] or the building of new blood vessels. Following surgery there is the need for tissue repair. This in turn requires the growth of new blood vessels to feed the healing tissues. This burst of angiogenic activity can also enable existing and possibly unsuspected metastatic tumours to develop and increase their own blood supply and has been shown to encourage distant metastases[249]. Furthermore, it is hypothesised that, *"...removing tumours could remove the source of inhibitors of angiogenesis or growth factors."* [250]

On the other hand, if the tumour is of a size that it is interfering with other bodily organs or processes, then its removal may be required. However, there has been evidence for several decades that radical surgery may not be any more helpful than conservative surgery for removal of the tumour itself in treating breast cancer[251, 252]. It may even do more harm than good as a result of the emotional and psychological effects[253] and of collateral tissue damage and the greater strain on the entire body[254]. This is now generally recognised in relation to mastectomies and is becoming recognised in relation to prostate tumours[255]. Arguably, removing a significant, space-occupying and obstructive tumour may then enable the body's own defence mechanisms, plus whatever sympathetic regimes you adopt, to be more effective.

CHAPTER 22

WHAT ABOUT CHEMOTHERAPY?

If you are considering having chemotherapy I strongly recommend that you read *'Questioning Chemotherapy'* by Ralph Moss first[256]. It is not the intention here to persuade you one way or the other about chemotherapy. Many people are convinced that it works, and that it is worth the pain, the damage to the rest of their body and toxic side-effects. Other people are convinced that it is totally inappropriate and that it should, and will eventually, some time in the future, be thought of as a barbaric form of treatment that should be relegated to the dark ages of medicine. With the placebo effect in mind, and a recognition of the effect and the power of your mind and convictions on physical outcome, a case can be made for doing whatever form of therapy you have the greatest belief in and conviction about. If you are at all undecided, then this is the time to gather all the facts you can. If you already have cancer your medical team is probably working hard to convince you of the benefits of chemotherapy, claiming great advances and minimal toxic effects. Moss's book will help to balance your information base.

Moss is an experienced and respected science writer in the cancer field who, though now working independently, began his career writing for the Memorial Sloane Kettering Cancer Centre, and so who, arguably, had the best possible inside information on the subject. He has reviewed this topic extensively. After pointing out that each new drug is first hailed as the new revolutionary breakthrough, only to be quickly forgotten as the results prove disappointing, at best, and the next new miracle drug hits the scene, Moss has this to say, *"...even if some few patients live longer [on chemotherapy] their 'success' is bought not only at the expense of their own toxicity but of all the other patients who do not benefit. Some of these may have had their lives shortened in the course of the treatment (so-called toxic or treatment deaths). Others may have experienced terrible side effects."* (p.xvii) After commenting on some of the biased reporting practices he concludes, in his introduction, that, *"...chemotherapy is not an effective weapon against the vast majority of solid carcinomas in adults."* (p.xix) and, *"The amount of toxic chemicals needed to kill every last cancer cell was found to kill the patient long before it killed or eliminated the tumour."* (p.29)

If you are not sure what to do, it may be tempting to be seduced into 'doctor knows best' and let someone else take over the decisions as to the nature of your health care, but that may be unwise. Ultimately, the decision has to be yours, even if that decision is to let someone else decide. In your own best interests, this is the time to gather all the facts you can.

Chemotherapy agents are highly toxic. The hope is that they kill the cancer cells before they kill you. People who are handling the drugs are warned that they should wear eye protection, head cover, overshoes and protective clothing to avoid serious eye and skin damage, and that the drugs create risks of liver problems, reproductive abnormalities, blood diseases and chromosomal damage. They are warned as to how to handle the drugs and advised not to eat, drink, smoke or apply cosmetics while preparing the drugs since accidentally touching them or inhaling them, during preparation for treatment, poses a serious risk[257]. Yet these are the chemicals that are going to be fed into your veins, or given to you to swallow. If you do decide to go ahead with chemotherapy you should keep the above instructions in mind if you are treating yourself at home.

There is also concern about disposing of chemotherapy drug-contaminated equipment and, from an environmental perspective, the dangers of pollution from contaminated faeces from the patient. So clearly, chemotherapy agents are highly toxic. Even more disturbingly it is well established, and has been so for over 25 years that they are also, themselves, carcinogenic[258, 259, 260, 261, 262, 263, 264].

Chemotherapy has certainly helped in the treatment of a number of relatively rare cancers, but ironically most of this success was achieved prior to 1971 and the declared war on cancer. The success stories include blood and related cancers such as lymphomas, including acute lymphocytic leukaemia, lymphosarcoma, Burkitt's lymphoma, Hodgkin's disease and multiple myelomas. Other successes include choriocarcinoma (cancer of pregnancy) and testicular cancer, Ewing's sarcoma and rhabdomyosarcoma, Wilm's tumour and retinoblastoma.

Since 1971 and the start of Nixon's war against cancer, tens of billions of dollars have been spent on cancer research. If a variety of 'massaging' techniques are removed from the figures, most studies show an improvement in the five-year survival rate as a result of chemotherapy of between 2.1 per cent (America) and 2.3 per cent (Australia) over the past thirty or more years[265].

Massaging techniques include:

- excluding people who die during the trial period;
- including people (as successes) who live for five years, even if they still have cancer or die soon afterwards;
- including the drop in lung cancer deaths without allowing for the drop in cigarette smoking;
- including non-melanoma skin cancers (which are rarely fatal): this achieved a one-off boost to the apparent successes.

How well is chemotherapy tolerated? The following example should give you pause for thought. A study of a high-dose regime of ifosfamide, carboplatin and etoposide, (ICE) used to treat ovarian cancer, metastatic breast cancer, non-Hodgkin's lymphoma and some other cancers, produced the following outcomes: In the low-dose patient group: 67% of the patients developed mucositis (painful inflammation and ulceration of the mucous membranes lining the digestive tract), and 39% developed enteritis (inflammation of the small intestine, causing abdominal pain, cramping, diarrhoea, dehydration and fever). In the medium-dose group 50% had central nervous system and lung complications. In the higher-dose group 61% experienced liver toxicity, 70% had kidney damage, 81% had ear damage, 90% had adverse pulmonary effects, and 94% suffered damage to their hearts. Eight per cent of the patients died of the effects of the chemotherapy trial. The authors stated that, *"..the dose-limiting toxicities of ICE were CNS toxicity and acute renal failure,"* and that this drug combination was, *"...well tolerated with acceptable haematopoietic side effects and predictable organ toxicity."*[266]

So give some thought to what might lie behind the various statements that chemotherapy might prolong your life (by how much, and where is the evidence?), that the drugs are well tolerated and that the side effects (what are they?) are negligible or minimal. Keep in mind that these are relative statements, measured against the common expectations, which are not always good, and which may in fact be very low indeed.

If you are told that a certain drug has produced a 'positive response' you may assume this to mean that the result has been a cure, or a very significant prolonging of life in a majority, if not all, cases. In fact, it could mean that a small percentage of patients had lived a few weeks longer, even though others had died sooner, and all had experienced serious toxic effects. So ask. If you are told that you need not worry, new treatments due on the market soon, or just recently on offer, have produced great improvement in results, ask just what those improvements are and what were the previous results, against which they are being measured. Ask your doctor for the evidence for what he is telling you. Science papers are now readily available on the Internet and are not that difficult to read, at least in so far as the abstract and conclusions are concerned. Try to find out exactly what his or her words mean. If you are seriously considering having chemotherapy it is important that you fully understand just what will be done to you, the full consequences, all the probable toxicities, and the real, un-hyped, possible benefits. Your practitioner, MDS or CAM, should be able to help you read and understand the research papers.

If you do not ask you may, later, wish that you had. When you find that you have become incontinent, have serious ongoing pain, can no longer do certain things, or have other symptoms, you may complain of them to your doctor, only to be told something like, *"It's only to be expected, after all, you have had such-and-such chemotherapy."* You may think then. *"If only I'd known..."*, but by then it is too late, the decision has been made and acted upon, the damage has been done. This will be especially tragic if you are also told that, *"...unfortunately, in your case, the treatment was not as successful as we had hoped..."*

Treatments like chemotherapy can certainly poison and kill cancer cells. However, many of the treatments are even more effective against oxygen-rich (healthy) cells than against oxygen-starved (cancer) cells. Thus, not only do these treatments kill cancer cells but they can have an even more devastating effect on healthy tissues and hence on you, the host. As your cells, organs and tissues become damaged they become progressively less and less able to defend you or to work against the cancer cells. Your immune system becomes weakened. Your hormones become imbalanced. Your body becomes laden with toxins, your liver is challenged and probably overloaded with them.

It is extraordinary, from a logical perspective, that you will almost certainly not be given advice as to how to remove the toxins from your body, after your treatment, if not before it ends. If the chemo is breaking down cancer cells then the debris has to be removed. Clearly you should therefore embark on a variety of different detox procedures to hasten the removal from your body of the toxic breakdown products of the tumour. At the latest this should be done once the course of chemotherapy has been completed. Arguably, procedures such as enemas, which remember, were part of the Medical Merck manual until 1971, should be started immediately so that the 'debris' is removed from your colon as rapidly as your liver puts it there and not be left sitting and available for reabsorption and autointoxication.

Chemotherapy is aimed at the most rapidly dividing cell types or tissues. These include your hair follicles and the cells of your bone marrow, immune system and the lining of your mouth and digestive tract. Once you have damaged your bone marrow you compromise your ability to make healthy new cells, red blood cells for your blood and white blood cells and others for your immune system. You may produce less healthy or fewer of the valuable stem cells that we have already discussed and that are important for tissue repair. It is known that, *"Long-term bone marrow damage, characterised by stem, progenitor and stromal cell abnormalities is a frequent occurrence after cytotoxic treatments."* [267]

Once you have damaged your digestive system, absorbing the essential nutrients that you need for both health maintenance and for recovery becomes compromised. Once you have damaged your liver, several hundred different chemical functions are compromised. Once you have damaged your kidneys, or other organs etc., it may become almost impossible to repair these organs, certainly after the damage that has been done to the rest of your body, and damage there will be, otherwise why would you have all those toxic reactions? These treatments lead to a number of other health problems, as witnessed by the toxic effects noted above and experienced during and following any treatment programme, from hair loss, through nausea to a range of other and more serious problems.

Behind the rationale for the use of either chemotherapy or radiation is the assumption that cancer cells are **weaker** than healthy cells and so will die sooner than healthy cells. The problem with this assumption is that both these two methods damage the mitochondrial respiratory enzymes. You will recall that these are present and active in all healthy cells, but not in fermenting or cancerous cells. So the net result is damaged respiratory enzymes in healthy cells and an increase in the amount of toxins present so that healthy cells become even more likely to turn into cancer cells, either at the time or in the future. You have, in effect, increased the likelihood of developing or encouraging cancer, not reducing it.

Chemotherapy can, itself, cause cancer, as can the inflammatory reactions it can induce. As tissues are damaged, just as there is after surgery, there can be serious attempts at healing which includes increased angiogenic activity in which there is an excessive formation of new blood vessels. You will recall that these new blood capillaries can help to rebuild the damaged tissue but they can also be taken over by, and used to feed, cancer cells and cancer cell clusters or tumours that remain.

Long-term toxic effects of chemotherapy include, among other problems, fatigue, neuropathy, post-menopausal symptoms, disrupted memory and thinking, heart failure, kidney failure, infertility and liver problems. Late onset toxic effects include cataracts, infertility, osteoporosis, reduced lung capacity and secondary cancers[268]. All these things should be thought about if you are considering accepting chemotherapy.

The following two tables list some of the actions and toxic symptoms of some common chemotherapy agents. The information is taken from Dr. Moss's book, which should be consulted for more details and lucid explanations. He takes it from many medical sources[269, 270, 271, 272].

Group	Action	Resistance	Carcinogenic	Likely toxic effects
Alkylating Agents	Damages or destroys DNA.	Readily develops	Yes	Cessation of menstruation, loss of sperm potency, mutagenic to the next generation.
Nitrosureas	Subclass of alkylating agents. Fat-soluble and highly reactive.			
Antimetabolites	Similar to a natural metabolite so interferes with the function of the latter.			Don't distinguish between healthy and cancer cells, so disrupts normal metabolism of whole body.
Antitumour Antibodies	Natural compounds from microbioal culture broths. Enter the nuclear DNA.		Some are thought to be, e.g. Dactinomycin	
Platinum Analogues	One of the most important groups.			
Plant-derived agents	Many are known plant poisons.			Mostly extremely toxic in their extracted and purified form and so of limited use.

Group or type	Agent	Usage	Toxic effects	Carcinogenicity
Alkylating agents	Mechlorethamine (nitrogen mustard)	Usually in combinations.	Blistering and inflammation (topically), nausea, vomiting, thrombophlebitis, venous sclerosis, dangerous if inhaled.	Yes, and next generation mutations.
	Melphalan (Alkeran) = Mechlorethamine plus phenylalanine (an amino acid)	Breast, ovaries, multiple melanoma.	Liver and kidney damage, damage to blood production, nausea, vomiting, hair loss.	Leukaemia.
	Chlorambucil (Leukeran)	Chronic lymphocytic leukaemia, (CLL microglobulinemia, some non-Hodgkin's lymphoma. Occasionally breast or ovaries.	Least toxic of the alkylating agents. Immune depression (reversible), nausea (mild). Skin rash, hair loss. Male sterility, liver damage, seizures. Proteinurea, decreased menstruation.	Secondary leukaemia.

Group or type	Agent	Usage	Toxic Effects	Carcinogenicity
	Busulfan (Myleran)	Chronic myelocytic leukaemia, acute leukaemia. Interferes with cell replication.	Suppression of bone marrow, scarring of lungs and heart, cataracts, skin darkening, decreased adrenal function, skin rash, dry skin, hair loss, weakness, jaundice. Seizures, liver damage.	
	Cyclophosphamide (Cytoxan, Neosur, Endoxan)	Non-Hodgkin's lymphomas, multiple myeloma, leukaemia, breast, ovarian.	Less GIT damage than other alkalysing agents, blood deficiencies, hair loss, nausea, vomiting, bleeding in GIT, mouth sores, skin and nail discolouration, lung disease, heart damage.	
	Ifosfamide (IFEX), usually in combination with carboplatin and etoposide	Testicles.	Mouth sores, intestinal inflammation, liver toxicity, hearing, CNS, hearing, heart (up to 94%) and lung damage. Disturbing or frightening hallucinations (when eyes closed).	

Group or type	Agent	Usage	Toxic Effects	Carcinogenicity
Nutrosoureas (a subclass of the alkylating agents)	Carmustine (BiCNU)	Brain, lymph gland, plasma cell cancers.	Suppresses bone marrow, reduces RBC and platelet counts, liver and kidney damage, nausea vomiting, lung scarring.	
	CCNU (Lomustine)	Lymphomas, brain cancer, Hodgkin's disease.		
	Streptozocin (Zanosar)	Inhibits DNA synthesis and glycolysis. Islet cell tumours of pancreas, adenocarcinoma of the pancreas, metastatic carcinoid tumours.	Severe nausea and vomiting. Damages beta cells of pancreas and kidneys.	
	Thiotepa	Early stage bladder cancer, breast, ovarian.	Mild nausea and vomiting. White blood cell damage, appetite loss, dizziness, headaches, hives, asthma-like symptoms, pain at injection site.	

Group or type	Agent	Usage	Toxic Effects	Carcinogenicity
Antimetabolites (something that closely resembles a normal compound in the body and so interferes with its function)	Methotrexate	Mimics folic acid. Cancers of the amniotic sac, blood, lymph glands. Childhood leukaemias, osteogenic sarcoma, non-Hodgkin's lymphoma, choriocarcinoma. Many other cancers, inc. breast, head, neck, brain.	Cell destruction, extensive sickness. Suppresses immune function.	

Group or type	Agent	Usage	Toxic Effects	Carcinogenicity
	Rescue Factor, leucovorin (folinic acid)		Damages immune system and mucous membranes. Reduced white blood cell count. Mouth sores, diarrhoea, elevated liver enzymes (so reduced function), live fibrosis (25%). Kidney damage, lung inflammation. Brain injections lead to inflammation, paralysis, malfunction of cranial nerve, seizures, coma, nerve cell demyelination, mental deterioration, spasticity, coma.	
	Fluorouracil (5-FU, Efudex)	Breast, rectum, stomach, pancreas, head, neck, skin, anus, oesophagus.	Sores of GIT, diarrhoea, ulcers. Nausea, vomiting, hair loss, anorexia, reduced white blood cell count, skin rashes and darkening. May suppress bone marrow in large doses.	

Group or type	Agent	Usage	Toxic Effects	Carcinogenicity
	Cytarabine (Cytosar-U, Ara-C)	Acute myeloid leukaemia.	Nausea, vomiting, diarrhoea. In high doses, bone marrow suppression, pancreatitis, brain dysfunction, slurred speech, confusion, coma, occasional fatalities.	
	Mercaptopurine (Purinethol or 6-MP)	To maintain remission in acute myeloid leukaemia.	Bone marrow suppression, GIT toxicity, nausea, vomiting, anorexia, mouth sores. Liver damage (30%) with jaundice and necrosis.	
	Thioguanine (6-GT)	Acute non lymphoblastic leukaemia.		
Antitumour Antibodies	Bleomycin sulphate (Blenoxane)	Squamus cells of cervix, head and neck, larynx, penis, skin, vulva, cancer of lymph glands and testicles.	Lung scaring, pneumonia (10%), allergic reactions, itching, fever, chills, vomiting, decreased appetite, weight loss, pain at tumour site. Hard and/or tender finger tips, nail ridges, skin discolouration, pruritic erythemia.	

Group or type	Agent	Usage	Toxic Effects	Carcinogenicity
	Daunorubicin hydrochloride (Cerubidine)	Inhibits DNA and RNA synthesis. Acute myeloid leukaemia.	Highly toxic to white blood cells. Mild nausea and vomiting, hair loss, red urine. Acute and chronic heart damage, abnormal ECGs, wild heartbeats. Congestive heart failure (up to 12%). Total heart failure following local radiation. Topically, skin irritation.	
	Doxorubicin (Adriamycin)	Inhibits DNA synthesis. Leukaemias, sarcomas, cancers of breast, bladder, lung, prostate, testis, thyroid, uterus and more.	Reduced white blood cells, near universal hair loss. Mild nausea and vomiting. Nail and skin discolouration. Heart muscle damage. Congestive heart failure (1-4%).	

Group or type	Agent	Usage	Toxic Effects	Carcinogenicity
	Idarubicin (Idamycin)	Leukaemia, Hodgkin's disease, an indolent form of non-Hodgkin's lymphoma. Advanced breast cancer.		
	Mitoxantrone (Novantrone)	Inhibits RNA and DNA. Lymphoma. Breast cancer.	Damages granulocytes. Nausea and vomiting (30%). Baldness (10-15%). Blue finger nails and urine.	
	Mitomycin (Mutamycin)	Interferes with DNA and RNA synthesis. Stomach, pancreas, breast, head, neck, lung, cervical. Activated preferentially in low-oxygen tissues such as tumours.	Nausea, vomiting, anorexia. Progressively destroys white blood cells. Pneumonia. Hemolytic-uremic syndrome. GIT bleeding and blood in urine, in children.	

Group or type	Agent	Usage	Toxic Effects	Carcinogenicity
	Dactinomycin (Actinomycin D, Cosmegen)	Interferes with DNA production. Combined with radiation for nephroblastoma, rhabdomyosarcoma, Ewing's sarcoma, Wilm's tumour.	Damages blood production. Nausea, vomiting. Diarrhoea, mouth sores, rectal inflammation. Acne-like skin. Hair loss.	
	Plicamycin (Mithracin)	Interferes with RNA synthesis, blocks PTH. Disseminated germ cells of the testes.	Major damage to bone marrow, liver, kidneys. Reduced red and white blood cell depletion, severely raised liver enzymes, proteinuria (kidney damage). Thick reddened and coarsened skin.	

Group or type	Agent	Usage	Toxic Effects	Carcinogenicity
Platinum Analogues	Cisplatin (Platinol)	Binds to DNA.	Kidney malfunction, nausea, vomiting, nerve damage, impaired sight and hearing, bone marrow suppression, occasional seizures. Cardiac arrhythmia, damage to brain tissue, glucose intolerance, pancreatitis. Peripheral neuropathy similar to B12 deficiency.	Leukaemia
	Carboplatin (Paraplatin)	Ovarian, cervix, small-cell lung, head and neck, bladder, testis, mesothelioma and brain cancers.	Similar to, but slightly less toxic than Cisplatin. Low blood count, nerve damage, hearing loss, kidney toxicity, nausea, vomiting, loss of appetite, diarrhoea, constipation, mouth sores, altered sense of taste.	
Miscellaneous	Altretamine (Hexamethyl-melamine, Hexalen)	Uncertain action. Breast, lymphomas, small-cell lung cancer.	Nausea, vomiting. Mood alterations, hallucinations, nerve damage.	

Group or type	Agent	Usage	Toxic Effects	Carcinogenicity
	Dacarbazine (DTIC-Dome)	Metastatic melanoma.	Causes the most severe nausea and vomiting of all cytotoxic drugs. Fever, malaise, muscle aches and pains. Diarrhoea. Sun exposure leads to burning. Facial flushing, loss of sensation, light-headedness. Acute liver poisoning.	
	Hydroxyurea (Hydrea)	Action mechanism unknown. Certain blood cancers. Head and neck, ovaries.	Bone marrow suppression. Reduced red blood cells and platelets. Irritation of the mouth, nausea, vomiting, diarrhoea, constipation, skin rash, burning sensation on urination, hair loss, drowsiness, headache, seizures, decreased kidney function.	

Group or type	Agent	Usage	Toxic Effects	Carcinogenicity
	Mitotane (Lysodren or o,p'-DDD)	Closely related to DDT. Blocks the synthesis of adrenocorticol hormone in healthy and malignant cells. Palliative treatment of cancer of the adrenal gland.	Liver and kidney impairment. GIT disturbances, visual disturbances, lethargy, depression. Maculopapular rash (e.g. hives) (15%).	
	Procarbazine (Matulane)	Brain, Hodgkin's disease.	Immune suppression, moderate nausea, decreased appetite, leucopoenia and thrombocytopenia. A mild hypnotic. Tyramine foods and drinks must be avoided. With alcohol it causes sweating, flushing, headaches. I.V. may cause confusion or coma. Lung problems, maculopapular rash.	Teratogenic. Carcinogenic in monkeys.

Group or type	Agent	Usage	Toxic Effects	Carcinogenicity
	Asparaginase (Elspar)	All.	Allergic reactions. Anaphylactic shock with hives, swelling of voice box lung spasms, low blood pressure (50% of children). Possible clotting difficulties, haemorrhages. Brain dysfunction, confusion, stupor and coma (in 25% of children).	
Plant-Derived Agents	Vincristine sulphate (Oncovin) from Periwinkle	As a herb: Astringent, sedative, diarrhoea remedy. Derived drug: lymphocytic leukaemia, Hodgkin's disease, non-Hodgkin's lymphoma, Wilm's tumour, Ewing's sarcoma, childhood rhabdomyosarcoma.	Drug form: Suppressed bone marrow, reduced white blood cells. Very irritating, has to be given IV. Nerve damage, loss of various sensations. Palsy, constipation, abdominal pains, bowel obstruction.	

Group or type	Agent	Usage	Toxic Effects	Carcinogenicity
	Vinblastine sulphate (Velban), From Periwinkle.	Derived drug: Destructive to proteins and DNA. Hodgkin's disease, testicular cancer. Relieve symptoms of breast cancer, choriocarcinoma, Kaposi's sarcoma. Damaged white blood cells.	Mild nausea. Frequent constipation and mouth sores. Hair loss, rashes, light sensitivity. Continuous infusions can lead to hepatitis. Possible estravasation.	
	Etoposide (VePesid),	Extracted from mandrake. Hodgkin's lymphoma, germ cell malignancies, leukaemias, small-cell lung cancer.	Reduced white blood cells. Nausea, vomiting (30%). Severe allergic reactions (2%). Nerve damage at high doses.	

Group or type	Agent	Usage	Toxic Effects	Carcinogenicity
	Teniposide (Vumon, VM-26)	Related to Etoposide. Hodgkin's and non-Hodgkin's lymphomas, germ cell malignancies, leukaemias, bladder and small-cell lung cancers.	Similar to Etoposide.	
	Paclitaxel (Taxol)	Stops cell division by altering the shape of cellular microtubules, metastatic breast cancer. Prostate, ovarian, metastatic breast cancer.	White blood cell damage, nerve damage, numbness, altered sensations in hands and feet. Hair loss, nausea, vomiting, inflamed mucous membranes, myalgias, phlebitis, rapid heart beat, diarrhoea.	

CHAPTER 23

WHAT ABOUT RADIATION?

Let's first consider the rationale for using radiation as a treatment. An obvious reason is that radiation destroys cells. If you are focused solely on removing a tumour, radiation can do this. It is easy for your medical team to tell you that radiation can destroy the tumour and that without a tumour you are not considered to have cancer. Thus, they can reassure you and you can relax, even if this supposed safety is an illusion, for as you will know from reading this far, cancer is an entire process, not just the tumour. The radiation beam cannot be seen and the treatment does not hurt. Thus, many patients are further reassured.

From the medical perspective, radiation is big business with a big income potential, and once an expensive treatment unit has been set up it is obviously commercially desirable to keep it functioning as near to non-stop as possible. The equipment can be 'manned' by a technician, which keeps the costs down.

Radiation treatments

Different cancers respond differently to radiation therapy. Cells that are rapidly killed by low doses of radiation are known as highly radiosensitive cells. Those that can withstand considerable amounts of radiation have low radiosensitivity. In general, cell radiosensitivity is directly proportional to the rate of cell division, in other words, rapidly dividing cells are the most susceptible to radiation. Radiosensitivity is inversely proportional to the degree of differentiation of cells, so that the most undifferentiated cells are the most radiosensitive. In addition, if cells have a high metabolic rate and/or are well nourished they are also prone to being radiosensitive.

Radiation measurements are slightly complicated as there are two systems, the System Internationale (SI) that derives from the metric system or the conventional system still used in the United States.

- Emitted radiation is usually measured in Becquerel (Bq) or curies (Ci) after Marie Curie, in the two systems, respectively.

- One Bq is equivalent to one atomic disintegration per second; one Ci is equivalent to 37 billion (37×10^9) disintegrations per second.

- Radiation that an individual absorbs, i.e. the amount of energy taken up by human tissue, is measured in grays (Gy) or rads (radiation absorbed dose). One Gy equals 100 rads.

- Biological risk of exposure to radiation is measured in sievert (Sv) or rem. One Sv equals 100 rem.

- Many different types of particles can be emitted from an atom, they include alpha and beta particles, gamma rays, x-rays etc., and they all have different effects on the body. They are assigned a Quality Factor (Q).

So risk (i.e. the amount of energy deposited in human tissue) is:
$$rem = rad \times Q$$

To put this into perspective, it is estimated that during the Chernobyl disaster a total of 81 million Ci of radioactive caesium was released.

Cosmic radiation during a five-hour plane flight
= 3m rem or 0.03m Sv.

One dental x-ray = 4 to 15m rem or 0.04 to 0.15 Sv.

One chest x-ray = 10m rem or 0.1m Sv

One mammogram = 70m rem or 0.7m Sv.

One year of exposure to natural radiation (from soil, cosmic rays etc.) = 300m rem or 3m Sv (where m = 1,000).

Highly radiosensitive cells include: Those of the lymphoid organs, bone marrow, blood, intestines, ovaries and testes.

Those with fairly high radiosensitivity include: Those of the skin and epithelial linings such as are found in the cornea of the eye, the mouth, oesophagus, rectum, vagina, cervix, uterus, ureters, urinary bladder and urethra.

Moderate radiosensitivity is shown by cells of the lens of the eye, the stomach, fine blood vessels, growing cartilage and bone.

The next lowest groups, with fairly low radiosensitivity are the cells of mature bones and cartilage, salivary glands, lungs and bronchial tubes, liver, pancreas, kidneys, and the pituitary thyroid and adrenal glands.

Those with the least radiosensitivity are in the muscles, brain and spinal cord[273].

Thus, leukaemia, lymphoma cells and germ cell tumours are most susceptible to radiation. However, radiation is rarely successful against leukaemia as the cells are dispersed throughout the bloodstream and so throughout whole body. Radiation against leukaemias also produces side effects including secondary cancers[274] and subsequent leukaemia[275]. It can be more successful with lymphomas if they are localised. Epithelial cancers, or solid tumours, on the other hand, have much lower radiation sensitivity and need a much higher dose, usually in the range of 60 to 70Gy. Kidney cancers and melanomas are essentially resistant to radiation treatments. Cancer types that are considered to be amenable to radiation treatment include anal, cervical, head, neck, non-small cell lung, prostate, and skin cancers.

Once a cancer has metastasised, radiation is of little use because, as with leukaemia, it would be necessary to treat the whole body, and this is too dangerous. Radiation is less successful on large tumours than on small ones and so, for large tumours, the radiation may be preceded by surgery or chemotherapy, aimed at reducing the tumour size or increasing its radiation sensitivity.

Radiation risks

From a CAM perspective there are at least three problems with radiation treatment for cancer:

- it does harm, it causes a large number of toxic side-effects that can vary from mild to life-threatening;
- it can cause further cancers;
- it does not address or aim to correct the initial problem(s) that caused the cancer in the first place.

But what about the risks versus the benefits? They are discussed in more detail below, but here are some of the main points:

- radiation kills healthy cells as well as cancer cells;
- radiation can cause cancer, probably by damaging DNA and causing cellular mutations[276];
- radiation can kill immune cells in the blood as they pass through the radiation beam, thus leaving you more susceptible to infections;
- immune cells cluster round tumours in their efforts to attack it and they are killed by the radiation, thus disproportionately weakening your immune system. You already know that an underactive immune system can contribute to the occurrence of cancer [Chapter12];
- radiation destroys phospholipids[277] and these are the essential components of cell membranes which are vulnerable to oxidative damage[278, 279] and so the cell membranes themselves, including those of red blood cells and so the cells of the immune system passing through the radiation beam are susceptible to radiation damage;
- radiation destroys some of the enzymes involved in the Krebs Cycle, such as succinic dehydrogenase, and the cytochromes, where energy from the Krebs Cycle is converted into high energy ATP;
- x-rays using as little as 0.2Gy can destroy the mitochondria in cells. Healthy cells contain hundreds of these organelles and, as you will recall, they are essential for both healthy aerobic energy production and for appropriate apoptosis, two activities that threaten cancer cells. Radiation treatment for most solid tumours uses up to about 1.8Gy

and is repeated 30 times. Clearly this can do immense damage to your mitochondria and so to your energy production;

- The same x-rays increase the level of nitrogen in mitochondria and both reactive oxygen species (ROS)[3] and reactive nitrogen species (RNS)[4] are detected within minutes of exposure to ionising radiation[280]. Keep in mind that there are usually many fewer functioning mitochondria in cancer cells than in healthy cells and it is worth considering what damage could be being done to healthy cells by this procedure. Even at low doses of 0.25-0.5Gy, radiation destroys the lymphocyte defence wall around the tumour and so cancer cells can more readily escape and metastasise;

- radiation, in so far as it is successful, causes massive tissue destruction. There is specific tissue debris, there is also a massive release of free radicals, reactive oxygen species, l-lactic acid, hydrogen peroxide, and many other toxic species. These seriously overload the body's toxic handling capacity, yet patients are almost never given any advice on how to deal with this, whereas CAM practitioners would be advising a thorough detox procedure [See Chapter 26].

See *'Chemotherapy cures cancer and the world is flat'* by Lothar Hirneise[281] for further comments on this topic (references in German).

Toxic side effects

There are countless examples of toxic side effects from radiation, too many to list here, so the following are just a few examples. Radiation for prostate cancer can lead to proctitis[282] or inflammation of the anus and rectum, and bleeding. In the brain, side effects include visual deterioration which develops noticeably between three and six years after treatment; pituitary dysfunction, plus a variety of other changes within the brain, commonly leading to pituitary dysfunction or tumours.

---

[3] Reactive oxygen species (ROS) are small molecules that have unpaired electrons and so are highly reactive. They can damage cell structures and lead to oxidative cell stress. They are one of the reasons why you need anti-oxidants to protect your health.

[4] Reactive nitrogen species (RNS) are small molecules, generally made from nitric oxide and the superoxide radical. They too can cause cell damage and, in this case, nitrosative stress.

If you have once had such radiation you can never relax and be sure that you won't have a recurrence. For instance, following such treatment one patient had a clival (part of the cranium) tumour, with the radiographic appearance of a meningioma, 30 years post-irradiation for acromegaly. At least one study reported several delayed significant consequences from radiation treatments for benign brain tumours that were considered to be safe[283].

Is radiation carcinogenic?

One of the things we know for sure about radiation is that it is carcinogenic and can cause cancer. This has been well known, extensively researched and frequently reported in medical literature for many decades. In a review article published in 2000 Little describes the cellular and molecular mechanisms by which radiation affects individual cells[284]. He reviews the research into cancer-causing ionizing radiation and describes the effect of radiation on oncogenes and tumour suppressor genes and the loss of cell-cycle check points.

Your oncologist may tell you that radiation is safe because they can target it directly at the cancer cells, but can they, and is that sufficient safety? Little makes several points. Radiation that falls on the cytosol of cells (as opposed to the nucleus) can increase the frequency of mutations, so its effects go beyond the direct action on the nucleus. Radiation-induced damage, including mutations, is known to occur in cells that have not received direct nuclear irradiation, since radiation can induce a type of genomic instability in cells that increases the rate of mutations and other genetic changes and these can arise in the descendants of irradiated cells many generations later. What is called the 'bystander effect' involves cell-to-cell communication via the gap junctions between cells, and this affects the p53 damage response pathway. You will recall that protein 53 (p53), a tumour suppressor protein, is a major part of your defence against cancer, sometimes referred to as the 'master watchman' or the 'guardian angel gene' referring to its role in conserving stability by preventing genome mutations[285]. However, if it is mutated it becomes an oncogene and encourages cancer. Since these gap-junctions exist between cells, there is little to be done to block this knock-on effect and, as a result, damaging or mutating your p53 gene can have serious negative (cancerous) consequences for your health.

Other studies have shown that mutation of the protective p53 gene is an early step in the damage caused by irradiation and that the consequences are passed on to daughter cells[286]. This effect can be seen in humans who can be at increased risk of many types of cancer, even thirty years after their initial exposure to radiation[287]. The consequences of the (cellular) bystander effect include the production of secondary cancers, alteration to tissue control mechanisms, genomic instability and either immediate or delayed mutations in tissues outside the irradiation zone[288].

There is an enormous amount more that could be said about the damage caused by irradiation at the cellular level, but it is time for us to focus on some of the clinical effects. An example of the delayed effect of irradiation is shown by the increased incidence of lung cancer, ten years after radiation therapy for breast cancer in non-smokers, and an even greater risk in smokers, the lung cancer occurring on the same side as the previous breast cancer[289].

In the twenty year period between January 1973 and December 1993, 220,806 women who were diagnosed with breast cancer were followed up. Among those who had had radiation therapy for their breast cancer, the relative risk for oesophageal squamous-cell carcinoma increased to 5.42 (95% CI, 2.33 to 10.68) and the relative risk for oesophageal adenocarcinoma increased to 4.22 (CI, 0.47 to 15.25) ten or more years after radiation treatment. There was no increased risk for either type of carcinoma among women who had not had radiation treatment[290].

So remember, whatever treatment your doctor or oncologist recommends, you would be wise to ask them for the evidence base for their recommendations and for real figures as to the likely outcome. One woman [pers. comm.] was told that radiation would reduce her risk of a recurrence of her cancer by 10 per cent. When pushed, her oncologist had to acknowledge that he had no evidence that it would prolong her life, but that he 'intuited' that it would. In spite of describing some shocking side effects he insisted that it would also improve her quality of life, but, when questioned further could provide no details as to what this meant or provide evidence for the statement.

Long-term toxic effects from radiation treatments include fatigue and skin sensitivity. Late onset toxic effects include cataracts, cavities and tooth decay, heart problems, hypothyroidism, infertility, lung problems, intestinal problems, memory deterioration and secondary and primary cancers[291].

CHAPTER 24

WHAT YOU CAN DO TO HELP YOURSELF

If you have read this far you are almost certainly interested in doing what you can to help yourself. Equally, cancer should not be underestimated and it is strongly recommended that you find professional help of a type that suits you. Some things you can do for yourself. There is a lot more that professionals can do for you and you should endeavour to enlist their support and persuade them to work *with* you.

With all the self-help books and Internet reports that are available it is too easy to assume that you can do it all yourself. You cannot. Alternatively, it may seem that there is not a lot more that you can do for yourself and that only the professionals can understand what is required. Clearly this is true if you elect to follow the MDS route, but not if you incorporate the CAM approach. So enlist professional help, of a type that appeals to you, and combine that with doing your own research. You can do a lot for yourself, and you can use the following ideas whatever other therapies, CAM or MDS, that you elect to use. *"You don't know what you don't know"*, and not exploring professional avenues could cost you dear. So let's get started.

When planning the foundations of an anti cancer programme there are some aspects of what you can do that are common to the majority of cancers, certainly to the majority of solid tumour cancers. Then there are additions that may be indicated depending on the unique features of your own cancer. There are two aspects of these unique features. One aspect relates to the location of the cancer and the tissue type, i.e. whether it is lung, breast, prostate or colon cancer, for instance. The other aspect relates to specific biochemical and physiological aspects of your own particular cancer, independent of its location and tissue type. Your overall strategy should be made up of a combination of these, and for the latter aspects you will need professional help.

In brief: Your Recovery Programme = Your Self-Help Lifestyle Programme + Professional therapies in relation to (a) the location or type of your cancer and (b) the results of tests that alert you to unique aspects of your own particular chemistry.

Your Self-Help Lifestyle Programme

There are two layers to this programme:

Step 1
Firstly, there are all the ideas discussed in *'Vital Signs for Cancer'*. All the suggestions found in that book, and discussed briefly below [Chapters 25-27] are aimed at preventing cancer, preventing a recurrence of cancer, or improving your chances of recovering from cancer if you currently have it. These aims are achieved by doing all you can to restore or maintain optimum homoeostasis and optimum health.

This layer involves following a good diet [Chapter 25] and doing the various tests necessary to ensure that you have no nutritional deficiencies, that you remove toxins and improve liver function [Chapter 26]. Attention should be paid to stress and your adrenal glands, your thyroid gland, blood glucose balance, correct hormonal balances and a healthy immune system. On top of all that it is important to recognise the emotional factors that can impact on your health. In short, this layer involves testing for and removing or minimising all the Predisposing Factors [Chapter 27].

Step 2
Secondly, you will want to incorporate the suggestions made here. You will want to do the tests described in these pages and make the appropriate additions to your programme. You should incorporate the ideas described in earlier chapters. This involves recognising Dr. Otto Warburg's hypothesis that oxygen deficiency and mitochondrial dysfunction are causative in cancer; improving the health and function of the cell membranes with the fatty acids, as described by Dr. Budwig; attending to stress, adrenal exhaustion and the adverse production of l-lactic acid as hypothesised by Dr. Fryda; providing the pancreatic enzymes as postulated by Dr. Beard and practiced by William Kelley and

by improving your immune function as suggested by Dr. Abo. These topics are discussed below in Chapters 28-34.

You should also develop your own unique supplement and remedy programme. This should be done with the help of your CAM practitioner. Do not rush off and buy first this product and then that product as you read or are told about one, then another. Cancer is much too serious a problem for such an ad hoc approach. Supplements or remedies that may help one person may have the opposite effect on another, so take advice [Chapter 34].

Your Professional Programme

As already indicated, there are many other tests that can be done and that can give valuable information as to the specific details of your metabolism, the state and function of your tissues, and the strengths and weaknesses of your cancer cells. A full understanding of these features can dictate a very specific and personalised therapy for you. This can be immensely powerful, but it absolutely does need professional guidance. As an example, in Chapter 15 you learnt about a test for p53 and a component of the corrective response to that that could be included in your programme. This is a powerful tool. There are tests that can provide information as to the strength of your extracellular matrix (which, if weak can encourage metastasis), the possible excessive growth of new capillaries (which could be feeding cancer cells), the possible presence of a protein coating to the cancer cells (which can make it more difficult for chemicals to reach and damage the cancer cells and so should be removed), whether or not there is sufficient apoptosis (the death or suicide of old or damaged cells) and more. Once you and your practitioner have this information they can help you to plan a recovery programme for you that focuses on the most effective remedies and therapies that are uniquely for you.

Other important information can be obtained from tests for the balance of your various neurotransmitters, the individual molecules, produced mainly by your brain, that instruct the rest of the cells throughout your body. These are part of the total communication within your body and all should be in balance if you want to achieve optimum health. Your immune system is vitally important and there are many tests that can provide useful information. Put simply, there are two halves to your immune system and they should be in balance. If they are not, and tests can readily show this, then altering this balance in the right direction is crucial. Again, the results of these tests provide useful information, both as to the possible metabolic errors that allowed cancer to develop in the first instance, and to the appropriate path to take to restore good health.

You will no doubt note that all these tests and all these suggested avenues for recovery are focused on just that, on restoring and recovering your health and on perfecting your body chemistry and physiological harmony and function. The aim is not focused, as is the MDS system, on destruction, on destroying the tumour while at the same time trying, not always very successfully, to do as little collateral damage as possible, and yet recognising and admitting that a significant amount of collateral damage almost always occurs.

Whatever other treatment or management programme you plan you will almost certainly benefit from instigating the CAM protocols outlined here. As previously stated, in almost all cases, this can all be done in conjunction with MDS treatments if you so wish. You should consult with your practitioners as to any possible unwanted interactions. Keep in mind though that the MDS treatments will often work somewhat against the CAM programme. In relation to your physical health you can think of the possible treatments, simplified, as shown in the following table.

System	Possible harm	General health	Toxins	Detoxing	Removal of cause, future prevention	Tumour
MDS system	Toxic effects, damaging general health.	No input.	Adding toxins.	No attempt made.	None or limited.	Killing cancer cells.
MDS + CAM	Damaging general health (MDS) and possibly reducing benefit of some CAM procedures.	Some improvement to general health (largely CAM-related). Possibility of some synergistic benefit.	Adding toxins (MDS components).	Some detoxing (CAM).	Some (CAM).	Killing cancer cells.
CAM system	None.	Significant improvement to general health.	Removing toxins.	Detoxing.	An important focus of the protocols.	Cancer cells dying.

Remember that in addition to whatever physical and chemical treatments or supplement and lifestyle changes you apply, you should also attend to emotional issues. Doing this will help, whichever physical therapies you choose or which treatment system.

Some of the questions that I am commonly asked relate to the cost of CAM remedies and protocols. It is true that the tests, the supplements and remedies and the various pieces of equipment that are recommended can be costly. They may cost a lot less than MDS treatments but, unfortunately, they are rarely covered by your health insurance regime, whatever that may be, while the MDS costs remain largely hidden from you. So I make the following suggestions:

If the budget is very small

1. Determine your Metabolic Type and eat only the foods recommended for you. Focus on the recommended foods that are also indicated in the chart in Chapter 25.

2. Do buy organic, that is important. Organic food may not be perfect but you must do all you can to eliminate all possible toxins, and buying organic foods is one way to reduce your toxic load. In general, organic foods tend to contain more vitamins, minerals and other nutrients than do foods produced by other methods. They may cost somewhat more than conventionally produced foods but are often a lot more satisfying, so you may need to eat less, and should decrease your need for supplements.

3. Organically grown foods also contain more phytoalexins than do foods that have been chemically treated during growth. Phytoalexins are antimicrobial substances synthesized by plants to protect themselves from plant pathogens. They are chemically varied, broad spectrum pathogen inhibitors and include many compounds that are also beneficial to humans, such as resveratrol. They are rarely produced (or needed) by chemically protected fruits.

4. Eat at least 75% of your diet raw, more if you can. (This will reduce your cooking bill.) Make sure vegetables and berries constitute 75% of your diet, including green vegetable juices. (This will cut out some costly low-nutrient foods.)

5. Determine your pH using inexpensive pH paper strips and aim to increase your early morning salivary pH to 7.

6. Use the Budwig mixes (see below) for protein and to increase oxygen into the cells. This will give you low–cost, high-quality and well-absorbed protein.

7. Follow Dr. Fryda's treatment with d-lactic acid (inexpensive). Soak in a very hot bath each day and add 100gms of sodium bicarbonate (inexpensive). Details below.

8. Follow all the detox methods described in Chapters 26 and 32 (almost all of them are inexpensive).

As the budget increases

1. Take pancreatic enzymes and supplements, as recommended by your practitioner.

2. If you don't already have them, buy a food processor, a powerful blender and a top quality juice extractor – it is worth the outlay and will allow you to make your own foods, such as humus, nut butters and smoothies and thus produce savings in the long run.

3. Buy a food dehydrator.

4. Do some of the basic tests described in *'Vital Signs for Cancer'* and repair the damages as indicated by these test results.

5. Have the CA Profile test done and use the results to monitor your progress.

Budget permitting

1. Do the extra tests suggested by your CAM practitioner.

2. Take all the remedies and follow all the recovery suggestions as their need is indicated by the test results. Your professional therapist will recommend these.

3. Repeat the tests at regular intervals. This may be monthly at the start and then at increasing intervals as the results improve.

4. Buy a Far Infra Red sauna sleeping bag (or equivalent).

5. Explore other therapies, such as hyperthermia, intravenous vitamins, inpatient visits to residential clinics and so forth. There are many options available out there if you do some relatively easy searching.

It is now time to look at these suggestions in more detail.

CHAPTER 25

DIET – GENERAL

The first and foundation layer of any recovery programme is the correct diet for you. What you eat dictates, to a large extent, what your body is made of and how it functions. Never underestimate the power of your diet for generating health or disease.

Your individual needs will depend on your genetic make-up, but this you cannot change. Your diet, however, is something over which you do have control. Eating the right diet for you means eating the diet that is right for your own individual metabolism. There are two methods you can use to determine this. Have a hair sample analysed by American Research Laboratories, or by Trace Element Inc. [See Resources]. They will assess your metabolism via the ratios of calcium, magnesium, sodium and potassium. Alternatively, you can go to www.healthexcel.com, check the box that asks if you want to determine your Metabolic Type a third of the way down on the left side of the Home Page. Then click on *"Which diet is right for you? Take the test now."* Go to the bottom of the next page. Click on *"Let's begin."* Pay their fee, answer the questions and wait for the results to land in your email inbox. These will include your metabolic pattern and a page indicating foods that are (a) very good for you; (b) good for you; (c) only to be eaten occasionally; and (d) to be avoided. Work within these guidelines. You will also receive information as to the extent to which you are a Fast Oxidiser, Slow Oxidiser, Balanced Oxidiser, Sympathetic Dominant, Parasympathetic Dominant or Balanced Dominant type. There is more on the site but it can be costly and overwhelming and this is the essence of what you need.

Most people with cancer (but not all) are either Sympathetic Dominant or a Slow Oxidiser. For these two groups red meats and dark poultry should be avoided and the diet should be mainly vegetables with some fish or white poultry meat. This is the basis of the alkaline residue diet recommended for most people with cancer. However, if you are Parasympathetic Dominant or a Fast Oxidiser you may still get cancer, although in general this is less likely; if so the rules are different and you can eat more flesh foods. One diet does not fit all.

The important thing is to eat the foods that, on this basis, are right for you, not the foods that other well-meaning friends, helpful books or other people tell you to eat. William Kelley [Chapter 16] found that the Sympathetic Dominant diet suited him perfectly and gave him the best benefit. He then encouraged his family to eat the same way, especially his wife, who was not well at the time. He was surprised to find that her symptoms got worse on the diet he advised for her. When she reverted to a Parasympathetic Dominant, high meat, diet, her health improved.

Within the foods that are listed for your Metabolic Type make the following choices:

Food	Include	Quantity	Avoid
General	All food should be organic and fresh. Frozen is occasionally acceptable.		Tinned food, processed food or food with added (non-food) chemicals.
Vegetables	Almost all vegetables – 75% raw food including juiced. The rest lightly steamed. Homemade soups – blend raw or very lightly steamed vegetables. Do NOT overcook.	75% of your diet.	Potato, parsnip. Tinned vegetables. Fried or roast vegetables or vegetable chips.

Food	Include	Quantity	Avoid
Fruits	None at the start, then introduce gradually as advised, fresh or frozen berries. When there is overall improvement you can add in other fresh fruit including apples, apricots, cherries, berries, figs, papaya, pineapple. Goji berries, may be acceptable. Avocados (technically a fruit) are beneficial and can be included from the start, as can olives.	250gms+ of berries every day. One piece of other fruit when permitted. Avocados, use freely, on their own or to improve other combinations.	Bananas (contain sucrose). Frozen fruit (other than berries). Tinned fruit, sweetened fruit or fruits in syrup or with added sugar. Pale coloured fruits (few phytonutrients) such as pears, white peaches etc. Dates (too sweet).
Drinks	Generous quantities of fresh vegetable juices made from greens, carrots, beetroot, broccoli, celery, red cabbage etc. with ginger. Nut milks (without vegetable oils or sugar). Herb teas, especially green tea. Dandelion coffee (max 1 cup/day). Purified water.	1 litre of vegetable juices. 1 litre of total fluid for every 25kgs of body weight.	All soft drinks, carbonated drinks (including sparkling mineral water), fruit juice drinks, pre-made fruit juices, coffee, alcohol. Any drinks with sugar. Even fruit juices give too much sugar, too quickly and without any fibre.

Food	Include	Quantity	Avoid
Fats and oils	Flaxseed oil (stored in deep freeze once opened), olive oil, hemp oil. Coconut oil for its anti-viral, anti-fungal and anti-bacterial actions. Avocados and tahini make good spreads. Small amounts of organic butter (preferably not from cows) may be acceptable.	Flaxseed oil 50-90ml per day. Use coconut oil when you do cook.	Other nut and seed oils. Vegetable oils. Sunflower oil. Commercial mayonnaise or salad dressings. Animal fats, shortening, margarine, alternative butter spreads. Rancid fats.
Seeds and kernels	Chia, linseeds, pumpkin, sesame, sunflower. Apricot, nectarine, peach and plum kernels, apple seeds. All raw.		Roasted, fried or salted seeds and kernels.
Nuts	Fresh raw nuts, soaked first. Raw nut butters with no additions, freshly made in small quantities and kept refrigerated.		Peanuts. Fried, roasted or salted nuts and nut butters. Rancid nuts.

Food	Include	Quantity	Avoid
Seasonings	Freshly and freshly dried herbs and spices. Especially basil, chives, coriander, garlic, ginger, parsley, rosemary, cayenne, cinnamon, cumin, turmeric, kelp. Black pepper. Potassium salt.		Salt. Commercial sauces and flavourings. Seasoning mixes containing sugar, salt or added chemicals.
Grains and Cereals	None at the start. Small amounts when there is significant improvement. Choose from millet, buckwheat, brown rice, amaranth, quinoa.	Limited.	Wheat in any form. White flour, white pastas, white rice. Probably best to avoid barley, oats and rye as well.
Dairy	Organic sheep's, goats' or buffalo natural yoghurt, kefir, quark or cottage cheese, all made from raw, unpasteurised milk		Milk. Butter. Hard cheeses, cheese with more than 40% fat. Cows' milk or milk products. NO non-organic dairy products.
Breads	None at the start. When permitted, choose from sprouted grain breads made from permitted grains (above), yeast-free breads.	Max 1 slice a day.	Wheat bread. Breads with refined (white) flour.

Food	Include	Quantity	Avoid
Beans and sprouts	Alfalfa and other seeds and beans, sprouted.		
Eggs	Organic, lightly boiled or poached.	2-3 per week.	Fried, or scrambled eggs, omelettes. Commercial or free range eggs (unless also organic) in any form.
Meat and fish	High omega-3 fish, organic salmon, preferably wild. Small amounts of organic red meats from grass-fed (not grain-fed) animals, and organic poultry ('free range' is not enough), depending on Metabolic Type.		Shellfish and crustaceans. Smoked, salted, fried or processed meats. Processed meats with any additives including nitrates, antibiotics, hormones.
Sweets	Xylitol, ribose, mannose, stevia. Carob powder. Later, pure organic cocoa powder in small amounts.		Sugars, under any name, in anything: sugar, evaporated cane juice, agave, malt, dextrin, rice maltodextrin, corn syrup, glucose, fructose, levulose, fruit sugar etc. All artificial sugar substitutes, saccharine, cyclamates, sucralose, aspartame etc.

All foods should, of course, be organically grown and produced. If you cannot find an organic food of your choice, then choose a different food that is available in organic form. Remember that not only do organic foods come with far fewer toxins than conventional foods, but they can also provide greater amounts of nutrients, or of beneficial substances such as resveratrol, known to be protective.

Many significant facts lie behind each of these individual dietary suggestions. Here are just a couple of examples:

- avoid all heated and processed fats that might contain trans fatty acids, they are known to be associated with an increased risk of cancer[292];
- avoid fats that have been heated in association with carbohydrates. Examples include chips, potato, corn or other crisps, roast potatoes and burnt toast. The combination creates compounds called acrylamides which are recognised carcinogens[293, 294].

Eating raw

The instruction to 'eat almost everything raw' does not limit you to an endless diet of lettuce, tomato and cucumber salads. Juices count as part of your raw food intake and I strongly recommend the purchase of a good juicer with a screw mechanism, rather than a centrifugal grating basket or overly high-speed juicer. With this you can make your own humus, nut butters and many other items. However, if funds are restricted then start with the cheaper style. You will find (in Appendix 7) places where you can buy the good quality (auger) juicers, and a list of books (in Appendix 4) on raw food preparation that may open your eyes to a lot of unsuspected possibilities.

I strongly recommend the purchase of a dehydrator. This is a small, square cabinet with either five or nine shelves (five is almost always enough unless you are part of a dedicated and very large family of raw food eaters). The temperature control allows you to spread food combinations on the trays and raise the temperature to no more than 40.5°C. At this temperature the foods still count as 'raw' and there is little if any loss of the food's precious enzymes, vitamins or other phytonutrients, but it allows you to make 'cookies', crackers and a variety of other tasty foods, all made from the permitted list of foods. The products have the advantage of being 'dry' and easy to carry with you for snack foods.

While it is true that you can obtain a large amount of vitamins and minerals in supplement form, there is growing evidence that the best source of nutrients is your diet. When you eat nutrient dense foods such as vegetables and berries, you derive many benefits:

- vitamins and minerals are present in different forms to the forms obtained from a synthetic supplement;
- these forms may be absorbed much more readily than the supplement forms;
- the nutrients are present with many of their cofactors;
- they frequently come in physiologically beneficial ratios;
- not only do you obtain known nutrients, you obtain many other plant ingredients with possibly, as yet, unsuspected benefits;
- there are many hundreds of phytonutrients, only a relatively few of which are ever added to manufactured supplements;
- you reduce the amount of non-nutrient binders and fillers that you consume with tableted supplements.

For all these reasons, and more, you are encouraged to make your diet as nutrient dense as possible. This is one of the many benefits of having a large amount of vegetable juices each day. Juicing is one way of obtaining a large amount of macronutrients in a readily absorbable form.

Vegetables and fruit

We are all exhorted to eat our 'five-a-day'. This is a start, but it is not nearly enough, especially if that five includes foods that are low in phytonutrients and have a high glycemic index, such as bananas, potatoes or crisps, chips, sweetcorn, other low nutrient fruits and vegetables, and wine. In general, the most helpful and nutrient-rich vegetables and fruits are the most brightly coloured ones. But even of these, 'five a day' is not enough. In fact, the World Cancer Research Fund in 1997 recommended seven-a-day for cancer prevention[295], and it is now recognised that this is minimal and doubling these figures would be a more helpful goal. There have been many studies showing benefit from acting on this advice.

One study showed that by increasing your vegetable or fruit intake by only 150gms a day you could reduce your risk of developing cancer by 2.5%[296]. Those who are quick to criticise anything outside the conventional wisdom were quick to say that this benefit was minimal, but is it? It is estimated that the current incidence of cancer in the UK is 250,000 per year. Two point five per cent of this is 6,250. Is preventing this many cases of cancer insignificant? If a medical drug could achieve this outcome would we applaud it? Almost certainly so. Keep in mind that the dietary change was only the addition of 150gms of vegetables or fruit, equivalent to one large apple or two medium sized tomatoes. The figures get better and better with further increases in the intake of vegetables and fruits. They also improved if you consume fresh raw vegetables rather than overcooked vegetables, and probably also improve if the vegetables are organically grown. People had hoped for better results from this study. However, you cannot expect a few overcooked vegetables to compensate for a poor lifestyle in other respects. If you truly want to be healthy, your entire lifestyle should be improved as well as this increased consumption of vegetables and fruit.

Many phytonutrients work better in combinations than when consumed separately. For instance, an *in vivo* study of implanted tumours found that tomato on its own reduced tumour growth by 34%, broccoli on its own reduced tumour growth by 42%, but in combination they reduced tumour growth by 54%[297]. You are much more likely to consume beneficial combinations if you eat ten or more servings a day than if you consume only five. Later, you will learn that Dr. Abo recommends eating small amounts of 36 different foods every day, rather than larger amounts of only a few different foods. By increasing the variety of the foods you consume, you increase the probability that you will get a much larger range of nutrients and beneficial plant combinations. Keep in mind that the strength of any chain is its weakest link, and one of those less common phytonutrients could be the weakest link in your chain.

Nearly every CAM protocol for helping people with cancer involves a high intake of vegetables and a limited or moderate intake of fruits. The limit on the intake of most types of fruit is due to their relatively high sugar content. As you know, sugar feeds cancer cells preferentially to healthy cells and encourages their growth. The worst sugars in this regard appear to be commercial fructose (commonly derived by processing corn syrup, also the basis of agave) and sucrose[298]. There are many claims that, since fructose is found in fruits, this is a 'healthier' sugar, but this appears to go against the evidence. It is possible that the fructose in fruits is less harmful than the commercially produced variety, but it also underscores the admonition to eat only limited amounts of fruit and not to drink fruit juices. At least when you eat fruit, rather than extracted fructose, on its own you are also getting the beneficial phytonutrients that are present in the fruit.

The list of vegetables and fruits below is not intended to be comprehensive. It is, however, a list of some of the foods that are nutrient dense or contain valuable anti-cancer nutrients. It is given to add weight to the emphasis we place on eating lots of vegetables. Once you realise the many hundreds of benefits they confer it is easier, at least for many people, to stick to this dietary advice. The information is put here for that reason.

The various foods contain components that are helpful in terms of your general health, optimising your health, preventing cancer, either primary or secondary, or in helping to support your recovery from cancer. Some of the suggestions are well supported by thorough research or clinical trials. Others are indicated by fewer laboratory studies or clinical outcomes, but not rigorously trialled. Others contain components that themselves have been shown to offer some health benefit. Clearly there is very little research money to be found for such research as the results are not patentable, but this should not deter you from paying attention to the clear hints, signs and suggestions that are available.

All of the foods listed below are relatively common, and are, at worst, harmless, certainly when compared to many of the highly processed foods of commerce with their added chemicals and altered metabolites. At best they have a lot of benefits to offer based on their various components. They are foods you should bring into your diet to replace any of the processed foods you may be eating.

In regard to fruits, keep in mind that, even though they contain some valuable nutrients, they do contain significant amounts of sugar, even if it is fructose, and that they should only be eaten in moderate amounts. The exception to this are the berries. These are high in particularly valuable nutrients and contain relatively small amounts of sugars. Also consider making the most of, and extending, the flavour and pleasure of fruits by adding them to vegetable dishes. Examples of this would include adding apples to raw cabbage coleslaws, instead of eating them on their own, or adding very thinly sliced oranges to a salad of red onions and tomato.

The common vernacular talks of 'fruits and vegetables'. I suggest changing this to 'vegetables and fruits', thus emphasising the preference that should be given to vegetables over fruits.

Salt

Eating heavily salted foods can increase your risk of developing cancer[299].

The term 'salt' as commonly used in the kitchen, means sodium chloride, and this salt remains sodium chloride whether it is rock salt (mined from rock deposits that are usually the residue of ancient oceans) or sea salt, obtained by evaporating sea water from today's oceans. In chemical terms a salt is the combination of a positive, metal ion or cation, such as sodium, potassium, calcium or magnesium, with the negative anion half of an acid such as sulphate, nitrate, or chloride. Thus, potassium chloride is also, chemically a salt. From a kitchen perspective it also tastes just like sodium chloride salt and can be used interchangeably with it.

When considering the role of salt in the diet it is important to consider the roles of both sodium and potassium. For the millennia during which we were hunter-gatherers we had a food supply (mainly plant foods) that was high in potassium and low in sodium. This gave an evolutionary advantage to those of our ancestors whose kidneys could hold on to all the sodium in the blood, and let the excess potassium go, into the urine. This lies behind the enormous value placed on salt (sodium chloride) deposits, when they were found, or in salt when it was brought into Europe from the East and commanded a high price – in fact it is the basis of the word 'salary'. All worked well until (sodium) salt became so readily available.

When you consume potassium it flows round the body, is taken up by any cells that need it, and then, still in the blood, flows through the kidneys. The kidneys retain little of it and so it is lost in the urine. Now we are left with kidneys that hold back sodium (of which most people now eat an excess) and let go the valuable potassium (of which we have a relatively inadequate supply).

The recommended daily intake for sodium is 1,500mg which is equivalent to 3,780mg of sodium chloride, and for potassium is 4,700mg which is equivalent to 8,920mg of potassium chloride salt. You derive some sodium from the foods you eat (before processing or salt is added). The amount of potassium you obtain depends largely on the amount of vegetables and fruits that you eat. However, the foods of commerce give you considerably more sodium and very little potassium.

Cancer cells thrive on sodium. A high sodium intake increases the amount of acid wastes produced, and this benefits cancer cells which thrive in an acid environment.

In your tissues, potassium is found mainly inside your cells and sodium in the extracellular fluid. Most carcinogens alter the potassium to sodium ratio of your cells, decreasing the amount of potassium and increasing the amount of sodium. Most of the protective agents or anticarcinogens do the opposite. As you grow older, the level of potassium inside your cells falls and the level of sodium increases, as does your risk of developing cancer. Furthermore, among people suffering from diseases associated with excess potassium (such as Parkinson's disease and Addison's disease) there is a below average incidence of cancer. Conversely, among people suffering from diseases associated with a deficiency of potassium (stress, obesity, alcoholism) there is an above average incidence of cancer[300].

There are several actions you can take:

- reduce your (sodium) salt intake to an absolute minimum. Over time you will gradually come to appreciate the flavours of the foods themselves more, and lose your taste for salt;

- avoid foods with added salt, and this includes almost all processed foods, including those that are organic, and otherwise healthy;
- if you do want the flavour, use potassium chloride salt instead of sodium chloride. It is available from most health food stores;
- increase your use of fresh herbs and spices.

Pepper

No, I am not going to suggest you give up pepper, in fact I am going to encourage you to use it liberally, particularly freshly ground black pepper. Black pepper comes from the whole peppercorn, in contrast to white pepper which comes from the inner part of the seed only. Whole, or ground, black pepper corns contain piperine and this is valuable in relation to your absorption of curcumin, a recognised anticarcinogen derived from turmeric. In fact, adding 20mg of piperine, in human trials, increased the absorption of curcumin by 2,000 per cent[301].

Herbs and spices

There are many culinary herbs and spices that are known to have protective actions in both the prevention of, and recovery from, cancer as well as other health benefits that help to reduce predisposing factors. They include, basil, caraway seeds, cayenne or chilli, chives, coriander, cumin, garlic, ginger, parsley, rosemary, sage and turmeric. If you put the name of any of these herbs and the word 'cancer' in a search engine you will find a goldmine of information. Many other herbs, such as oregano, marjoram, thyme and others have general health benefits, all of which can help in prevention and recovery, at least indirectly. So use herbs and spices as often as you can. Herbs are best when used fresh, but are also excellent if they have been carefully dried and are used within a few months.

Vegetables and fruits

In general they are all important, but some are more so than others. Potatoes and parsnips have a high glycemic index, raise your blood glucose level and provide negligible amounts of trace nutrients. Avoid them. Choose the dark and brightly coloured sweet potatoes instead.

Always choose brightly coloured vegetables and fruits rather than the white or pale coloured options. Thus you would choose spinach rather than iceberg lettuce, and apricots rather than pears. However, all of these are better than white bread, white rice, white flour, white pasta, chips, crisps, sugar and many of the foods of commerce that contain these foods.

Below are just a few of the beneficial foods and some of their relevant active ingredients or activities. Sometimes the research available relates specifically to the individual food, other studies have focused on specific components found in a food, thus there are gaps in the referenced information in the table. I repeat, the list is not intended to be comprehensive. It is a guide as to the benefits of eating a wide variety of vegetables and fruits. There are, of course, many other active ingredients in these foods and herbs than those mentioned here.

There is no claim that any one of these foods will 'cure cancer'. However, they can all contribute, to a lesser or greater extent, to a recovery programme. Hopefully this information will encourage you to add even more of these valuable foods to your diet, and reassure you that the effort to include them really is worthwhile.

Apples contain ferrulic acid which is anti cancer[302], pro-apoptotic[303], antioxidant, and inhibits the damaging effects of ROS (reactive oxygen species). They also contain polyphenols and procyanidins which are apoptotic[304], and ursolic acid (see below) especially in the peel.

Globe artichokes contain silymarine, which reduces tumour promotion[305] and inhibits angiogenesis[306], and polyphenols which are antioxidant and induce apoptosis[307].

Avocados contain procyanidins and pigments, glutathione, lutein and other carotenoids, and beta-sitosterol which are antioxidants[308] and contribute to cell cycle arrest and apoptosis[309].

Beetroot contains carotenoids and betacyanin which are anti-inflammatory[310] and anti-tumour[311].

Broccoli in particular and the cruiferous family in general (cauliflower, dark green cabbages etc), contain Indole-3-carbonyl (I-3-C). I-3-C is converted into di-indolyl methane (DIM) in the body and this in turn is effective at correcting any imbalances in the ration of 16-oestrogen to 2-oestrogen and thus helping to reduce the risk of oestrogen associated cancers. Sprouted broccoli seeds contain many times more I-3-C than do broccoli florets, so look for these in your local organic shop. You may find them on their own or combined with alfalfa sprouts. Similarly, sprouting broccoli is better than a head of it as it is younger and higher in general nutrient content.

Citrus fruits contain limonene, a powerful anticancer agent[312]. However, it is not the juice that is so powerful but the skin. Blend the entire fruit and think of it as raw marmalade without the sugar. Adding the safe sugar, xylitol, can sweeten it.

Green tea contains catechins, a group of compounds that includes epigallocatechinn-3-gallate (ECCG), which is the most abundant catechin found in green tea. Research results are not conclusive but it is thought that the mechanism of action of the benefit of green tea is due to the inhibition of proteases, certain kinases, that interfere with receptor-mediated functions, all of which can lead to reduced cellular proliferation, cellular growth, angiogenesis, invasion and metastasis and to increased apoptosis[313].

The onion and garlic family, which includes all forms of onions, leeks, garlic and chives has been found to be beneficial in a wide range of cancer types. Garlic is particularly helpful[314]. These vegetables contain diallyl sulphide, S-allyl cysteine and allicin which help in the repair of damaged DNA, reduce the formation of carcinogenic nitroso compounds, reduce cellular reproduction and increase apoptosis[315].

Raspberries, cherries, pomegranate and grapes contain ellagic acid which helps to reduce the effect of carcinogens such as benzopyrene[316] and 4-nitroquinoline 1-oxide[317].

Grapes can contain resveratrol. Resveratrol blocks the three phases of cancer development (initiation, promotion and progression), it inhibits angiogenesis and metastasis and promotes apoptosis[318, 319, 320]. Thus, it is a very protective substance for humans. When the grapes are stressed by a fungus such as *Botrytis cinerea*, they produce this resveratrol.

However, when grapes are commercially grown and sprayed with fungicide chemicals they are not stressed by the fungus and so do not need to produce resveratrol. So to maximise your intake of resveratrol your grapes should be organically grown. One usually thinks of eating organically grown foods to avoid toxins, in this case it is to make sure you get some beneficial compounds that would otherwise be lacking in the food.

Red onions and cranberries are sources of quercetin which has been shown to inhibit cancer growth and stimulate apoptosis[321]. Quercetin is also found in a variety of nuts (but not peanuts or cashews).

Many herbs, including basil, oregano, peppermint, rosemary and thyme, plus fruits such as bilberries and papaya contain ursolic acid. This acid inhibits several types of cancer[322], including multiple myeloma [323], and is the starting material, in the body, for a number of other anti-cancer and anti-tumour agents[324].

Tomatoes contain lycopene, a red carotenoid. It is antioxidant, cardioprotective, anti-inflammatory, anti-mutagenic and anti-carcinogenic. Tomatoes and tomato products have been shown, *in vitro* and *in vivo*, to have anticancer benefits. The mechanisms behind this are thought to include scavenging dangerous reactive oxygen species (ROS), increasing detoxification, reducing cell proliferation, inducing gap-junctional communication, inhibiting cell cycle progression and modulating signal transduction pathways[325].

Selenium is an important element in the management of cancer, helping to reduce oxidation and improving immune function[326]. It can replace the sulphur atom in a number of organic compounds, if the vegetables are grown on selenium-rich soils. This is particularly true of garlic, the onion family in general and the brassicas[327]. Selenium is also found in brazil nuts.

There are hundreds of other examples that could be given here, but these should be sufficient for you to decide to commit to the '75% vegetable plus berries' guideline.

Protein

In general, red meats and dark poultry meats should be avoided by people with cancer. People for whom these foods are suitable are less likely to be the ones with cancer. If you do eat these meats make sure they are organic, come from grass-fed animals and are unprocessed, and that they are cooked slowly at only moderate temperatures. Fats should not be eaten if overheated, crisped or burnt.

Fish in general remains one of the best protein sources. If you choose the oily fish this has the advantage of giving you increased amounts of a variety of different omega-3 fatty acids. One of these fatty acids is DHA. Recent research shows that supplementing the diet of experimental rats with this has reduced tumour formation by two-thirds[328]. Fish oil added to the diet has reduced the formation of many types of cancer, including breast cancer[329, 330, 331], colon cancer and cancer of the small intestine[332], colon cancer[333, 334], prostate cancer[335], lung cancer[336], papillomas[337] and sarcomas[338]. Omega-3 fatty acids have also been shown to reduce the rate of progression of tumours of the breast[339], prostate[340] and kidney[341]. By contrast, corn oil has been shown to increase the risk of tumour development[342].

Prevention is always better than cure and it is clear that DHA supplementation, and increased intake from fish, is more effective in prevention than in correction[343].

Eating fish may be a problem if you are a vegetarian, but when you discover your metabolic type, you may well find that fish is positively indicated for you. If you still decline it then you would be wise to supplement your diet with DHA. Although this is generally extracted from fish, it is now also available extracted from algae.

There are some basic biochemical steps that you need to understand if you are to understand the relative importance of the different omega-3 fatty acids in your body and their sources. Put simply, when you eat these fats there is a multi-step process leading to the ultimate active and beneficial compounds which include DHA and prostaglandins of the 3 series (PG3). These are the beneficial compounds that are anti-clotting and anti-inflammatory and so very good for your health. The main steps are as follows:

Alpha Linolenic acid (ALA) (omega-3) → eicosapentaenoic acid (EPA) → docosahexaenoic acid (DHA) → PG3

Or: ALA → EPA → DHA → PG3

The intermediate steps involve desaturases (enzymes that catalyse the removal of hydrogen from the fatty acid, making it less saturated) and elongases (enzymes that catalyze the addition of pairs of carbon atoms to the fatty acid chain, making it longer). These enzymes require vitamins B3, B6 and C and minerals such as zinc and magnesium as coenzymes if they are to work efficiently.

The richest plant food source of omega-3 fatty acids is flaxseed oil, lesser sources include a variety of nuts and seeds. However, these only provide ALA and not EPA or DHA, whereas fish provide ALA, EPA and DHA. The conversion steps can be very slow in some people[5, 344] and even slower if you are deficient in the coenzymes. In some people the steps can be so slow as to render them PG3 deficient unless they eat fish or take DHA as a supplement[345]. These people cannot rely on flaxseed oil to boost their PG3 level.

A number of factors can reduce your conversion of ALA to DHA and they include:

- a diet high in linoleic acid (LA). This is the common fatty acid of most common vegetable oils that pervade the general diet of commerce, including corn oil, sunflower oil, safflower oil and others. It can reduce the activity of the enzymes (the desaturases and elongases) by 40%. This is true even if they are organic and cold-pressed;

- trans fatty acids, as found in many vegetable oil 'spreads', hydrogenated fats and over-heated or processed fats and vegetable oils;

---

[5]   15% ALA converts to EPA and 5% to DHA

- a deficiency of any of the coenzymes listed above;
- alcohol;
- diabetes;
- ageing.

Dairy products are generally thought of as a good protein food. However, the majority of milk protein is casein and this has been shown to encourage cancer in experimental animals. Casein is a fat-soluble protein and so is concentrated in hard cheeses. The remaining milk protein is water-soluble and is found in the whey fraction. Thus, whey protein isolate, which can be obtained as a powder, is casein-free. Non-protein milk products, such as cream and butter are unlikely to contain much casein.

Cows' milk contains the growth factor IGF-1[346,347] and this, in combination with the casein content, commonly used as a tumour stimulant in experimental animals, is reason enough to avoid such dairy products. The milk is also rich in hormones. This is true even if they are not given to the cow via feed or treatments as the cows are kept in an unnatural state of almost permanent lactation or pregnancy.

Superfoods

There are certain 'derived' foods available from your health food store that can improve your diet even further. These include items such as lecithin granules, which is good for your heart and liver and improves the health, flexibility, oxygen absorbing ability and communicating ability of your cell membranes [Chapter17].

Camu camu powder. Also known as *Myrcieria dubia,* Camucamu, Cacari, and Camocamo, this is a small bushy tree that grows in the Amazon rainforest. It is related to Jaboticaba (*Myrciaria cauliflora*) and the Guavaberry or Rumberry (*Myrciaria floribunda*). The fruit, red to purple in colour and somewhat like a cherry, is one of the richest sources of vitamin C, second only to the less readily available kakadu plum from Australia. Camu camu contains 21,000 to 500,000ppm of vitamin C compared to acerola at 16,000-172,000ppm, and oranges at 500-4,000ppm. The fruits also contain bioflavonoids, anrocyanins. It also contains beta-carotene, vitamins B1, B2, B3, the minerals calcium, iron and phosphate and the amino acids, leucine, serine and valine, in addition to a small amount of protein. Other components include anthocyanins, which make up the red skin pigments, flavonoids, flavanols, flavonols, catechin, delphinidin 3-glucoside, cyanidin 3-glucoside, gallic acid, ellagic acids and rutin, and hydrolysed tannins such as gallo- and/or ellagitannins[348]. In brief, camu camu is an excellent fruit and can also be consumed as a nutritional supplement in powder or capsule form.

The **goji berry** is thought to be the richest source of carotenoids of all known foods, it contains about 500 times the amount of vitamin C as is contained in a similar weight of oranges, and contains several other immune supporting components. These include polysaccharides which fortify the immune system and a powerful secretagogue; as such it stimulates the pituitary secretion of human growth and is a strong antioxidant.

Traditionally, goji berries have been regarded as a longevity, strength-building, and sexual potency food. When studies were done with elderly people given the berries daily for three weeks it was found that in 67% of them there was a tripling of their T-cell transformation functions and a doubling of the activity of their white cell interleukin-2 level, all indicating a boost to their immune function. At a lifestyle level their spirit and optimism increased significantly, 95% of them experienced improved appetite and better quality of sleep and 35% of them experienced partial recovery of their sexual function. The berries can be eaten on their own, as a snack, but you should eat only moderate amounts as they do contain fruit sugar. In combination with raw nuts they make a tasty and satisfying snack. Goji juice can be bought, but again, be careful of the fructose content and only consume small amounts at a time. It is much better to eat the whole berries.

There are many **green powders**. They include Barley Greens, Wheat Grass powder, Vital Greens (which contains a wide range of added vitamins, minerals and other nutritive substances), chlorella powder, spirulina powder and blue-green algae powder. They are generally all an acquired taste, but if you come to enjoy them they are very beneficial. They are alkalising, help in the elimination of toxins and are generally very good for your health.

There are also **red** and **purple powders**, made from a variety of fruits and vegetables of these colours. They should not replace fresh vegetables and fruits in your diet, but they can be helpful additions, providing a range of phytonutrients.

Lecithin is usually derived from soy, although it is also present in egg yolks. It is difficult to find an organic source, but do make sure that what you buy is non-GM. Lecithin is a source of essential fatty acids and nutrients that support brain and liver function. It is an emulsifying agent and so helps in the digestion of fats, especially if your liver needs assistance or if you have had your gall bladder removed. It can be added to sweet or savoury foods. If you add it to oil and vinegar dressings it will hold the two in an emulsified form and prevent them separating. Add to a variety of foods, sweet (including Budwig mixes) and savoury, such as sauces and salad dressings. Up to a tablespoon a day is helpful.

Linseeds are also known as flaxseeds. Their oil is a rich source of omega-3 fatty acids. The seeds absorb liquids and set into a gel. As such they can be added to fruit juice to make a soft fruit jelly. Within your digestive tract they have the effect of holding water in the stool, increasing the bulk of your stool and so preventing constipation. The seeds can also be used to treat diarrhoea as in that case they absorb the excess liquid in the stool and help to firm it up, thus slowing down the over-short transit time. They can be eaten sprouted, whole or ground and can be added whole to a variety of vegetable or fruit dishes. If you grind them first, be sure to eat them soon afterwards, otherwise the oils the seeds contain will be oxidised.

Pectin (unmodified) is found in many fruits, including citrus fruits. It is what is used to make jam set, and is found mostly in the pips and the pith of citrus fruits. It is estimated that a diet that contains about 500gms of vegetables and fruit would provide approximately 5gms of pectin, but this will vary somewhat with the nature of the fruits and vegetables chosen.

Pectin is a large, complex carbohydrate molecule made up of galactose and uronic acid molecules joined together by bonds that are not broken down within your digestive tract. As such it is not absorbed into your bloodstream but operates as a non-digestible carbohydrate, or soluble fibre, for short. In this mode it helps to prevent constipation. It also combines with a number of compounds within the gut including many toxins, and it reduces the (re)absorption of cholesterol from the colon and so helps to lower the blood cholesterol level[349]. Pectin has been shown to slow the rate of development of prostate cancer[350], to be useful in the treatment of melanomas, and to reduce the risk of metastasis[351, 352].

It is thought that modified citrus pectin (MCP) may reduce the ability of travelling cancer cells to bind together or to attach to distant tissues. MCP is available in health food stores, or from supplement suppliers as a fine powder. This can be added to many different foods, from Budwig mixes, to salad dressing, from smoothies to a variety of desserts.

Pure **slippery elm powder** (with no added sugar, milk powder, flour or other additives) is helpful if you have any irritation or damage to the digestive tract, including ulcers, Crohn's disease or irritable bowel syndrome. It combines with water and, in effect, covers the damaged area, putting an internal bandage over it. It is a mild aperient and thus very gently helps to reduce the risk of constipation.

Whey protein isolate should not be confused with whey powder which contains a large amount of milk sugar. Whey protein isolate is a valuable and inexpensive protein source. It is free from casein (the milk protein that causes concern) and lactose (milk sugar). It can be blended with Budwig mixes, or added to salad dressings, sauces and other foods.

There are several **safe sugar alternatives** and most of them are generally available from health food shops. FOS or fructo-oligosaccharide is a slightly sweet powder. Its main use is as a prebiotic. It helps re-establish any probiotics. It can be added to anything where sweetness is appropriate. Use up to one teaspoonful a day.

Mannose is a safe sugar in that it is not converted into glucose in the bloodstream, and does not feed cancer cells. It helps to prevent urinary tract infections and is one of the active ingredients in cranberries. Add up to three teaspoonfuls a day where sweetness is appropriate.

Xylitol tastes just like sugar and can be used instead of sugar. It fights oral bacteria and improves calcium absorption. It is a five-carbon sugar alcohol and is not metabolised to glucose (a six-carbon sugar) and so does not raise the blood glucose level or feed cancer cells. Some of it is metabolised to ribose, needed for DNA and RNA synthesis. Very occasionally and at high intakes it may cause mild diarrhoea.

Ribose is another five-carbon safe sugar. It is a component of RNA and of the high energy compound ATP. A small amount helps to balance the intake of xylitol.

CHAPTER 26

TOXINS, DETOXING AND YOUR LIVER

It is commonplace to assert that cancer is caused by carcinogens and, by definition, a carcinogen is anything that causes cancer, at least in some people some of the time. But that simply takes us round in a circle. In fact we can think of a carcinogen as any substance or energy field that triggers or leads eventually, over time, to any of the metabolic errors and failures of Phase One of the Cancer Process that in turn lead to some or all of the above failures that constitute Phase Two of the Cancer Process and directly precipitate one or more tumours.

When viewed from a CAM perspective, cancer, like any health problem, has at least two components: the health and resources of the individual, including their genetic make-up, versus the external insult. For instance, carcinogens can damage your cells, a deficiency of antioxidants and other essential nutrients can weaken your immune system. Your body might be able to withstand either of these two problems on their own. But when you are both exposed to carcinogens and deficient in essential nutrients that you need to avoid damage to mitochondrial function, the effect is very much worse and your chance of developing cancer is greatly increased.

There are many thousands of carcinogens. All of them can be considered to be toxins, though not all toxins are necessarily or directly carcinogens. This is one of the reasons that you will, or should, find that any cancer recovery programme, certainly any CAM one, places a huge emphasis on a detox programme as an integral and essential part of the total programme. It is unfortunate that the MDS system almost never includes any such suggestion.

It is impossible to live in the twenty first century without being exposed to toxins. If you live in the Western world the problem is worse than if you live in some other parts of the world. If you live in an urban setting, especially in a large and busy city, the problem is generally, though not always, worse than if you live in a rural setting.

If you have any type of health problem you will almost certainly have toxins in your body. Some may have caused the problem, either directly or indirectly. Others will have been produced as your system tries to fight the problem. Certainly, if you have any type of cancer you have toxins in your body. Cancer itself generates toxic compounds. If you have had surgery, chemotherapy or radiation you will have more toxins to deal with.

Whole books have been written on the nature of the toxins in our environment and I recommend that you read up on this topic. You will find references in Appendices 4 and 5. Once you know which are the worst ones, which ones are already in your tissues, and where they come from, you can take steps to minimise your exposure to or your intake of them.

In *'Vital Signs for Cancer'* I considered the subject of toxins in detail. I indicated a number of tests that you can do to determine what toxins you carry in your body. You can do tests for some or most of the various types of toxins. Some of the tests are direct. Others are indirect, and detect the toxins by the consequences of their presence. The more tests you do to pin-point the problems the more effective your detox programme will be. Alternatively, you can simply start on some serious detox programmes, in which case, the more detox methods you incorporate into what you do the better are your chances of a positive outcome. Some methods are discussed in Chapter 32.

You do not have to be the passive victim of the toxins. Do what you can to minimise your exposure. You can do this in a general way. You can also focus your efforts if you have done the tests and identified some of the toxins that are in your tissues. At the same time you should improve your defences. A lack of essential nutrients, such as antioxidants, can increase your vulnerability to toxins and even lead to the creation of more toxins, such as the oxygen free radicals mentioned above [Chapter 7].

There are many categories of toxins or ways of allowing toxins to be present and do harm. The list is extensive, but they include:

(1) substances that are specifically toxic;
(2) substances that are specifically mutagenic;

(3) substances that are specifically carcinogenic;

(4) substances that you need but that can be harmful in excess or in the wrong place, such as oestrogen;

(5) nutrient deficiencies that lead to the failure of protection from toxins;

(6) nutrient deficiencies that allow the creation and continuance of toxins within the body, such as LDL (bad) cholesterol;

(7) a failure of the body's detox system, such as:

   i)   poor cellular clearance of waste products;

   ii)   poor (cellular) matrix clearance of toxins;

   iii) poor lymphatic drainage;

   iv)   poor liver detox function to eliminate toxins;

   v)   poor kidney function;

   vi)   constipation and poor colon clearance;

   vii) dry skin and lack of sweating;

   viii) poor lung function and clearance;

   ix)   A detoxing process, such as hydroxylation which makes a substance more water soluble so it can be carried to the liver, but that actually converts a mild toxin into a more dangerous toxin. This constitutes an excess of Phase 1 detox over Phase 2 detox within the liver [353].

(8) Stress. There are many types of stress. They all weaken your immune and adrenal systems and lead to both an increased need for essential nutrients and the creation and output of toxic compounds.

   i)   Even good stress (eustress), derived from pleasant and exciting stressors can put a strain on the body. Excitement can lead to fatigue, headaches or even increased blood pressure and heart attacks;

   ii)   bad stress (distress) can do considerably more damage;

   iii) prolonged stress, the type where you think you are coping whereas in fact you are using up your capital resources can fool you into thinking you can continue to cope indefinitely;

   iv)   overload occurs when you have to do more than is within your capacity and when excessive demands are being made on your time and energy;

   v)   toxic stress, the type where you feel helpless and hopeless about a situation you cannot change is arguably the worst and most damaging type of stress.

Other toxic states may be self-inflicted, you may even be poisoning yourself. This can be done simply by failing to clean your teeth thoroughly and regularly. Poor teeth hygiene in general and the presence of root canals in particular are serious Predisposing Factors. A recent paper has underscored the dangers or poor oral hygiene to your heart[354] as well as to the risk of developing cancer and other diseases. It was found that in a study of 11,869 men and women, those who never or rarely brushed their teeth, had raised C-reactive protein (CRP) and a significantly increased risk of cardiovascular disease.

One of the serious and almost ubiquitous group of toxins you will probably have to deal with is the mould or fungi group. The blame is commonly placed on *candida albicans* although the true diagnosis could more accurately be called a general state of gut dysbiosis (or wrong organisms) as a wide range of mould and fungi species could be involved. If you didn't have an overgrowth of these moulds or fungi before you developed cancer you have probably developed one since. That is the clinical experience of most practitioners who work in this field. If you have had surgery you will have been given a large quantity of antibiotics and this increases the probability that you will develop the problem. Cancer itself creates an environment in which fungi thrives. You should consider going on an anti-fungal programme.

Heat

Hot baths and far infra red (FIR) saunas are beneficial and can be had at home. Cancer cells are vulnerable to heat. Applied hyperthermia is even more powerful. Whole body hyperthermia or local hyperthermia, both of which would be done in a clinical setting, not only damage cancer cells but help to mobilise toxins and encourage their loss in sweat.

CHAPTER 27

DEALING WITH OTHER PREDISPOSING FACTORS

You cannot regain your health by focusing totally on the tumour and on 'having cancer', which for most people means 'having a tumour'. Cancer is a whole body problem and so it is the whole body that merits your attention. It is a process that starts out with changes to a single cell and progresses, possibly over a period of years, until a detectable tumour is identified. Do not be content to accept minor problems as a part of life, or a part of the ageing process. Every fault or health issue in your body, no matter how small should be investigated and corrected. They can all have unexpected knock-on effects or be indicators of other, and deeper, symptomless problems.

In brief:

• Your diet and toxins have already been considered.

• Check for nutrient deficiencies and make good any that are detected, either by direct analysis, or by the effects of their deficiency such as indicated by the ONE test[6]. It is impossible to get all the nutrients you need from the modern diet, no matter how good, so at the very least take a basic all-purpose supplement.

• Consider having a stool analysis done to determine how well your digestive system is functioning. Three bowel motions a day is the optimum if you want to avoid auto-intoxication. Make good or correct any errors that are found.

• Check your blood glucose level, for both hypoglycaemia and diabetes, either actual or incipient. The number of people with hypoglycaemia, insulin resistance and other blood glucose management problems is growing at an escalating rate. Any problem that leads to even temporarily raised blood glucose levels runs the risk of stimulating cancer or feeding cancer cells.

---

[6] Offered by Genova Diagnostics, see Appendix.

- Check out the status of your adrenal glands and manage your stress levels. You may be able to reduce the stressors, you may not, but you can certainly change your attitude to them. Stress is almost certainly one of the major problems and one of the largest triggers for the start of Phase Two of the Cancer Process.

- Test the levels of the two major forms of oestrogen, oestrogen-2 and oestrogen-16 and make sure that your ratio is correct. An oestrogen imbalance is behind a large number of the oestrogen-related cancers. If your ratio is not correct, take the appropriate action. The test report will usually provide guidelines as to how to do this and your practitioner can help you.

- Check your thyroid function with the simple underarm temperature test you can do at home. A sluggish metabolism will not help you when you need to martial all your defences to eliminate cancer cells and restore your health.

- Check out your immune system; your CAM therapist will be able to help you with this. If you 'never get a temperature' even when you have the flu, this is not a good sign and suggests that you need to stimulate your immune system into better activity.

- Neurotransmitters are the important messenger molecules, coming mainly from your brain, that 'instruct' your cells how to behave. A simple urine test can tell you about yours, and any imbalances should be corrected[7].

- Check for signs of inflammation, for example by measuring CRP in your blood. Inflammation is a ready trigger for cancer, predisposing you to it if or when other insults are added.

- Correct any other health problems. The fact that they may not be mentioned specifically here does not mean they are unimportant in relation to cancer. Keep in mind that cancer is a whole body problem and all errors merit attention.

- Arthritis, for instance, suggests an acid system and the need to alkalise it; cancer thrives in an acid system and general health improves when your system is alkaline. Inflammation, as in inflamed joints, is a contributing factor.

- Skin problems may suggest digestive disorders, toxins or hormone imbalances; all of these can be part of Phase One.

---

[7] Offered by Neuro-Lab in the UK and Neuro Science in the US (by post).

- Migraines, headaches, eczema, asthma, food cravings etc., suggest allergies and food sensitivities. These should be detected and then avoided.

- The existence of allergic reactions suggests that your immune system is over-stressed; this will leave it less able to deal with the challenges faced when you are stressed and subjected to pathogens that may in turn be predisposing factors to Phase One of the Cancer Process, or carcinogens that can trigger Phase Two.

- Fatigue suggests nutrient deficiencies and a variety of other problems. If you do not have the energy you want you should determine why, and then make the appropriate corrections. The chances are your cells do not have sufficient energy either and this could indicate mitochondrial malfunction, a Predisposing Factor.

- Herpes, warts and verrucas all indicate viral problems, another Predisposing Factor.

The list is almost endless. It pays to be vigilant and to right any wrongs that you recognise.

CHAPTER 28

OXYGENATION

Since, according to Otto Warburg, and others since his time, lack of oxygen is a primary cause of cancer, an important step in your recovery programme should be to do all you can to increase both the supply of oxygen to your cells and your cellular uptake of oxygen. This latter is not always easy, along the lines of taking a horse to water but not being able to make it drink – if it is not so inclined.

There are several ways you can contribute to a positive outcome in this regard, and you would be well advised to incorporate all of them. They can generally be divided into three groups:

(1) those that increase the level of oxygen in your blood;
(2) those that facilitate the entry of oxygen across the cell membranes;
(3) those that facilitate the use of oxygen within the mitochondria and thus the utilisation of oxygen.

The first group includes exercise, deep breathing, oxygen and other nutritional supplements.

Exercise

Even a small amount of daily exercise can make a large and significant difference to your health. If your current state of health permits it then aim to do half an hour of brisk walking each day, as fast as you can comfortably manage. Alternatively, you may to choose to swim, bicycle or exercise on a rebounder. If you are relatively immobile then at least practice doing exercises with the muscles you can use.

Breathing

Healthy deep breathing should be even easier to do than exercise. Stop reading now, and monitor your breathing. Are you taking in only small shallow breaths? Or does each breath take in a sufficient volume of air that your chest walls and diaphragm have to move to accommodate it. If the latter movement does not occur then you should aim to achieve this on a regular and automatic basis. After all, without taking in sufficient air you will not deliver sufficient oxygen to all your cells. Simply increasing the availability of oxygen will not necessarily ensure its uptake by the cells, but it is a first step and an essential prerequisite.

Oxygen supplements

Oxygen supplements are available from suppliers such as health food stores. They generally come in liquid form. While they may seem like a good idea, keep in mind that getting oxygen into your blood is only a first step, the vital one is getting it into the mitochondria, and that needs further action. Some people claim that the same is true of various hyperbaric oxygen procedures[8], that you cannot simply force the oxygen into your cells, even under pressure. On the other hand, people have reported good results from the careful use of hyperbaric oxygen chambers, or from breathing in oxygen enriched air while exercising.

Essential nutrients

For oxygen to be carried through your blood you need to have sufficient haemoglobin and a lack of haemoglobin can cause anaemia. There are many different types of anaemia, several of them due to a lack of essential nutrients. The most obvious one is iron, the mineral atom at the core of the haemoglobin molecule. Anaemia is often associated with cancer[355], however, and if you are concerned about cancer you should only take iron supplements if you are certain you are deficient in it. An excess of iron can feed cancer cells[356, 357]. Other nutrients are also required to prevent anaemia, including vitamin E, several of the B group vitamins and vitamin C. This is one of the many reasons why nutrient deficiencies constitute one of the Predisposing Factors to cancer.

---

[8] Hyperbaric oxygen medicine is the medical use of oxygen administered in a compression chamber at above atmospheric pressure, leading to increased level of oxygen in tissues and organs.

The second group, getting the oxygen into the cells, includes the use of flaxseed oil as described by Dr. Budwig, and taking MSM as a supplement.

Flaxseed oil
For more on the use and benefit of flaxseed oil see Chapter 17 and Chapter 29 on the Budwig Protocol. Dr. Budwig recommended taking at least a tablespoon of flaxseed oil a day, preferably combined with the sulphur in the amino acids cysteine, cystine and methionine found in many protein-rich foods. She recommended yoghurt or quark. The rationale for using this is the expectation, based on her experience, that it improves the health of the cellular membranes, improves their communication capacity and their oxygen-uptake. For people who have had cancer or are endeavouring to recover from cancer she has recommended up to 90ml of the oil be consumed daily.

MSM, or methyl sulphonyl methane, releases oxygen when metabolised within the cells; it releases two oxygen atoms for each molecule of MSM. It is also alkalising. MSM is often recommended for people with arthritis, to help the connective tissues. It is also thought to help reduce the incidence of metastasis[358].

Zeolites, formed from volcanic rocks immersed in water for a very long time, can absorb and release large amounts of oxygen[359]. They have been recommended for a number of medical uses[360] including the delivering of oxygen into the cells.

The third group includes trace minerals and vitamins that improve the utilisation of oxygen within the cells.

Trace nutrients
You already know that several trace nutrients are needed as coenzymes, both for the enzymes required for the Krebs Cycle and for oxidative phosphorylation. As a reminder, these include, but are not limited to, vitamins B1, B2, B3, B5, lipoic acid and biotin, together with trace minerals such as copper, iron, magnesium, manganese and zinc. I say 'not limited to' because on a regular basis we continue to recognise the increasing roles of these and other trace nutrients in many different

cellular reactions, and it is unlikely that we yet know all the trace nutrients that are required for optimum cellular health.

Lipoic acid is one of the necessary cofactors of the Pivotal Step that enables the acetyl groups from glucose to enter the mitochondria and start on the aerobic phase of energy release from foods.

Coenzyme Q10, or CoQ10, is needed in the mitochondria for the respiratory chain. You will recall that this is the sequence of reactions by which high energy compounds derived from the breakdown of glucose release their energy in ever smaller quanta of energy until this energy can be readily handled and managed. This amount of energy is just sufficient to convert low energy ADP into high energy ATP which, in turn, can then be transported to any reactions where energy is needed. This conversion utilises oxygen to convert the hydrogen in foods to water. Without CoQ10 the mitochondria, and hence the cell, cannot utilise its oxygen and so, according to Warburg, the cell turns cancerous.

CHAPTER 29

THE BUDWIG PROTOCOL

We discussed earlier [Chapter 17] the benefits that Dr. Budwig ascribed to a high intake of flaxseed oil in combination with the protein from quark or similar dairy product. So the key part of the Budwig diet is the use of top quality organic flaxseed oil combined thoroughly with organic cottage cheese, yoghurt, quark or buttermilk derived from goats, sheep or buffalo, preferably raw and unpasteurised. It is essential that these ingredients are organic and free from chemical additives.

The aim is to ensure that you have a sufficient quantity of the omega-3 fatty acids to balance the omega-6 fatty acids you will be getting from the rest of your diet, from the nuts, seeds, avocados and olive oil, if you use it. You can determine your own levels of omega-3 and omega-6 fatty acids, and indeed of a range of other fatty acids, by a simple analysis of your red blood cells. Many laboratories offer this test.

For good results in relation to prevention, the whole of Dr. Budwig's diet can be followed unless you are already on a more strict regime. If you already have cancer a stricter version of her diet is recommended and is described below. Remember to drink sauerkraut juice or take d-lactic acid daily.

Flaxseed oil is unstable and easily oxidised so it is important that you buy the oil in small amounts and use it up within a few days. Bottles should be stored in the refrigerator until they are opened. Once opened they should be stored in the deep freeze between uses. Even when in glass bottles it can be stored in the deep freeze. The melting point of flaxseed oil is so low that it will melt within minutes at room temperature and be ready to use. If you are in a hurry, put the bottle of oil into some cold or lukewarm water; the oil will melt within a minute, there is no need to heat it by using hot water, and in fact this is undesirable and could increase oxidation. Once you have used the amount you want, put the rest back in the deep freeze.

You can help to preserve some of the oil by making it into the Budwig mix described below. This, once made, should be kept refrigerated and should be eaten as soon as possible, certainly within the day.

There are two major components to the Budwig regime. There are the Budwig mixes that involve flaxseed oil and ground flaxseeds, and there are the other foods that make up the rest of the diet. A full description and discussion of her regime can be found in her books that you will find detailed in Appendix 4 and via the website in Appendix 3, both at the end of this book.

There are several specific products for which Dr. Budwig provides recipes:

The Core Budwig Mix

The basic Budwig mix is flaxseed oil combined with cottage cheese or other soft dairy products. Dr. Budwig suggests that all healthy people wishing to prevent cancer should eat one tablespoon (15ml) of the oil a day. Someone with cancer should consume up to six tablespoons a day (90ml), eight tablespoons (120ml) if they are very unwell. The oil should be combined with the quark, cottage cheese or natural yoghurt. The ingredients must be thoroughly mixed together before they are eaten; use a blender or an electrical blending 'wand' and blend for 60 seconds. Then allow the mixture to stand for ten minutes before eating it. This enables important reactions to take place between the fatty acids in the oil and the sulphur of the amino acids in the protein source.

If you are incorporating whey protein isolate, add this after the strong blending and mix in gently, preferably with a fork so as not to denature the whey proteins. This is because some of the valuable ingredients in this protein are enzymes and their shape is an important aspect of the way they work, so they should not be damaged by vigorous mixing.

You can increase the proportion of flaxseed oil if that is appropriate, i.e. if the taste is acceptable, or if you are making a modified oil-and-vinegar dressing with it where more oil is appropriate. The proportions are not critical and vary somewhat in her writings. The flaxseed oil should be a high lignin oil, stored in a black or brown glass bottle and under an inert gas.

If you are concerned about the use of dairy products you can also add other protein powders, such as hemp protein powder or pea protein powder instead of using dairy products. If you use these then you should add a protein source rich in cysteine, such as CysteinePeP from Allergy Research Group. Although this is derived from whey protein it is very rich in cysteine and so you need less of it. Sesame seeds are rich in the sulphur amino acids and so, if it is appropriate, such as in a salad dressing, you could use tahini as one of the ingredients.

Flaxseeds, ground, may be used in the mixtures instead of the oil, but in that case you will need three times as much seeds as the amount of oil you would otherwise use. The seeds should be ground in a coffee grinder and eaten within fifteen minutes of grinding. In this way you minimise the amount of oxidation that can occur.

The flaxseeds contain a large amount of soluble fibre, so blending them (either whole or ground) with liquid tends to produce firm jellies.

Linomel

This is made by combining ground flaxseed with a small amount of honey. You can also, if you wish, add some whey protein powder to this mix. If you are a vegetarian this is useful way of increasing the protein content of your diet. If you wish to omit honey (if you are avoiding all sugars) you can replace this with xylitol, FOS, ribose or mannose, all safe forms of sugar. This mixture can be sprinkled on a variety of dishes where a slightly sweet taste is appropriate, such as berries and the basic Budwig mix that you might have for breakfast or a dessert.

Oleolox-fat

Butter and margarine or similar spreads are excluded on this regime. Oleolox is used instead and can be spread on vegetables. It is delicious and is made as follows:

Ingredients:

250gms of coconut oil, 1 onion, 10-20 cloves garlic, 125ml flaxseed oil.

Method:
Chill the flaxseed oil in the deep freeze in a wide-necked container. Finely chop the onion and cook it in the coconut oil, gently, until transparent. Add the crushed and finely chopped garlic cloves and cook for no more than 3 minutes. Strain off the coconut oil and, when cool, blend it into the flaxseed oil, mixing well. Keep refrigerated. Do not use this for cooking, flaxseed oil should not be heated. The onions and garlic provide the necessary sulphur compounds. Add freshly ground pepper if desired (also contains sulphur).

Budwig recipes based on the oil/dairy combination

Budwig Cream

100gms yoghurt, 3 tablespoons flaxseed oil, 1 teaspoon xylitol or to taste.

Blend the yoghurt and oil together thoroughly for 60 seconds. Add the xylitol and blend until smooth.

Option: Add whey protein isolate.

Budwig Mayonnaise

2-4 tablespoons flaxseed oil, 4 tablespoons yoghurt, 2 tablespoons fresh lemon juice, plus mustard, herbs and seasoning to taste.

Blend the oil and yoghurt together thoroughly. Add the other ingredients and mix well. This can be sweetened slightly with a teaspoon of xylitol.

Budwig Spread

2 tablespoons flaxseed oil, 8 tablespoons low fat cottage cheese, herbs, spices, mustard, Liquid Aminos, or other flavourings, including Brocco-guard.

Combine the oil and cottage cheese thoroughly for 60 seconds. Mix in generous amounts of the herbs and spices.

Serve this with a salad or cooked vegetable dishes. Spread it on linseed crackers. Use it as a dip, using vegetable sticks as the dippers.

Nuts and Seed Butters
(These are not part of Dr. Budwig's original regime but can fit within it.)

A variation to the mayonnaise above can be made by adding a small amount of dark (unhulled) raw tahini or brazil nut butter instead of a small proportion of the yoghurt. They both contain the sulphur amino acids. You can also add ground sesame meal, however it is unlikely that you will accomplish the appropriate reaction between the sulphur amino acids and the fatty acids, and this is why I suggest using tahini, where the seeds are already very finely ground.

If you have a vegetable juicer that will allow you to make your own nut butters you can combine flaxseed oil with the nut butters you can make yourself from brazil nuts, almonds, macadamias, walnuts or pecans. This will be relatively runny (depending on the amount of oil you add) and can be made into a pleasant and savoury sauce for serving with steamed vegetables by the addition of Braggs Liquid Aminos. This latter is a liquid that tastes somewhat similar to soy sauce but is not made of soy and is not fermented so does not exacerbate any possible problems with *candidiasis* or other fungal problems.

The Budwig Daily Diet - if you have chosen to follow the full protocol

The original Budwig diet is excellent for health maintenance and for prevention. However, more recent research suggests that including fruits, fruit juices and grains can increase your blood glucose level to an unacceptably high level if you have cancer. This could be a mistake, certainly at the beginning of any recovery programme and at least until you are fully in remission. The following is a variation on the Budwig diet and takes these considerations into account.

First thing in the morning:

A glass of sauerkraut juice or acidophilus milk. This may be an acquired taste, but it is worth persevering. If you are not used to it, start with just a small amount. Alternatively, take 30 drops of d-lactic acid three times a day [Chapters 11 and 31].

Breakfast:

Muesli

Combine 50gms yoghurt and 15ml flaxseed oil thoroughly and use as a cream.

Place 2 tablespoons Linomel in a bowl. Cover with 250gms fresh berries, or fresh fruit in season (but preferably berries).

Pour the Budwig cream over this. Add chopped nuts for decoration and texture.

Morning snack:

Humus made with olive, hemp or flaxseed oil, in combination with pureed sprouted chickpeas.

Vegetable pieces such as slices of carrot, sticks of celery or segments of tomato.

500ml of freshly made vegetable juice based on green leaves, ginger, carrot and celery with other additions to taste. Drink slowly, throughout the morning.

Lunch:

A large raw vegetable salad. Dress this with Budwig mayonnaise.

Lightly steamed vegetables, using mainly above ground vegetables. When they cool, a small amount of Oleolox can be dotted over them for flavour.

Dessert: Fresh berries with Budwig cream or spread. Or blend frozen berries with Budwig cream, ice cubes and xylitol to make Budwig ice-cream.

Afternoon snack:

1-2 tablespoons of Linomel.

500ml fresh vegetable juice (as above).

A glass of champagne is permitted if you are very unwell. This has a serious purpose. It is used to improve the absorption of the flaxseed oil. It is NOT to be included if you are sufficiently healthy to be able to absorb and digest meals well.

Evening meal (6.00 pm):

This should be light, such as a raw vegetable salad or other 'raw' food meal.

In general: Include nuts, especially brazil nuts, almonds, macadamias and walnuts, both as snacks and with meals. Have several cups of herbal teas in the day, especially green tea.

There is a practical problem with the vegetable juices if you are making them for only one person. Ideally you should drink about a litre a day. Juices should be drunk within fifteen minutes of making them so that there is minimum loss of nutrients due to breakdown or oxidation. Yet they should be taken in small amounts, over several hours, so as not to raise your blood glucose level. Clearly there is a contradiction in this set of instructions, unless you are to be permanently in the kitchen, making yet one more 100 ml glass of juice, every hour. One way round this is to freeze some of the juice until you are ready to drink it.

When starting on this diet the following regime should be followed for the first day

Have no nourishment on this day other than 250ml (8.5oz) of flaxseed oil with honey, plus freshly squeezed fruit juices (no sugar added!). If you are very ill champagne may be added on this first day in place of the juice and is taken with the flaxseed oil and honey. Champagne is easily absorbable and has a serious purpose here.

Then follow the instructions above.

Dr. Budwig reported great improvement in the majority of people she treated with her diet. She also reported what she considered to be miraculous improvement in the very ill and even people with terminal cancer. At the very least, many of them reported decreased pain and improved quality of life. She also reported many terminally ill patients whose health improved enormously on this diet.

Dr. Budwig suggests that you will have to remain on this diet for at least 5 years (and preferably your entire life). She stated that in a few years the tumours often disappeared. She also found that people who broke the rules of this diet, (i.e. who went back to eating preserved meats, high temperature heated fats, chips and other acrylamide-rich foods, sweets and other forbidden foods) sometimes grew rapidly worse and often couldn't be saved after they had gone off the regimen and then returned to it in an attempt to repeat the benefits.

If you follow this stricter version of Dr. Budwig's at the start, once you are in full remission (as shown by the tests indicated here) you may be able to add in more variety, such as some fruits and small amounts of whole grain products.

In 1967, Dr. Budwig broadcast the following sentence during an interview over the South German Radio Network, describing her incoming patients with failed operations and x-ray therapy: *"Even in cases when surgery, radiation and chemotherapy failed, it is still possible to restore health in a few months at most. I would truly say 90% of the time."*

There has, inevitably, been debate as to how much can be achieved by this regime alone. However, it is clearly the basis for a good diet and makes a sensible foundation to the rest of your prevention or recovery protocol.

For further information on the diet see Appendices 3 and 4 for the website and books.

In view of what we have learnt in the decades since she published her diet details, and especially in the most recent decade, it is worth considering and commenting on the changes made here, to her original diet.

Dr. Budwig was renowned in her field. However, research and current knowledge has moved on.

(a) Her diet, which includes generous amounts of fruits and whole grains, is an excellent one to follow for people interested in prevention of serious degenerative diseases.

(b) For use in active cancer, her diet is probably too rich in fruits and grains to achieve optimal results.

(c) William Kelley initially included generous amounts of fruit in his diet, but in later years he came to believe that this might have been a mistake and that fruits should be largely omitted because of their high sugar content. The fruits that are acceptable are raspberries, blueberries, strawberries and other more exotic berries such as acai, amla and pomegranate, when available. These are relatively low in sugar but high in phytonutrients. Eating a minimum of 250gms of raspberries, rich in ellagic acid, each day can be helpful.

For completeness it is worth emphasising the following:

(d) Cancer cells love sugar. They are at least six times as efficient at taking glucose out of your bloodstream than are your healthy cells (and possibly a lot more than). Sugar feeds cancer.

The carbohydrates in vegetables are broken down slowly over time in the digestive tract because of their high fibre content. They then release glucose (from the starches they contain) only slowly into your bloodstream, over an extended period of time. Vegetable juices should be drunk 'little and often' to avoid this surge in blood glucose level and should consist mainly of above ground vegetables (preferably green or dark red/orange). Vegetables also contain very high levels of beneficial phytonutrients which constitute a worthwhile trade-off against the slow-release glucose from the vegetable starches.

Grains generally release their glucose more rapidly than vegetables, and they contain only modest to negligible levels of phytonutrients (depending on their level of processing). This is especially true of refined grains such as white flour, pastas and rice, which must be avoided altogether, but also partially true of whole unrefined grains.

Thus. the aim is to keep a steady BSL and to alkalise the body. Hence the diet should:

(a) be 75% vegetables (as said above);

(b) be rich in phytonutrients; and

(c) consist of 75% raw food (including the vegetable juices);

(d) be chosen from the foods indicated for your Metabolic Type;

(e) include the Budwig mixes (the cream, mayonnaise and spread, Linomel and Oleolox-fat).

If you feel the above (a) to (d) is too big a change to make initially then follow the full Budwig diet (see her books), including the mixes. Although this may not lead to such positive results the diet is almost certainly a significant improvement on your current diet and as such will be beneficial. You should still choose the positive foods for your Metabolic Type, provided they are also included in this programme.

CHAPTER 30

CORRECTING YOUR ACID ALKALINE BALANCE (pH)

You have learnt that cancer cells thrive in an acid environment and struggle to survive in neutral to alkaline environments. Most people, on the typical Western diet tend to be too acidic. So part of your recovery protocol should be to increase your cellular pH as indicated by your salivary pH first thing in the morning.

The common diet of today leaves a highly acid residue in your body. The foods that contribute to this are proteins, starches and sugars plus animal fats and refined and processed vegetable oils, soft drinks and alcohol, almost everything, in fact, except fresh vegetables and fruits. In addition, most toxins are acidic or leave an acidic residue and, as we have seen, cancer cells produce l-lactic acid, making your system even more acidic. Thus, you are far more likely to be too acidic than either neutral or too alkaline.

It is important that your bloodstream maintains a neutral pH and is neither too acid nor too alkaline. To ensure that this balance is maintained a variety of paired reactions, called buffer systems, are active. As a result of these, if your blood becomes too acidic, acids are pushed out of your blood and into your cells, making them and your organs, in turn, more acidic.

So many researchers have stated that relatively little benefit will accrue from your supplements and remedies until you have increased your pH that this is now a commonplace. This does not mean you should not use supplements, or try to make other positive changes, right from the start. It does mean that you should make increasing your pH to be a top priority. This process can take many weeks or months, particularly if you already have cancer and have to deal with the cancer-produced lactic acid as well as toxins and acid-residue foods, often in the form of carbonic acid, in your body.

The need to increase your pH is one of the reasons that it is suggested that 75% of your diet should be vegetables and (a few) fruits. The more fresh vegetables, green juices and green powders you consume the better.

It may seem contradictory to suggest an acid for the purpose of increasing alkalinity, but betaine hydrochloride is an exception. Hydrochloric acid is the essential acid produced in your stomach. It helps to ensure the complete breakdown of protein in your stomach. Betaine is the delivery system for this acid in supplement form. You produce less and less stomach acid with age and this can lead to a variety of health problems. Betaine hydrochloride has been found to work well when potassium is also given. Since this acid improves digestion it reduces the amount of pancreatic enzymes needed for protein digestion and this can release these enzymes for systemic activity against cancer cells [Chapter16].

Coral calcium is, as the name suggests, produced from coral. Corals are colonies of marine organisms that secrete a calcium rich external 'skeleton'. When the animals within this calcified structure die, their 'skeletal remains' are a rich source of organically derived calcium, magnesium and other minerals. Because of its organic origins the minerals are thought to be much more readily absorbed than many other forms of mineral supplements. Because of the high concentration of alkali minerals, it is also alkalising.

Zeolites, such as Natural Cellular Defence, can also help to alkalise your tissues.

Dr. Fryda takes this concept a major step further, as we will see in the next chapter.

CHAPTER 31

LACTIC ACID AND
DR. FRYDA'S PROTOCOL

You will recall that Dr. Fryda [Chapter.11] states that cancer cells produce the harmful form of lactic acid, l-lactic acid and that this is both indicative of cancerous activity and a trigger for the increased mitosis and the growth of more cancer cells. She advocates taking the d-form of lactic acid to neutralise the l-form, and suggests that doing this should be a first step, either before or with anything else you choose to do from the start.

Remember, the d- form and the l-form can be thought of as mirror images of each other. When swallowed and absorbed, the d-form combines with the l-form to make a biologically inactive mixture. Once there is sufficient d-lactic acid to neutralise the l-lactic acid your body can revert to normal metabolism, repair of the adrenal glands can take place, adrenalin output potential can build back up to normal levels, and other therapies can become effective.

Fryda suggests a dose of 30 drops of d-lactic acid three times a day. This, she asserts, will gradually cause your cells to dump their toxic waste into your bloodstream and will eventually bring your venous blood pH down to below pH 6, a result that is normally reached on the 35th day. After a further three days of following this procedure your venous blood, she states, normally returns to the correct pH value of 7.4.

If you follow this plan, you should remember that during these three days, from day 35 to day 38, you may feel ill as a result of the amount of toxic acid that is being washed out of your tissues, into the bloodstream and then metabolised or excreted. Feeling bad on these days should be a cause for rejoicing, as it suggests that this crossover is being achieved. Your various bodily excretions such as urine, faeces and sweat, may have a strong and unpleasant smell. This is a crossover time, when the body is changing from the old, harmful metabolism back to normal, healthy metabolism. She notes that in people of average health, those with allergies, and those with no cancer the crossover time generally starts after 15 days. This protocol is simple and inexpensive. However, although it is something you can do for yourself, it is better to do it under supervision, particularly as it is very easy to fail to recognise the symptoms on days 35 to 38 as those of crossover, even though you are expecting them, for the symptoms themselves change your attitude to what is occurring.

Fryda states that after the crossover time there is likely to be a new burst of health, possibly even leading to a state that leaves you feeling better than you have done for years. Once this state is achieved, and not before, according to Fryda, the other therapies can be fully effective. Also, the tumour is now in an environment where its metabolism is made more difficult.

She has found that it is possible that therapy with d-lactic acid should be continued for months or even years. The necessity for this will depend on the extent to which your stress level can be reduced on the one hand and the suggested lifestyle changes can be implemented on the other. It will depend on the extent to which your adrenal glands and immune function, plus your overall health can be improved and thus an environment maintained in which no further cancer cells can grow.

You can add further to this therapy by putting 100gms of sodium bicarbonate in a hot bath and lying in this for half an hour once a day. This, Fryda suggests, helps to draw the lactic acid out of your body.

Exercise

Fryda also stresses the importance of physical activity. Exercise helps to burn up the excess glycogen that she states is engorging the cells, it also leads to the production of the valuable d-lactic acid. There are many studies that have shown that when exercise is combined with almost any other therapy, the latter becomes more effective [361]. Exercise can reduce your risk of developing cancer [362], it can help to reduce the fatigue associated with cancer[363], and it can boost the activity of your immune system[364], for instance by increasing the activity of your Natural Killer cells[365].

CHAPTER 32

PANCREATIC ENZYMES AND WILLIAM KELLEY'S PROTOCOL

William Kelley based his recovery programmes, for himself and for people who consulted him, on the following:

(1) correct diet, both in general and in relation to your Metabolic Type;

(2) an extensive detoxification programme;

(3) supplements and specific remedies;

(4) body work;

(5) resolving emotional issues and reducing stress;

(6) pancreatic enzymes.

1.   Diet was discussed in Chapter 25.

2.   An overview of detoxing was given in Chapter 26. The following is detoxing the Kelley way:

Detoxing the colon and helping the liver:

Days 1-3

Do the Colon Cleanse with Epsom salts for three consecutive days once a month. This purges the colon. See below.

Days 4-6

Fast for three days on nothing but water and vegetable juices diluted 1:1 with water.

Days 1-30

Do a coffee enema every morning.

Days 1-14

Do a bacteria (probiotic) enema each evening. Simply add half a teaspoon of powdered bifidobacterium (bifido) to a retention enema made using either coffee or green tea. This will be the second enema if you do two in close succession (back-to-back enemas).

Week 3-52

Do a lemon enema twice a week, in the evening, using the juice of one lemon in a litre of water.

Months 2-10

Do coffee enemas morning and evening. Add Bifidobacterium (bifido) powder to a retention enema once or twice a week, more often if you pass wind, at all.

Months 1-3

Do a weekly colonic if available. Once a month do a liver flush.

For the Colon Cleanse, dissolve 1 tablespoonful of Epsom salts in purified water and drink this first thing in the morning. Repeat this twice more at half hour intervals. Make an alkalizing punch by juicing 12 oranges, 6 grapefruit and 6 lemons. These must all be organic, and thoroughly washed. Add water to a total volume of 5 litres. Two hours after the first dose of Epsom salts, start drinking this punch. Drink 500mls every half hour.

There is no need to discard the pith and peel, and besides, they contain even more valuable nutrients than do the juice and pulp. The pith and peel can be dried in a dehydrator and then ground to a fine powder. This can then be added to salad dressings, deserts, Budwig mixes or any other dish in which the citrus flavour (without the acidity) would be appealing. The pith and peel can also be blended with a small amount of the juice and eaten (again, thinking of it as raw marmalade).

You can help to detox via the kidneys by drinking diuretic herbs such as dandelion coffee, drinking hot water with a slice of lemon in it, and making sure that you drink, daily, one litre of water for every 50lbs body weight.

You can eliminate significant amounts of toxins through your skin. This can be done using a Far Infra Red sauna. The most convenient of these looks like a sleeping bag. Whether you shower or bath, use a skin brush and give your body a vigorous rub, all over. This helps to eliminate dead cells and to improve peripheral circulation. The bicarbonate baths already referred to [Chapters 11 and 31] will also help. Twice a week rub your whole body with an olive oil and castor oil mix, then soak in a hot bath for 15 minutes to allow the oil to soak in. Wrap yourself in towels and go to bed to sweat it out for one hour. Take a shower afterwards.

You can also eliminate toxins via your lungs. If your nose is blocked, sniff salt water.

Be sure to practice, and make a habit of, regular deep, abdominal breathing.

Gentle aerobic exercise, up to the level of which you are capable, will be of benefit.

Aim for half an hour of brisk walking each day if you can.

3. Body work should include work, such as chiropractic or osteopathy, which aims at correcting errors of your physical structure, but it should also include aims to release emotional issues.

4. Resolving emotional issues may come out of the body work that you do. However, a course of psychotherapy will almost certainly be helpful. You can also work with books on stress release[366, 367]. See also Book 4 of this series, on emotional issues and their relation to cancer.

5. Pancreatic enzymes are the vital component of Kelley's programme and a component that is often omitted by other practitioners. With regard to these he made the following suggestions:

For cancer prevention he suggested that people take 1.6gms of pancreatic extract with each meal and 0.8gms with snacks. These will help to improve general digestion. More importantly, they will destroy any cancer cells as soon as they form and help to prevent the building of a tumour.

For people who have had cancer, but whose HCG and other test results are all now normal, and who are therefore in full remission, he suggested taking 2.4gms with meals and 1.2gms with snacks. Keep in mind that the absence of a tumour can only be regarded as partial remission if your tests results show that there are still problems at the cellular level. In this case you should continue with your full protocol.

For treating cancer, the usual dose of pancreatic extract is 25 to 45gms a day, spread over six to seven doses and taken an hour away from meals with one dose being taken between 3.00 and 4.00 a.m. if you wake at that time. You should also take 0.8gms with meals. The quality of the pancreatic extract is vitally important and you should select a product that has been specifically prepared for this purpose. Capsules usually contain approximately 400mg each and so the above doses mean taking between 60 and 106 capsules a day. If you use capsules at double the strength you will only need to take half that number but they will be twice the size and you may find them difficult to swallow.

The lower amounts are generally sufficient for Fast Oxidisers and those who are Parasympathetic Dominant. The higher amounts are generally necessary for those who are Slow Oxidisers or Sympathetic Dominant. The former group tend to have more active digestive systems and a greater output of digestive and pancreatic enzymes than the latter group. If your Metabolic Type test showed you to be either a Mixed Oxidiser or a Balanced Dominant type then your amounts could be midway between the above figures.

In fact, the actual amount that you need will depend on many factors, including your Metabolic Type, the extent of your cancer and other individual considerations. However, these figures provide good guidelines. It means taking a very large number of capsules, but most people get used to it and it is important to keep in mind the seriousness of the health problem you are facing if you have cancer.

Kelley found that people got good results if they took the enzymes (or pancreatic extract) for twenty five days a month, during which time the cancer cells are being destroyed, and then stopped for five days, during which time healthy tissues can repair and any accumulated toxins can be released. The five enzyme-free days provide a good opportunity for you to focus particularly strongly on any detox procedures that you may not be doing routinely. This is a good time, for instance, to do your monthly liver flush.

Kelley noted that if you have extensive cancer you may feel ill, progressively, during the twenty five days of taking the enzymes and while cancer cells are being broken down. If this is mild, continue for the full twenty five days. Kelley considered that to be a good sign and an indication that the cancer cells are being destroyed, leading to the toxicity that is causing the symptoms. If the symptoms of tumour lysis become excessive, then stop for five days and allow for both the elimination of the released toxins and the repair of healthy tissue to continue, then resume. Never stop for more than five days as this would give the cancer cells a chance to start rebuilding [Dr. N. Gonzalez, pers. comm.].

Most people feel better during the repair five days but if you feel bad during that time too (with symptoms that will be somewhat different to those you experience when taking the enzymes) then he suggested that that means you need to keep taking the enzymes, and should continue to take them without stopping. After a further fifteen days try to come off them again. However, if you experience these problems you should certainly get professional guidance from someone experienced in this method.

CHAPTER 33

IMMUNE FUNCTION AND DR. ABO'S PROTOCOL

Dr. Abo [Chapter12] defines his four rules for overcoming cancer:

(1) re-evaluate your lifestyle patterns;
(2) overcome your fear of cancer;
(3) don't blindly agree to any treatment that suppresses immunity;
(4) stimulate your PSNS.

In relation to Rule Number 1 it is important that you do what you can to reduce your external stressors. Make what changes you can in the aspects of your life that stress you. Change your job, move house, follow an interest that you have suppressed, clarify your goals, what you really want out of life, and then go for it. If you do have cancer, this is not the time to postpone your goals. Aim for them now. Read LeShan's book[368], already mentioned. In it you will find a host of examples of people who have done just that and achieved positive outcomes. You will also find a significant number of self-tests and searching questions you can use to unearth some of your true desires, concerns, fears, insecurities and more, and ways to determine how you can resolve whatever issues you have in a way that is positive for you and for those you care about. Read my own book on the subject[369], and read as many other books as appeal to you, books that relate to ways you can reduce not only the stress in your life but your inclination to focus on the stressful aspects of any given situation. Above all, make whatever positive changes are indicated by your research and explorations.

Rule Number 2 may seem difficult to follow given the general fear that cancer induces in most people today. However, just as much fear was induced back in the 1820s, and before, by a disease that struck just as unexpectedly and frequently lead to death. It started, for no apparent reason, with symptoms that included burning sensations of the tongue, intermittent constipation and diarrhoea, poorly localised abdominal pain, then loss of appetite followed by weight loss. These symptoms were followed by nerve problems such as numbness and tingling and a generalised loss of co-ordination. 'Ankle drop' came next so that tripping on uneven surfaces or steps was common, with loss of vibratory sense in the legs and loss of positional sense. Accompanying mood changes included depression, irritability, paranoia and delusions, with a progressive fatigue to the point of total exhaustion and finally death.

This was a recognised progression, as feared then as cancer is now. The cause was not known but many possibilities were suggested. All the known chemotherapy of the day was tried, often with devastating consequences, but with only occasional and seemingly random success. Top experts studied the problem to no avail. No matter what the doctors tried, no successful cure was established. For most people the disease was overpowering and the eventual outcome was death. It was a disease bigger and more powerful than the medical profession. The symptoms were known, the cause was unknown and the treatment was horrendous and also unsuccessful. The disease was greatly feared. Sound like cancer today?

Finally some 'quack'[9] came along and started giving his patients chopped up raw liver. Did the doctors laugh? Was the man ridiculed? Of course he was. How could something as simple as eating chopped raw liver be adequate to eliminate all those terrible symptoms? When others started doing the same thing they too were ridiculed and told they were fools. Fortunately, the doctors of the day were not licensed and so those broad-minded doctors that adopted this innovative technique had no licence to lose; they could continue with their chopped raw liver treatment. In time the conservative and critical doctors were forced to recognise that this crazy 'alternative cure' worked. Eventually, the treatment was recognised and even later it was realised that no virus, bacteria or other parasite caused this frightening and often fatal disease, nor was it genetic. Instead,

---

[9] The word 'quack' is used here for its current meaning, as a term of disapprobation or implied ridicule. A couple of centuries ago it was actually a complementary term, applied to doctors who were considered to be at the forefront of their profession and who used mercury or 'quicksilver' in medical treatments, a practice we now know to be highly toxic. It is worth keeping this in mind before praising to-day's doctors who espouse the use of highly toxic chemicals.

it was a nutritional deficiency disease. It was caused by either a deficiency of vitamin B12 in the diet, or by inadequate production of intrinsic factor from the parietal cells lining the person's stomach. Intrinsic factor is needed for the absorption of vitamin B12, and its production generally declines with age, often in parallel with a reduced production of stomach acid, or due to other problems affecting the parietal cells. The disease is now known as pernicious anaemia. It is totally and easily treatable and has lost its threat. Something that feared is now no longer frightening.

A similar scenario could be described for a number of other health problems that were once thought of as both frightening and life-threatening, yet which were eventually solved by relatively simple lifestyle changes. So never underestimate the power of improving your (total) lifestyle in relation to the prevention of, or the recovery from, cancer, and before you ridicule this, saying that cancer is much more complex and dangerous than pernicious anaemia, remember this. It fooled the top doctors of the day, as does cancer now. It was solved by a lifestyle change, as CAM therapists advocate now for cancer. It was more than a simple nutritional deficiency, it was indeed a lack of an essential nutrient, but one with physiological complications as well. CAM therapists of today would say much the same about cancer. It is easy to look back now and consider those doctors, and perhaps people in general, two hundred years ago, to be naive and short on knowledge, compared to what we know today. It will, surely, be just the same for people in general and doctors in particular decades ahead, when they look back on the doctors of today and the way they treat cancer.

It is my belief, and that of many of my colleagues, that within the next few decades we will know so much about the causes of cancer, such as all the Predisposing Factors and all the carcinogenic substances and activities we have recently incorporated into our lifestyle, that it will no longer be feared. At worst, like diabetes, we will have learnt to manage it. At best, we will have learnt how to avoid it and, possibly a more difficult accomplishment, we will have changed our lifestyles in such a way that we can avoid it. Along with this scenario will go a recognition that surgery, chemotherapy and radiation 'treatments' were (seen from this vantage point in the future), totally inappropriate, unnecessary and counterproductive.

In my experience, people with cancer who choose to become involved in their own health care, generally do extensive reading and become self-educated to a greater extent than anyone with any other health problem. As you explore all the possible constructive, helpful and harmless CAM ways of dealing with cancer you may be surprised by the richness of positive options open to you. As a result, you can build an appropriate optimism as to the outcome you seek, and in this way you can reduce your fear and manage your stress. So one vital aspect of any prevention or recovery protocol is to learn as much as you possibly can, and then, most importantly, put what you learn into practice. This is the way to follow Rule Number 2.

In Rule Number 3, Dr. Abo states not only that you should not blindly agree to any treatment that suppresses your immunity, he also adds, *"...if you've already begun such treatment, stop immediately."* This is a serious suggestion and one to which you should give a lot of thought. In the end it is your choice. As we saw back in Chapter 22, there is a lack of proven or guaranteed success in treating solid tumours with chemotherapy. Much the same can be said for surgery and radiation, and all three methods compromise your immune system. However, for many people the risks and the toxic effects of chemotherapy and radiation are minor compared to their conviction that these are the right methods to follow. Such is the power of the mind, as illustrated by the placebo effect, that whatever you are absolutely convinced is the best method for you to follow, probably is[10].

Rule Number 4 involves stimulating your PSNS. This can be done in several ways.

- Eat. Digestion is, after all, one of the main functions of the PSNS. But don't overeat, or eat to get fat. Follow all the rules for a good diet, already given, and eat large amounts of vegetables, preferably raw. The Japanese diet, as followed and endorsed by Dr. Abo for dealing with cancer, has much in common with the dietary suggestions given above. It focuses on a high proportion of vegetables and the incorporation of a range of types of mushrooms

---

[10] This information and these ideas are for educational purposes only. They should not be taken as a suggestion from the author that you stop any medical treatment already prescribed for you.

and seaweeds. He does recommend brown (not white) rice. Although this is high in starch, it is also a source of fibre, trace minerals and B group vitamins and is probably the best, and most alkaline, of all the grains to incorporate. Even so, only small amounts should be included so as not to reduce the intake of vegetables and all the nutrients they contain.

- He recommends organic food, locally grown, and in keeping with your own origins. Eat small amounts of a large number of different types, up to 36 different foods a day. In this way, of course, a wide variety of nutrients is obtained.

- Eat slowly and chew your food thoroughly, up to twenty or thirty times a mouthful. This aids your PSNS.

- Avoid stimulants, such as coffee.

- Stimulate blood flow by doing gentle exercise. If you are not well and exercise is difficult, just do what you can. Even half an hour's gentle walking each day can make a positive difference. Yoga and tai chi are also recommended. While they may not be considered as aerobic exercise they do stimulate the flow of blood and lymph.

- Take long, deep and slow breaths. These stimulate the PSNS. Shallow, short breaths and rapid breathing stimulate the SNS.

- Smile and laugh as much as you can, even if you are pretending, initially, just doing it, even just forcing your mouth into the smile shape, will help your PSNS (and improve your mood and optimism).

- Avoid anti-inflammatory drugs, pain killers, tranquilisers and sleeping pills. According to Dr. Abo these all stimulate the SNS.

- Keep warm. The enzymes of your immune system become increasingly active with increasing body temperature. For many of them, particularly those that operate in acute conditions, the optimal temperature is above that of body heat. Far infra red (FIR) therapy is beneficial, for many reasons. It is partially useful for the heat it produces as cancer does not thrive at raised temperatures, but in addition it stimulates lymphocyte activity. Hot baths, in the range of 39°C to 42°C (102°F to 107°F) stimulate the PSNS. Above that temperature the SNS is stimulated. However, few people can enjoy baths much hotter than 42°C. Hot baths induce a sweat that helps in the elimination of toxins. The sweat induced by an FIR sauna is even more efficient at carrying toxins out of the body.

- Meditate, or practise other relaxing procedures such as the Emotional Freedom Technique (EFT), Autogenic Training or relaxing visualisations. You will be able to find a range of books and tapes to help you with these.
- Do what makes your heart sing. Bring joy into your life. Be creative. This also implies that you are balancing your astral and etheric energies [Chapter19].

Foods that stimulate the PSNS	Neutral foods	Foods that stimulate the SNS
Green vegetables	Brown rice	Salt
Mushrooms		Red meat
Seaweeds		Poultry
Miso, natto and tamari (fermented soy products)		Eggs
Sesame		Greasy foods
Beans		
Whole fish (he suggests these are better than fillets of a larger fish)		
Yoghurt		
Umeboshi plums, pickles (no sugar)		Salt
Vinegar		Coffee

If you are familiar with the macrobiotic diet you will recognise many of these recommendations, although in the suggestions given here there is a much greater emphasis placed on vegetables than on rice. You will also notice that this is essentially similar to the diets suggested above by Dr. Budwig, William Kelley and many others.

Dr. Abo wisely points out that healing achieved in this way generally takes longer than the seemingly quick, though possibly temporary, results that are sometimes achieved by drug medicine, certainly in relation to other health problems, if not always to cancer. This is because CAM methods are working at a much deeper level and are aimed at bringing about a much more fundamental change to your entire being, to your body, emotions and mind, or as some would say, to your body, soul and spirit. Once achieved, however, the result is correspondingly more powerful and long lasting. The extent to which this is achieved will depend on the extent to which you make the appropriate changes.

In the West, CAM therapists recognise and are familiar with 'healing reactions', sometimes referred to as a 'healing crisis'. These symptoms are brought about by tumour lysis, the elimination of toxins, and changes that are occurring within the body. Calling them 'kouten hannou', Dr. Abo describes them as follows:

- fever, mild headache, fatigue and mild cold-like symptoms. These result when your immune system tries to increase the flow of blood and lymph in an attempt to remove toxins and supply needed nutrients to damaged tissues. This requires energy output and so you feel tired;

- inflammation, the symptoms of which are redness (as there is increased blood flow to the area), swelling (due to the increased blood flow) and pain (as the various reactions occur);

- diarrhoea, or altered bowel habits, as the stimulated liver increases the output of both bile and toxins. This liver detox pathway can be encouraged by enemas, by the liver flush described in 'Vital Signs for Cancer', and by the supplements that support improved liver function[370].

While these symptoms indicate general change and improvement, and so should be welcomed, they should only be mild. It is rarely appropriate to make such drastic changes that your body's coping mechanisms are overwhelmed. If, for instance, you mobilise toxins faster than your liver can deal with them and faster than they can be eliminated, either in your urine or stool, you will leave them circulating throughout your body, free and available to cause problems elsewhere. Make sure you are doing all you can to avoid bottlenecks in the elimination process.

CHAPTER 34

SUPPLEMENTS

However good your diet, it is not possible in these days to get all the nutrients you need from it, particularly if you have cancer. Even if you eat only one hundred per cent organically grown food, locally grown, picked fresh and eaten within hours, and almost no-one does this, you will not get sufficient. You will not, for instance, get as much nutrition as our ancestors could have achieved millennia ago. There are many reasons for this. In particular:

- plants grown wild contain more nutrients than plants farmed, year after year, on the same land, which gradually becomes depleted of minerals and other nutrients;
- your needs today, compared to those of your ancient ancestors, are greatly increased. Compared to them, your body has to deal with the toxins and challenges of twentieth century living.

In fact your diet will not be that good, no matter how hard you try:

- even if you have your own plot of land and grow everything yourself, it is unlikely that you eat only fresh home-grown food;
- you will almost certainly eat out from time to time and not all that food will be fresh and organic;
- even if all your food is organic, some of it will have been picked at some distance from where you purchase it, picked before fully ripe, transported and stored;
- even if you eat most of your food raw, some of it will almost certainly be cooked, and so will have lost some of its nutrients by heat destruction;
- even if you mean to eat only organic food, unless you never eat in a restaurant, snack bar or with friends, then at least some of your diet will not be organic.

The list could continue.

An essential part of your recovery is to 'make your heart sing'. While you should eat the best possible diet (most of the time) and avoid eating out unnecessarily, this is no time to shut yourself away from your friends, hermit-like, and feel miserably and totally deprived. A balance is required. Perhaps you can take your meals with you when you go visiting, but in most instances this is not appropriate. So do the best you can, then accept that you will need to compensate with supplements and detox programmes.

As already indicated, the best supplements are those that are 'food-based', meaning that the nutrients in them are derived from foods, food concentrates or a variety of nutrient-dense plants. There are several brands that have at least some food-based supplements. You would be well advised to purchase a multivitamin and multimineral supplement of this variety.

When considering antioxidant-rich foods it is also valuable to asses their antioxidant capacity. This can be measured, and this is done by determining their ORAC, which stands for their oxygen radical absorbance capacity. Oxygen radicals are highly oxidising and the more of them a food or substance can absorb the higher is their antioxidant potential. WHO gives a list of the ORAC value of 100gms of many of the common foods that are antioxidant rich[371]. Other assays determine the trolox equivalent antioxidant capacity (TEAC) or the ferric reducing antioxidant power (FRAP).

Vitamin C supplements, for example, should be derived from acerola berries, amla or Indian gooseberries, camu camu, berries such as blueberry, raspberry and cranberry, fruits such as cherry, rose hips and citrus. Consider the benefits described below and then decide whether you would rather get your vitamin C from a combination of extracts of the active ingredients of these foods, albeit from dried foods or from supplements containing these foods if not available fresh, or from chemically-synthesised ascorbic acid.

Acerola, or *Malpighia emarginat (*Malpighiaceae) is a tropical shrub or small tree whose berries or fruit contain 1677.6mg of vitamin C in 100g of fruit[372], over thirty times the amount found in oranges[373]. It is rich in antioxidants, with the highest TEAC score of eleven domestic fruits[374].

Amla berries, also known as Indian gooseberry, come from *Phyllanthus emblica* (or *Emblica officinalis*) a deciduous tree of the Euphorbiaceae family. The berries are claimed to be rich in vitamin C, a variety of antioxidants[375], including tannins and polyphenols[376], ellagic acid, flavonoids, gallic acid and kaempferol[377].

Whether it is the vitamin C or the other antioxidants they contain, amla berries have been found to be antiviral and antimicrobial[378], to induce apoptosis and to modify gene expression in cells involved in rheumatoid arthritis and osteoporosis[379]. Extracts of the berries, leaves and bark have shown benefits in relation to experimental cancer, inflammation[380], some kidney diseases[381], and diabetes[382]. Human studies have shown cholesterol-lowering effects[383], and improvement in liver function[384].

Camu camu (*Myrcieria dubia*) is a small Brazilian tree, which gives a red or purple fruit something like a cherry and is related to the guava berry. It is up to 3 times richer in vitamin C than Acerola, but more acidic. The red pigments of the skin are thought to be due to anthocyanins. It contains significant amounts of flavonoids, flavonols, flavanols, catechins, gallic acid, ellagic acid and tannins[385]. As a result it is antioxidant, anti-inflammatory and supports the immune system.

Blueberries, in spite of their name, are false berries. They grow in cooler climates than true berries and are hardier. They have an extremely high ORAC value of 6652, are rich sources of vitamins B6, C and K and of manganese and fibre[386], anthocyanins, antioxidants and related phytochemicals thought to help reduce the risk of a variety of diseases including inflammatory disorders[387]. Recall that inflammatory states are a predisposing factor to cancer. They increase apoptosis [388, 389, 390] and have shown benefit in a number of types of cancer including colon[391] and prostate[392].

Raspberries. Raspberries contain many powerful antioxidants (ORAC value 4882), including polyphenols, anthocyanins, quercetin, gallic acid, ellagic acid, cyanidins, pelargonidins, catechins and keampferol. WHO figures show raspberries to be a rich source of vitamin C, manganese (provided it is in the soil) and fibre, and a good source of B1, B2, B3, B5, B6, and folic acid[393]. Their ellagic acid is particularly valuable[394]. This acid is known to inhibit certain carcinogens and protect against chemical damage[395]. It inhibits the cell cycle whereby new cells are formed, and induces apoptosis in a variety of cancer types including cervical[396].

Cranberries are best known for their help if you have cystitis. They have a moderate amount of vitamin C but are strongly antioxidant with an ORAC value of 9584 per 100gms. They are a rich source of quercetin[397], anthocyanidin, flavonoids, cyanidin and peonidin, and the cranberry polyphenols have been the subject of much study in relation to cancer. Like many other berries they have been shown to stimulate apoptosis[398] and inhibit tumour growth lines[399].

Rose hips have a long tradition as a supplement source of vitamin C, containing up to 20mg per gram of dried extract.

Citrus fruits were among the first to be recognised for their vitamin C content. They also contain a number of citrus bioflavonoids, and have an ORAC per 100gms of 1238 (white grapefruit), 1512 (pink grapefruit), 1225 (lemon juice), 823 (lime juice), 1785 (oranges), and 1620 (tangerines). These figures are considerably lower than those found in some of the above fruits.

Clearly these are useful additional components of a food-sourced vitamin C supplement and provide far greater health benefits than simply using chemically-produced ascorbic acid or some other form of synthetic vitamin C.

In a similar way, B complexes or multivitamin supplements can be made from a wide range of dried extracts of vegetables, fruits, sprouted grains, herbs, and other biological sources. In general, these have smaller amounts of the specific vitamins than many of the stronger supplements made from individual synthetic vitamins, but they also contain a large number of other compounds, many of which act synergistically, and provide a product that is more readily digested, absorbed and utilised by your body. Of course this is not always the case, and there are times when you will need the high concentrations of the regular supplements, but even then, I suggest that you combine them with ones based on extracts of foods and herbs.

Minerals are generally more difficult to absorb than vitamins. This is particularly true when they come as pure minerals. Frequently, they are better absorbed when they come bound with animal or plant compounds. Coral calcium, already mentioned, for instance is a particularly well absorbed form of calcium and associated minerals.

Specific Supplements

You already know from Chapter 8 that several of the B group vitamins and related cofactors are needed for the function of the Krebs Cycle. There is now a growing amount of experimental evidence to show that supplementing with these vitamins can improve mitochondrial function and health. The vitamins include thiamine or vitamin B1[400], riboflavin or vitamin B2[401], niacin, niacinamide or vitamin B3[402], pantothenic acid, calcium pantothenate or vitamin B5 and lipoic acid[403]. Minerals such as manganese and magnesium are also helpful. If there is any risk of mercury toxicity you will need chlorella to help detox and remove this element. You need biotin to ensure an adequate amount of oxaloacetate to accept the acetyl groups from the Pivotal Step leading into the Krebs or Citric Acid Cycle.

Coenzyme Q10 has been discussed already, as being essential for the respiratory chain that is part of the energy release of the medium high energy products that come from the Krebs Cycle (FADH and NADH) and have to be used to produce the lower and more manageable (but still relatively high energy compound) ATP. CoQ10 levels tend to fall with age. CoQ10 had been extensively used in the treatment of damaged or diseased mitochondria and has also been shown to reduce the level of lactic acid in the blood[404]. Idebenone, an analogue of CoQ10, works similarly but also quenches the many free radicals that are produced constantly both by the mitochondria itself and by the respiratory chain of reactions that occur within its inner membrane[405].

Other compounds decline with age and compromise mitochondrial function. These include **acetyl-L-carnitine,** necessary for the beta-oxidation of fatty acids[406], and N-acetyl cysteine needed for oxidative phosphorylation[407], [408] and best taken as the supplement **NAC**.

Cardiolipin is one of the phospholipids that make up the cell membrane and is important for several of the mitochondrial transport proteins. It too declines with age and or disease and can impair mitochondrial function.

These and other factors contribute to a decrease in mitochondrial membrane potential (function) by as much as 40 per cent[409] and possibly more.

You have almost certainly been told that exercise is helpful. One of the benefits occurs at the cellular level. It has been found that exercise increases the availability of manganese superoxide dismutase and glutathione peroxidase in cells[410]. Both of these enzymes are vital for eliminating the damaging oxygen free radicals that can harm the mitochondria and can prevent lipid peroxidation, another source of harm to the mitochondria

Even herbs can help to protect the mitochondria, one of which is gingko biloba[411].

Remedies

This chapter is only meant to be indicative. It is a foundation on which you can build. There are literally hundreds of nutrients, supplements and remedies that can assist you in overcoming cancer and rebuilding your health. Selecting the correct ones for your specific needs is a specialised job. It should certainly be based on professional experience and preferably on the basis of the results of various tests that can be organised for you. 'Evidence-based' in this case can be taken to mean 'based on the results of tests and of considerations pertaining to you as a specific and unique individual'. As said so often, throughout this book, take professional advice. This is a self-help book, not a do-it-yourself book. Supplements and remedies that may be good for one person may actually do you more harm than good, so ask for guidance.

CHAPTER 35

SUMMARY, THE WAY FORWARD AND YOUR 10-STEP PLAN

I have put forward the proposition that cancer is not simply a tumour or a collection of cancerous or transformed cells, it is a whole body, system, process, a two phase process. In Phase One of the Cancer Process your health is gradually degenerating, a process that may have taken many years. Your body has moved from generally good health at birth to worsening health at the present. This process, as you age, may be happening in ways you think of as negligible. Alternatively, there may be some obvious signs of failing health, either an accumulation of problems you think of as minor, such as digestive upsets, headaches, frequent colds, reduced energy, or else more serious problems such as diabetes, more serious digestive problems, arthritis, heart and circulation problems, and so forth. The accumulation and the worsening of these predisposing states gradually increases the probability that you might develop cancer when exposed to the ultimate stressor, carcinogen or other triggering factor.

Phase Two of the Cancer Process starts when you have permanent transformed or cancerous cells, ready to multiply at the slightest provocation, or possibly already in a state of steady multiplication and the growth of one or more tumours. The results derived from the CA panel of blood tests offered by American Metabolic Laboratories, and including the assays for your levels of HCG and PHI, can give you what is probably the earliest possible warning that you have crossed over from Phase One to Phase Two of the Cancer Process.

We have covered a variety of theories and suggestions as to the way cancers may start and how you may have entered Phase Two. It is worth noting that, while there are many different suggestions as to the ultimate cause of cancer, they can all, in fact, be built into one coherent and rounded hypothesis. Repeatedly, we have discovered that they are all a part, greater or smaller, of a coherent whole. This should provide confidence that we are on the right track to both prevention and recovery.

We can derive further positive endorsement from the fact that, although they all suggest slightly different recovery protocols, in fact the differences are indeed only slight, and often only a difference of emphasis. This too should provide confidence that we are on the right track.

The fundamental theories included Dr. Warburg's theory that cancer is due to oxygen deficiency and induced mitochondrial dysfunction, and that these are related to a lack of the functional groups that we now recognise as vitamins and minerals.

Dr. Fryda's theory, that cancer is due to adrenal exhaustion, adrenal deficiency, reduced circulation and increased glycogen storage, all of which reduce the availability of oxygen to the cells, interrelates with the ideas of Dr. Warburg.

Dr. Abo's theory, links in with that of Dr. Fryda, in that he too focuses on adrenal exhaustion, but he then brings in the adverse effect this has on immune function as a major contributory cause of cancer.

Dr. John Beard focused on the fact that the cancer triggers lead to the production and multiplication of trophoblastic or transformed cells, now recognisable as transformed or damaged adult stem cells.

A century later Dr. Biava supported and extended this concept. He was one of the first to report on the unique advantages of the zebra or rerio fish and we have been using the remedy derived from this for some time.

It now seems clear that you can increase the number and activity of healthy adult bone marrow stem cells by improving our diet and lifestyle and that their level in the blood is inversely correlated with the risk of developing cancer [Dr. Etienne Callebout, pers. comm.].

Both Dr. Beard and William Kelley recognised that these damaged cells would normally (a) be unable to live in a healthy, neutral to slightly alkaline, well oxygenated environment with efficiently functioning mitochondria; and (b) be killed off or destroyed by the proteolytic enzymes from a healthy pancreas.

Dr. Biava has suggested that even if genes are involved, if the cancer is thought to be 'genetic', this accounts for less than seven per cent of all cancers and thus that over 90% are due to diet and lifestyle.

Dr. Budwig recognised the role of cell membranes and the importance of restoring their natural fluidity and efficiency.

It used to be taught, in medical schools, that your genetic makeup was fixed and irrevocable. We now know that you can up regulate or down regulate (increase or decrease the expression activity) of these genes by making changes in diet and lifestyle, in your total environment, and that this is true even of such genes as BRCA 1 and 2 whose expression (not presence) has increased from 25% to 89% in recent decades [Dr. Etienne Callebout, pers. comm.].

There are, of course, all the various mutagens, carcinogens and other toxic agents that set off problems within the cells. These can lead to the production of mutated genes, including both the production of transformed or mutated cells and of mutated genes that, in their healthy state, would have helped to prevent the occurrence or survival of cancer cells. Part of your prevention programme should include avoiding, or minimising your exposure to, these mutagens and carcinogens. If you are not sure about this you should re-read the chapters on toxins and read other books on the same subject and that go into it in much greater detail than has been possible here.

I have already pointed out that these combined theories as to the ultimate cause of cancer have led to what amounts to a unified foundation for a recovery programme. On the basis of these ideas we have evolved a basis for a rational protocol by which you can support your body's recovery. This foundation can be the basis of your future approach to improved health whether you choose, ultimately, a MDS approach to tumour treatment or further layers of CAM protocol taking you towards recovery from cancer at the whole body level.

This whole process should not be considered as 'cancer treatment'. It is much more than that. It is the basis for healthy living for now and the future and a foundation for recovery. To this foundation you will need to add whatever specific strategies are appropriate for you. These should come from your health care practitioner, be they MDS or CAM.

In short:

There is so much that you can do to prevent and recover from cancer that cancer need not be the feared disease that it is today. The major fear, around cancer, is the fear of the unknown, particularly the fear that a recovery programme is unknown, that you are helpless and that there is a high likelihood that you will soon die of the disease. In fact, there is a huge amount that is known about what you can do to aid your recovery and return to good health and the sooner you put this into practice the sooner you can work towards better health.

Your step-by-step programme

1. Get oxygen into your cells, exercise, deep breathe, use the Budwig mix incorporating flaxseed oil. Take PQQ to increase your mitochondrial function.

2. Improve your diet. All the people discussed in this book have suggested a relatively similar diet: mostly vegetables, mostly raw, all organic, with small amounts of appropriate protein including both flesh foods such as fish, and plant sources such as nuts, seeds and sprouted seeds. The diet should be low in carbohydrate rich foods, totally devoid of sugars other than those in vegetables and berries, with increased amounts of oil-rich foods such as nuts, seeds and avocados, as well as flaxseed oil.

3. Ensure an adequate supply of all the essential nutrients (functional groups). Do the various tests to determine any deficiencies. Take supplements with the aim of improving the quality of your total diet and nutrient intake, not substituting for a good diet. Your first choice should be food-based supplements.

4. Do the tests for toxins that may already be present in your body. Avoid all harmful practices, toxins, mutagens, carcinogens, etc. Incorporate a thorough detoxification programme.

5. Deal with, transform or eliminate all toxic thoughts. Change your mental outlook, resolve emotional issues, explore some of your deeper needs and fears and deal with them.

6. Based on the work of Beard and Kelley, take large amounts of pancreatic enzymes.
7. Test for, and where necessary, eliminate or deal with all the Predisposing Factors.

Much of the above you can do on your own. However, you will need a practitioner to help you to organise the tests and to interpret not only the individual tests but the overall picture when all the results, symptoms and signs are integrated. In fact, it is important to work with a practitioner and absolutely vital that you do so if you have cancer.

These strategies will provide you with a firm foundation on which to build. If you do decide to use medical methods, surgery, radiation or chemotherapy, all the above will improve your health and maximise the benefit you may get from these and minimise some of the damage they can inflict.

If you decide to eschew current medical methods and rely totally on CAM therapies then these ideas are the foundation on which your CAM practitioner will build. Your body and your cancer are unique. Further testing can provide vital clues as to the most useful tools for you to use. This should be your way forward.

8. Work with a practitioner who is keeping up with the research. New information, new research, and new products that result from this research, are becoming available on a frequent and regular basis.
9. Find a practitioner with whom you feel comfortable and in whom you have confidence, and then work closely with them. But do not leave it all up to them. Take control of your health and your life and take (guilt-free) responsibility for all you are doing.
10. Build on the above basis by doing, or requesting, the tests that assess the detailed characteristics of your specific cancer (in addition to its location) and the biochemistry and cellular function of your tumour cells. The results of these tests will help your practitioner to determine the most appropriate corrective procedures to apply.

Finally, and importantly, work with your body, not against it. Work with your intuition and instincts. Do not let other people persuade you to do things with which you are uncomfortable or of which you are doubtful and afraid. Therapies work best when you embrace them and feel wholeheartedly positive about them. Never underestimate the power of your mind and your subconscious and the ability of these to harness your healing energies. Become better informed, read all you can get hold of, share these ideas with your practitioner so they can be incorporated into your protocol or discarded, as is appropriate for you personally, learn all you can about each step along the way. Knowing why you are doing things, making lifestyle changes, altering your diet, taking supplements and remedies and following therapies, makes it easier to stick to the changes you are making.

Then the success is yours. Good Health.

APPENDICES

APPENDIX 1: GLOSSARY

Acetylcholine	A neurotransmitter that also performs other functions.
Acetogenins	Phytochemicals found in pawpaw twig and Graviola (*Annona muricata*) that help to reduce blood supply to cancer cells and inhibit the growth of MDR cells.
Acrylamides	Carcinogens and mutagens, formed by heating starches, found in doughnuts, chips and crisps.
ACTH	Adrenocorticotrophic Hormone, produced by the brain and acts on the adrenal glands to stimulate cortisol secretion.
Adipose tissue	Fatty tissue where lipids, mainly as triglycerides, are stored.
ADP	Adenosine Diphosphate, a low energy compound is the product of ATP dephosphorylation.
Adrenalin	A hormone produced by the medulla (centre) of your adrenal glands. It is produced in response to stress and a fall in blood sugar level. It acts as a neurotransmitter.
Adipose tissue	Fatty tissue. Adipocytes are cells that store fat.
Aerobic	Oxygen rich.
AIF	Apoptosis Inducing Factor, causing cell death and involved with mitochondrial and cell membranes.
Amino acids	Small compounds containing a few carbon atoms plus oxygen and nitrogen and at least one amino (nitrogenous) group one acid. They are constituents of protein but also play roles in the body as individuals.
Amylase	A starch-splitting enzyme found in the saliva and produced by the pancreas that catalyses the breakdown of starch into sugar.

Amylopectin	A form of starch, the outer portion of a starch granule.
Amylose	A digestive-resistant form of starch found to be an effective pre-biotic.
Anaerobic	Without oxygen.
Angiogenesis	The process of building a new blood supply.
Antibodies	Chemicals produced by B-cells in response to antigens.
Antigens	Foreign or toxic substances, perceived, by your immune system, to be harmful. In auto-immune diseases this antigen may be a part of your own body.
Antineoplastic	Inhibiting or preventing the development or growth of cancerous cells.
Aperient	A gentle bulking agent for the colon. A very mild laxative like prunes.
Apoptosis	Voluntary suicide as occurs in old or faulty cells, known as appropriate cell death.
Arterioles	Small blood vessels, smaller than arteries, that carry oxygenated blood to the tissues.
ATP	Adenosine Triphosphate, a high energy molecule used as a source of energy in many cellular processes, including biosynthesis, motility and cell division.
Autocrine	Autocrine signalling is a form of communication whereby a cell secretes a hormone or chemical messenger (called the autocrine agent) that binds to autocrine receptors on the same cell, leading to changes in the cells.
Avidin	A compound found in raw egg whites, but destroyed by heat. It combines with biotin in the digestive tract and thus prevents the absorption of the biotin. Biotin (B7) is an essential nutrient, made by intestinal bacteria. Thus eating raw egg whites can create a biotin deficiency.
BAD	A pro-apoptotic protein, encouraging appropriate cell death.

BID	A pro-apoptotic protein, encouraging appropriate cell death.
BAX family	Pro-apoptotic proteins, include BAX, BAK and BOK.
BBB	Blood Brain Barrier. This is not a structural barrier in the sense of a skin around the brain. Rather it is a chemical barrier that keeps unwanted substances out of the individual cells that make up the brain.
B-cells	B-lymphocytes. Cells of your immune system. Produce antibodies.
Bcl-2	A group of proteins that influence apoptotic cellular behaviours.
Bcl-2 sub-family	Anti-apoptotic. Includes Bcl-2, Bcl-XL, Bcl-w, Mcl-1 and A1.
bcl-2	An anti-apoptotic protein, discourages appropriate cell death.
bcl-X	An anti-apoptotic protein, discourages appropriate cell death.
BHS family	3 pro-apoptotic proteins, include: BAD, BID, BIK, Blk, Hrk, BNIP3 and BimL.
Blastocyst	Consists of 70-100 cells, formed from the morula and becomes, on implantation, the embryo. The inner embryoblast becomes the embryo and the outer trophoblast becomes the placenta.
BSL	Blood Sugar Level. A measure of the amount of glucose circulating in your bloodstream.
CA 125	A cancer marker for ovarian cancer.
CA 15-3	A cancer marker for breast cancer.
Cachexia	The wasting cycle by which cancer cells cause energy loss to the body.
Cadherins	Calcium-dependent adhesion molecules. They cross cell membranes and help to bind the cells together.
CAM therapy	Complementary, Alternative and Metabolic therapy. This is somewhat analogous to naturopathy.
Capillaries	The very fine blood vessels that carry the blood through the tissues and from which nutrients can flow

out into the tissues and waste products and other compounds can enter the blood to be carried away by the venules.

Carboxypeptidase   A protein-splitting enzyme produced by the pancreas.

Caspases   A family of cysteine protease enzymes involved in apoptosis.

Caspase cascade   A cascade of reactions involved in apoptosis

CEA   Cancer Embryonic Antigen, produced normally during foetal development, not normally present in adult blood.

Cell membrane   Cell wall, consisting of a lipid-lipid bilayer with embedded proteins.

Chelating agent   Chelé = claw (in Greek). An agent that combines with other molecules, usually mineral atoms.

Choriocarcinoma   A type of cancer that occurs during pregnancy if embryo growth does not slow down.

Chymotrypsin   A protein-splitting enzyme produced by the pancreas.

Coenzymes   Substances that work with enzymes to facilitate reactions. Usually vitamins, minerals or other essential trace nutrients.

Collagen   Fibrous proteins of connective tissues.

Corpus luteum   A temporary endocrine structure that produces progesterone to maintain the endometrium.

Cysteine   A sulphur-containing non-essential amino acid found in most high protein foods.

Cytoplasm   A collective term that covers the matrix inside the various cell organelles.

Cytosol   The matrix or intracellular fluid of the cell within which the various cell organelles and structures are located. Often used interchangeably with cytoplasm.

Cytotoxic   Literally 'cell death', a substance or process that kills cells.

Desaturase   An enzyme that catalyses the removal of hydrogen, such as in long-chain fatty acids.

DGLA   Dihomo-gamma-linolenic Acid which has anti-inflammatory metabolites.

DHA   Docosahexaenoic Acid, an omega-3 fatty acid.

DHEA   Dehydroepiandrosterone, a hormone produced primarily in the adrenal glands and ultimately converted into oestrogen and androgen (the male sex hormone).

Differentiated cells   Fully matured cells that have developed the appropriate specialised characteristics of the tissues of which they are a part. These cells have lost their ability to subdivide or multiply.

Disaccharides   Molecules made up of two single monosaccharides joined together. Examples include sucrose, maltose and lactose.

DNA   Deoxyribonucleic Acid, made up of your genes.

Dopamine   A neurotransmitter released in the hypothalamus with many important functions.

EDTA   Ethylene Diamine Tetra Acetic Acid, a chelating agent especially for mercury and lead.

EGFR   Epidermal Growth Factor Receptors that increase glucose uptake by cancer cells. See Chapter 18.

Elongase   An enzyme that catalyses the lengthening of a chain, such as a long-chain fatty acid.

E-M pathway   Embden-Meyerhof pathway.

Embryo   The name give to the developing foetus during the first ten weeks of life.

Embden-Meyerhof Pathway   The anaerobic pathway that occurs in the cell's cytosol and converts glucose to either lactic acid or pyruvic acid, resulting in energy in the form of ATP.

Endocrine system   Your hormone system based on a series of ductless glands which secrete hormones into the blood supply to regulate many functions such as mood, growth and metabolism.

Enteritis   Inflammation of the small intestine.

Enzymes   Biological catalysts. Their name usually ends in –ase and the start of the word provides information as to

	the compounds involved in the reaction or the type of reaction.
EPA	Eicosapentaenoic Acid, an omega-3 fatty acid.
Epidermis	Outer skin layer.
Epigenetic code	Factors outside the genetic code that can change the expression of the genes. They influence the way this code is read or functions.
Epithelial tissue	Tissue made up of the cells that line the cavities and surfaces of the body.
Excitotoxins	Toxins that damage brain cells, e.g. aspartame, MSG.
FIR	Far Infra Red with wavelengths longer than those of visible light with lower frequencies.
Fibroblasts	Cells that produce the fibres that hold connective tissues together.
FGF	Fibroblast Growth Factor involved in angiogenesis, wound healing and foetal development.
Foetus	The developing baby from week ten after conception to birth.
FOS	Fructo Oligosaccharide. A prebiotic that helps beneficial bacteria, such as lactobacillus acidophilus and others, become firmly established in your digestive tract.
Free radicals	Highly active and dangerous 'bits' of molecules, unlike ions and far more active, generally destructive.
GABA	Gamma Aminobutyric Acid, an inhibitory neurotransmitter.
Genetic code	Information in the genes of the individual's DNA that codes for the formation of specific proteins (usually enzymes) that in turn dictate cellular function.
Geographic tongue	A tongue that is not smooth and uniform but has irregular patches of varying colour or textures, possibly with fissures.
GLA	Gamma-linolenic Acid, an omega-6 fatty acid found primarily in vegetable oils.

Glands	Specialised tissues that produce hormones. Examples include the thyroid and adrenal glands.
Glycemic Index	An indication of the extent to which a food increases your blood sugar level. A food with a high glycemic index raises your blood sugar level higher than one with a low glycemic index.
Glycogen	The large macromolecule composed of glucose units synthesised in the liver and muscles. Sometimes called 'animal starch'.
Gluconeogenesis	Synthesis of glucose from non carbohydrates such as lactate, glycerol and glucogenic amino acids. Used, with glycogenolysis, to keep sugar levels from dropping too low.
Glycogenolysis	The breakdown of glycogen into glucose, occurring in the muscle and liver tissues.
Glycolysis	The breakdown of glucose via the Embden-Meyerhof pathway in the cytosol of the cell.
Glyconutrients	Biologically active carbohydrate complex including glucose, galactose, mannose, fucose, xylose, N-acetylglucosamine, N-acetylgalactosamine, and N-acetylneuraminic acid.
Golgi apparatus	The part of the cell where large molecules such as proteins and lipids are organised.
Glycoprotein	A molecule with a carbohydrate (e.g. glucose or fructose) and a protein part (or an amino acid group).
GTF	Glucose Tolerance Factor, contains chromium and vitamin B3 and helps insulin to trigger cellular uptake of glucose from the bloodstream.
HbA1C	A combination of glucose and haemoglobin, often raised in the blood of people with diabetes.
HCAs	Heterocyclic Amines, carcinogenic compounds found in meat, poultry and fish cooked to a high temperature.
HCG	Human Chorionic Gonadotropin. The hormone produce by early embryonic cells and cancer cells.

HGF	Hepatocyte Growth Factor, a major role in embryonic organ development, in adult organ regeneration and in wound healing.
Hydrogenation	Adding hydrogen to a compound, usually across a C=C double bond. Used to solidify oils into fats.
Hydrophilic	Water-loving, or water-attracting, substances that can dissolve in water.
Hydrophobic	Water-hating or water-repelling, substances that are generally more soluble in lipids.
Hypochlorhydria	Lack of hydrochloric acid production in the stomach.
IGF	Insulin Growth Factor, a protein with non-suppressible insulin-like activity.
Insulin	Pancreatic hormone that drives glucose into cells.
ITP	Insulin Potentiation Therapy, a non-diabetic use of insulin.
Krebs Cycle	A sequence of reactions that occurs in the mitochondrion and converts acetyl groups into energy.
Lauric acid	A fatty acid in coconut oil.
LDL	Low Density Lipoprotein, bad cholesterol particles.
Ligand	A molecule that binds to another molecule or to a cell.
Lipase	Enzyme that catalyses the breakdown of lipids (fats).
Lipid	Fats and oils, composed mainly (but not only) of fatty acids, substances that are 'oily' or 'greasy' to the touch.
Lysis	Breakdown or destruction.
MDR cells	Medical Drug Resistant cells.
MDS	Medical, Drug, Surgery.
Melanocytes	Skin cells that produce the skin pigment melanin, the primary skin colour determinant.
Melatonin	Hormone produced in the brain that improves quality of sleep, reduces ageing and is a brain antioxidant.

Micron	A unit of length. One millionth of a metre, with the official abbreviation of μm.
Mitochondria	Organelles within cells in which components of carbohydrates, fats and proteins are oxidised with the release of energy and carbon dioxide.
mmol/l	A unit to measure concentration, such as the amount of glucose in a litre of blood.
MMP	Matrix Metalloproteinase, capable of degrading all kinds of extracellular matrix proteins, but can also process a number of bio-active molecules.
Monosaccharides	Single sugars. Examples include glucose, fructose, galactose and ribose.
Morula	A cluster of cells at the earliest stage of embryonic development, made up of totipotent undifferentiated cells. Grows into the blastocyst, the inner part of which becomes the embryo.
MSM	Methyl Sulphonyl Methane, a metabolite of DMSO used for arthritic problems, etc.
Mucositis	Inflammation and ulceration of the mouth and digestive tract, commonly follows chemotherapy and radiation treatments for cancer. Extremely painful.
Mucous membranes	These line all body cavities which communicate with the air, not all of them secrete mucous.
Mycotoxins	Fungal toxins.
Naturopath	Someone who functions somewhat like a general practitioner but who follows the naturopathic philosophy and uses natural remedies instead of medical drugs.
Naturopathy	Definitions vary, but as used in Australia, where I trained, it was the umbrella term for nutrition, herbal medicine, homoeopathy and an extensive range of other natural therapies. It does not generally include chiropractic, osteopathy or Eastern medical disciplines.
Neutriceuticals	Analogous to pharmaceuticals but made up of beneficial nutrients.

NGF	Nerve Growth Factor, important for growth, maintenance and survival of certain neurons.
Nitrosamines	Carcinogens produced from nitrates in combination with proteins in the acid environment of the stomach.
Noradrenalin	A stress hormone produced, like adrenalin, in the adrenal medulla but also elsewhere in the body. A neurotransmitter responsible for the fight and flight response.
Nucleoside	Components of DNA and RNA.
Nucleotides	Components of DNA and RNA.
Neurons	Nerve cells.
Neurotransmitter	A chemical messenger molecule produced by and sent out by nerve cells and generally excitatory (e.g. Glutamate) or inhibitory (e.g. GABA).
Oestrogen	A group of several different hormones relating to female sexual characteristics and activities, produced by the female ovaries and the adrenal cortex (outer layer) in both sexes.
Oligosaccharide	Several single sugar units, such as glucose, joined together.
Oncogenes	Activated oncogenes can cause non-cancerous cells to turn into cancer cells. The process usually follows a trigger such as environmental factors, toxins, viruses, a mutation in another gene or by abnormal cellular oxygen metabolism.
ORAC	Oxygen Radical Absorbing Capacity. A numerical measure of the antioxidant capacity of a substance.
Organelles	The 'organs' with specific functions, within cells.
Organs	Specialised structures within the body such as the liver, kidneys or heart.
Orthomolecular	(Curing ill health by) restoring the optimum nutritional state of the body.
p53 gene and protein	A tumour suppressor gene and its protein, regulates growth and proliferation of cells, prevents reproduction of damaged cells.
Pathogen	Substance that causes diseased (pathogenic) state.

PDGF   Platelet Derived Growth Factor, a hormone that stimulates angiogenesis.

Peptides   Chains of a small number of amino acids, very much smaller than proteins.

Peptidases   Peptide or protein-splitting enzymes.

Peristaltic action   The muscular movement of the walls of your digestive tract that moves the food and food residues along.

Phytoceuticals   Plant remedies.

Phytonutrients   Nutrients found in plants.

PKG   Protein Kinase G, an enzyme that controls angiogenesis.

Pleomorphic   Organism that has many different states.

Polysaccharide   Large carbohydrate molecule made up of many saccharides, e.g. glucose built up into starch or glycogen.

PTP   Permeability Transition Pores, such as are found through the membrane of damaged mitochondria. They signal apoptosis.

Prebiotics   Substances, such as FOS, that help probiotics to establish and flourish.

Predisposing Factors   Risk factors, nutrient deficiencies, toxins, and a wide range of health problems, some major, some seemingly minor, which increase the risk of developing cancer.

Probiotics   Beneficial micro-organisms. Usually applied to those that inhabit your digestive tract.

Progesterone   A female hormone produced in varying amounts through the menstrual cycle.

Protease   Or peptidase. An enzyme that catalyses the breakdown of proteins.

Proteins   Large molecules made up of tens or hundreds of amino acids joined together by peptide bonds.

PSA   Prostate Specific Antigen, a protein produced in the prostate gland, elevated in disorders there.

Receptor site   An area of cell membrane, usually a protein embedded in the fatty membrane, that accepts messenger molecules arriving in the blood and pass on this 'message' to the inside of the cell. The protein may also form a channel through which compounds can enter or leave the cell.

RNA   Ribonucleic Acid – derived from DNA and made up of your genes.

ROS   Reactive Oxygen Species, can do dangerous oxidative damage.

PSNS   Para Sympathetic Nervous System. This deals with your internal housekeeping, promotes the flow of digestive enzymes, peristalsis (movement) along the digestive tract, the preparation and expulsion of waste solids and or urine. Blood is pooled in your abdomen for nutrient absorption. This system can only operate when your SNS is turned off.

Secretagogue   a substance that causes another substance to be secreted.

Serotonin   Or 5-HT. A neurotransmitter made from tryptophan, contributing to well-being.

SNS   Sympathetic Nervous System. This deals with fight or flight. Blood flows from your abdomen to your limbs, lungs and eyes so you are ready to deal with physical dangers. It is the normal stress response even though in modern society most stressors are mental rather than physical. When this system is active your PSNS cannot function.

Substrate   The starting material for the reaction, usually catalysed by an enzyme.

Totipotent cells   Undifferentiated cells that still have the potential to become any cell type throughout the body.

Trans fatty acids   Unsaturated fatty acids exist normally in the cis form. During processing of vegetable oils and cooking of many fats however, the structure is rearranged into the trans form which gives rise to a number of dangerous toxins.

Trophoblast   The outer layer of cells of the morula (or developing embryo) which forms the placenta.

Trypsin   Protein-splitting enzyme produced by the pancreas.

Tumour lysis toxicity Toxicity due to the compounds being released when a tumour is broken down

Undifferentiated cells Cells that still have the potential to develop into a range of cell types. These cells are capable to subdivide and multiply.

VEGF   Vascular Endothelial Growth Factor, a hormone that stimulates angiogenesis.

Venules   Small blood vessels, smaller than veins, that carry deoxygenated blood from the capillaries to the veins and so back to the lungs.

VLDL   Very Low Density Lipoprotein.

Xenobiotics   Substances that are foreign to your body and that should not be there.

Xenoestrogens   Altered oestrogens that are foreign to the body and act like free-radicals. Carcinogenic.

APPENDIX 2

ASSOCIATIONS AND SUPPORT GROUPS

By its nature, such a listing as this cannot be up-to-date, fully comprehensive and accurate. Ask around, perhaps using these contacts as starting points, and you will doubtless find more.

Anthroposophical Medical Association
Raphael Medical Centre, Hildenborough Independent Hospital,
Hollanden Park, Coldharbour Lane, Hildenborough, Tonbridge, Kent
TN11 9LE
Tel: 01732 833924
Email: info@raphaelmedicalcentre.co.uk

Anthroposophic Health, Education and Social Care
Provides addresses throughout the country. Includes mistletoe therapy.
Website: www.ahasc.org.uk

British Naturopathic Association and Oncology Group. An excellent referral source when you are looking for a practitioner in the UK.
Tel: 01458 840072
Website: www.naturopaths.org.uk

Canceractive
Website: www.canceractive.com

Gerson Group UK
P O Box 406, Esher, Surrey KT10 9UL
The helpline operates seven days a week on tel: 01372 464557.
Website: www.gersonsupportgroup.org.uk

Penny Brohn Cancer Care
Chapel Pill Lane, Pill, Bristol, BS20 0HH
Helpline tel: 0845 1232310
Website: www.pennybrohncancercare.org

Yes to Life
Unit 7 Block C, Imperial Works, Perren St, London NW5 3ED
Tel: 0845 257 6950
Website: www.yestolife.org.uk

Breast Cancer Haven
A community-based free resource focusing especially on information and emotional support.
London – Tel: 0207384 0099
Leeds – 0113 284 7829
Hereford – 01432 361061
Email: info@breasthaven.org.uk

New Approaches to Cancer
Cancer self-help support groups in Woking, Brighton, Worthing and Ashford.
Tel: 0800 389 2662
Website: www.anac.org.uk

Other support and self-help organisations can be found at:
www.cancernet.co.uk/supportgroups.htm

APPENDIX 3

SOME HELPFUL WEBSITES

Budwig protocol
www.alternativehealth.com.au/Articles/ DrBudwigdiet.htm

Dr. Fryda
Google: For more information on Dr. Fryda put 'Waltraut Fryda cancer' into a search engine. This will lead you to Dr. Fryda's excellent book on adrenal exhaustion, lactic acid balancing and cancer.

Kelley's enzyme therapy
Click on the picture and listen to the video, click on the book title for details on the therapy, see also William Kelley's book.
www.drkelley.com
www.whale.to/cancer/k/Contents.html

Dr. Gonzalez on enzyme therapy
www.herbtime.com/InformationPages/ CancerEnzymeTherapy.htm

Dr. Gonzalez on treatment
www.dr-gonzalez.com/history_of_treatment.htm

Tumour-localised chemotherapy with CAM treatments and information on several German clinics and procedures.
www.burtongoldberg.com/index.html

Moss reports and newsletters
www.cancerdecisions.com

Health matters
Although many of the resources of this site are US-based, the content matter will help you to understand what to aim for when planning your strategy to regain your health.
www.naturalcancer.net/FreeGuide.htm

Information on cancer
Leads to other sources, includes cancer and immune system.
www.keephopealive.org

Metabolic type
This website can help you find the diet that is best for you, personally.
Click on 'Find Out Your Metabolic Type' then answer the questions.
You will be told your metabolic type and given a number of files
including a table of nearly all the foods you commonly eat, coloured
according to their suitability for you.
www.healthexcel.com or
www.metabolictypingonline.com/default.aspx

Raw food
Transitions, recipes, equipment.
www.living-foods.com and
www.rawfoodsupport.com

APPENDIX 4

BOOKS

The following lists are not designed to be comprehensive. They are books the author has used, recommended to patients or found generally helpful.

Food and food preparation

Mike Anderson, *Healing Cancer from Inside Out* (2009)

Mike Anderson, *Rave Diet and Lifestyle* (2009)

Elizabeth Baker, *The Gourmet UnCook Book – The Elegance of Raw Food* (1996)

Richard Beliveau and Denis Gingras, *Foods to Fight Cancer*, Dorling Kindersley (2007)

Dr. J. Budwig, *Flax oil as a true aid against arthritis, heart infarction, cancer and other diseases*, Apple Publishing Company (1994)

Dr. J. Budwig, *The oil-protein diet cookbook*, Apple Publishing Company (1994)

Dr. J. Budwig, *Cancer, the problem and the solution*, Nexus Hirneise - Handels GmbH (2008)

Jennifer Cornbleet, *Raw Food Made Easy,* Book Publishing Co. (2005)

Brian Clement, *Hippocrates LifeForce*. Healthy Living Publications (2007)

Gabriel Cousens, *Conscious Eating*, North Atlantic Books (2000)

Gabriel Cousens, *Rainbow Green Live-Food Cuisine*, North Atlantic Books (2003)

Sandra Goodman, *State of the Art Nutrition and Cancer*, Positive Health (1998)

Jane Grigson, *Jane Grigson's Vegetable Book*, Penguin (1998)

Viana La Place, *Verdura: Vegetables, Italian Style*, Grub Street (2010)

Juliano with Erika Lenkert, *Raw, the Uncook Book – New Vegetarian Food for Life*, Harper Collins (2003)

Deborah Madison, *The Savoury Way*, Bantam (1990)

Deborah Madison and Edward Espe Brown, *The Greens Cook Book, Extraordinary Vegetarian Cuisine,* Grub Street (2010)

Julie Sahni, *Classic Indian Vegetarian Cooking*, Grub Street (2003)

Jane Sen, *Healing Foods Cookbook,* Thorsons (2000)

Naomi Shannon, *The Raw Gourmet*, Alive Books (2007)

Diana Store (ed.), *Raw Food Works*, Raw Superfoods (2009)

Jason Vale, *The Juice Master's Ultimate Fast Food*, Thorsons (2003)

Ann Wigmore and Dennis Weaver, *Hippocratic Diet and Health Program,* Avery (1983)

Ann Wigmore, *Wheatgrass Book*, Avery (1987)

Kate Wood, *Eat Smart, Eat Raw – Detox Recipes for a High Energy Diet*, Grub Street (2002)

The mind and emotions

David Feinstein, Donna Eden and Gary Craig, *The Healing Power of EFT and Energy Psychology*, Piatkus (2005)

Isy Grigg, *EFT in Your Pocket*, New Vision Media (2005)

Lawrence LeShan, *Cancer as a Turning Point*, Plume (1994)

Lawrence LeShan, *How to Meditate – A guide to self-discovery*, Little Brown (1974)

Barbel Mohr, *The Cosmic Ordering Service*: *A guide to realising your dreams*, Hodder Mobius (2006)

Andreas Moritz, *Cancer is not a Disease – It's a Survival Mechanism*, Wellness Press (2005)

Dermot O'Connor, *The Healing Code: One Man's Amazing Journey Back to Health and His proven Five-Step Plan to Recovery*, Hodder Mobius (2006)

Martin L. Rossman, *Fighting Cancer from Within*, Henry Holt and Co. (2003)

Robert Schwartz, *Courageous Souls*: *Do We Plan Our Life Challenges Before Birth?*, Whispering Winds Press (2006)

Xandria Williams, *Choosing Health Intentionally*, Simon Schuster (1990)

Xandria Williams, *From Stress to Success*, Thorsons (2001)

Dental work and toxins

Dr. Paula Baillie-Hamilton, *Toxic Overload: A Doctor's Plan For Combating Illnesses Caused by Chemicals in Our Foods, Our Homes, and Our Medicine Cabinet*, Avery (2005)

Paul Blanc, *How Everyday Products Make People Sick*, UC Press (2007)

Russell Blaylock, *Excitotoxins: The Taste that Kills*, Health Press (1997)

Rachel Carson, *Silent Spring*, Penguin (1962)

Theo Colborn, et al., *Our Stolen Future*, Plume (1997)

Wendy Duyker, *Detox your Home, Body and Mind*, BAS Publishing (2005)

Randall Fitzgerald, *Hundred Year Lie: How to Protect Yourself from Chemicals*, Plume (2006)

Gary Ginsberg and Brian Toal, *What's Toxic, What's Not*, Berkeley Publishing Group (2006)

Hal A. Huggins, *It's All in Your Head: The link between Mercury Amalgams and Illness*, Avery (1993)

Robert Kulacz and Thomas Levy, *The Roots of Disease*, Xlibris (2002)

Felicity Lawrence, *Not on the Label*, Penguin (2004)

Lynne McTaggert, *The WDDTY Dental Handbook*, Wallace Press (1993)

George E. Meinig, *The Root Canal Cover-Up*, Price-Pottinger Nutrition Foundation (1997)

Michael Rutledge, *Product of Misinformation: Demistifying Cosmetics and Personal Care Claims, Terms and Ingredients*, Tapestry Press (2001)

David Steinman and Samuel Epstein, *The Safe Shoppers Bible – Consumer's Guide to Nontoxic Household Products, Cosmetics and Food*, Wiley (1995)

Pat Thomas, *Living Dangerously*, Newleaf (2003)

Amanda Ursell, *What are You Really Eating?: How to Become Label Savvy*, Hay House (2005)

E. D. Weinberg, *Exposing the Hidden Dangers of Iron*, Cumberland House (2004)

Ruth Winter, *Consumer's Dictionary of Food Additives*, Three Rivers Press (2009)

Information and a list of relevant books can be obtained from www.price-pottinger.org or by contacting the Price-Pottinger Nutrition Foundation, 7890 Broadway, Lemon Grove, CA 91945, USA.
Phone 00-1-619-462-7600.

Detoxing

Kathryn Alexander, *Dietary Healing The Complete Detox Program*, Annexus (2007)

Stanley Burroughs, *Master Cleanser With Special Needs and Problems*, Stanley Burroughs (1976)

Sandra Cabot, *Liver Cleansing Diet*, Women's Health Advisory Service (WHAS) (1996)

Sandra Cabot and Margaret Jasinska, *Ultimate Detox*, Women's Health Advisory Service (WHAS) (2005)

Bruce Fife, *Detox Book*, Piccadilly Books (2001)

Patrick Holford and Fiona McDonald Joyce, *Holford 9-Day Liver Detox*, Piatkus (2007)

Bernard Jensen, *Dr. Jensen's Guide to Better Bowel Care*, Avery (1999)

Jacqueline Krohn and Frances Taylor, *Natural Detoxification*, Hartley and Marks (2000)

Sidney MacDonald Baker, *Detoxification and Healing*, McGraw-Hill (2003)

Andreas Moritz, *The Amazing Liver & Gallbladder Flush*, Ener-Chi.com, 2007

Sherry Rogers, *Detoxify or Die*, Prestige Publishing (2002)

Jane Scrivner, *Detox Yourself*, Piatkus (2007)

Norman Walker, *Colon Health*, Norwalk Press (1979)

Brenda Watson, *Detox Strategy*, The Free Press (2008)

Xandria Williams, *Liver Detox Plan*, Vermilion (1988)

Infrared, mobiles and EMFs

Bruce Fife, *Health Hazards of Electromagnetic Radiation*, Piccadilly Books (2009)

David and Ora James, *A Handy Way to Cook Your Brain? Mobile Phones: What's the Damage?*, Body Conservation (2005)

Lynne McTaggert, *The Environment Book*, WDDDTY (1997)

Lynne McTaggert, *Your Healthy House*, WDDDTY (2003)

Alasdair and Jean Philips, *Powerwatch Handbook*, Piatkus (2006)

Cancer

Lise Alschuler and Karolyn Gazella, *Definitive Guide to Cancer*, Celestial Arts, (2007)

Ty M. Bollinger, *Step Outside the Box*, Infinity 510 Squared Partners (2006)

Dr J Budwig, *Cancer, the problem and the solution*, Nexus GmbH (2005)

Kathleen Deoul, *Cancer Cover Up*, Cassandra Books (2001)

Dr. Waltraut Fryda, *Diagnosis Cancer*, Xlibris (2006)

Max Gerson, *A Cancer Therapy*, Totality Books (1958 and 1975)

Burton Goldberg (ed.), *The Alternative Medicine Definitive Guide to Cancer*, Future Medicine Publishing (1997)

James Gordon and Sharon Curtin, *Comprehensive Cancer Care*, Perseus (2000)

Edward Griffin, *World Without Cancer: The Story of Vitamin B_{17}*, American Media (1997)

Lothar Hirnetse, *Chemotherapy Heals Cancer and the World is Flat*, Nexus GmbH (2005)

Josef Issels, *Cancer: A Second Opinion*, Square One Publishers (2005)

Lynne McTaggert (Ed.), *The Cancer Handbook*, WDDDTY (2000)

Michael Murray, Tim Birdsall, Joseph Pizzorno and Paul Reilly, *How to Prevent and treat Cancer with Natural Medicine*, Riverhead Books (2003)

Ralph Moss, *Cancer Therapy: The Independent Consumer's Guide*, Equinox Press (1993)

Dr. David Servan Schreiber, *Anti Cancer: A New Way Of Life*, Penguin, (2007)

Colin Woollams, *Conventional Cancer Cures, What's the Alternative*, Health Issues (2005)

Lawrence Wilson, *Sauna Therapy*, L.D. Wilson (2006)

APPENDIX 5

ADDITIONAL READING

This is a list of additional, general and useful reading.

Balch, Phyllis A., *Prescription for Nutritional Healing (4th ed.)*, Penguin (2006)

Campbell, C.T. and Campbell T.M., *The China Study: The most comprehensive study of nutrition ever conducted and the startling implications for diet, weight loss and long-term health*, BebBella Books (2006)

Critser, G., *Generation Rx: How prescription drugs are altering American lives, mind and bodies*, Houghton Mifflin Harcourt (2005)

Diamond, J. and Cowden, W.L. with Goldberg, B., *Alternative Medicine, Definitive Guide to Cancer*, Future Medicine Publishing Inc. (1997)

Elias, T., *The Burzynski Breakthrough: The century's most promising treatment...and the government's campaign to squelch it*, General Publishing (1997)

Fox, C., *The Global Race to Capture and Control the Stem Cell*, W.W. Norton (2007)

Goldberg, B., Anderson, J.W. and Trivieri, L., *Alternative Medicine: The Definitive Guide (2nd ed.)* Future Medicine Publishing (2007)

Hauser, R., Hauser, M. A., *Treating Cancer with Insulin Potentiation Therapy*, Beulah Land Press (2002)

Jaffe, R. A., *Galileo's Lawyer: Courtroom Battles in Alternative Health, Complimentary Medicine and Experimental Treatments*, Thumbs Up Press (2008)

Mahmud, K., *Keeping a Breast: Ways to prevent breast cancer*, Strategic Book Publishing (2008)

Makinen, K.K., *Biochemical principles of the use of xylitol in medicine and nutrition: with special consideration of dental aspects*, Birkhauser Verlag (1978)

Moss, R., *Cancer Therapy: the independent consumer's guide to non-toxic treatment and prevention*, (1992)

Moss, R., *The Cancer Industry*, Equinox Press (1996)

Moss, R., *A Guide to Natural Remedies on the Internet*, Equinox Press (1997)

Moss, R., *Herbs against Cancer: History and Controversy*, (1998)

Moss, R., *Antioxidants against Cancer*, Equinox Press (2000)

Moss, R., *Questioning Chemotherapy*, ISBN 1-881025-25-X (2004)

Moss, R. and Beuth, J., *Complementary Oncology: Adjunctive Methods in the treatment of cancer*, Thieme Publishing (2005)

Moynihan, R., Cassels, A., *Selling Sickness: How the world's biggest pharmaceutical companies are turning us all into patients*, Nation Books (2006)

Murphy, C., *Iscador: Mistletoe in Cancer Therapy*, Lantern Books (2001)

Pert, Candace, *Molecules of Emotion*, Pocket Books, ISBN 0-671-03397-2 (1999)

Servan-Schreiber, D., *Anti-cancer: A New Way of Life*, Viking (2008)

Sinatra, S. and Bennet, C., *Sugar Shock! How sweets and simple carbs can derail your Life – and how you can get back on track*, Berkley Trade (2006)

Somers, S., *Knockout: Interviews with doctors who are curing cancer*, Crown (2009)

Wright, J.V., *Xylitol: Dental and Upper Respiratory Health*, Dragon Art (2003)

APPENDIX 6

LABORATORIES AND TESTING KITS

The majority of these laboratories will accept tests only if they have been requested by a practitioner. Their contact details are given here so that you can pass them to your practitioner.

UK

Acumen
John McLaren Howard,
P.O. Box 129, Tiverton, Devon, EX16 0AJ
Tel: 07707 877 174
Email: acumenlab@hotmail.co.uk
Test: DNA adducts and test for salivary epithelial growth factor (EGF).

BioLab
Stone House, 9 Weymouth Street, London, W1W 6DB
Tel: 020 7636 5959
Website: http://www.biolab.co.uk
Tests: A wide range of useful tests, both medical and CAM-appropriate. Ask them for their list.

BodyBio
Contact via Nutri-Link, Nutrition House, 24 Torquay Road, Newton Abbott, Devon, TQ12 1AJ
Tel: 01626 882 100, 0870 4054 002
Website: www.nutri-linkltd.co.uk
Test: Computerised analysis of the results of basic blood biochemistry.

BTS Service for the Dr. Hauss Laboratory, Germany, in the UK
P.O. Box 5279, Brighton, BN50 9DU
Tel: 0844 330 1909
Tests: Stool analysis.

Doctor's Data
Tel: UK: 0871 218 0052; elsewhere: 1-630-377-8139
Website: www.doctorsdata.com
Tests: Hair mineral analysis.

Genova Diagnostics Europe
Parkgate House, 356 West Barnes Lane, New Malden, Surrey, KT3 6NB
Tel: 020 8336 7750
Email: infoUK@GDX.net
Website: www.GDX.net
Tests: Nearly all the tests for PDFs, in Part One, particularly useful for CAM-related tests, including the Optimal Nutrition Evaluation, or ONE, test.

Manifest Health Ltd
Tel: 01235 838 551
Email: contact@manifesthealt.co.uk
Website: www.manifesthealth.co.uk
Tests: Heavy-metal testing kits,
Equipment: Enema kits and therapeutic coffee for enema use.

Neuro-Lab Limited
681 Wimbourne Road, Bournemouth, Dorset, BH9 2AT
Tel: 01202 510 910
Email: dntaylor@btconnect.com
Tests: Tests for d-lactic acid and l-lactic acid.

The Doctor's Laboratory (TDL)
55 Wimpole Street, London
Tel: 020 7307 7383
Tests: A wide range of medical and CAM-appropriate tests.

USA

American Metabolic Laboratories
1818 Sheridan Street, Suite 102, Hollywood, FL 33020
Tel: 001 954-929-4814
Website: www.caprofile.net
Tests: HCG, PHI, CEA, their full CA profile.

Analytical Research Laboratories
2225 W. Alice Avenue, Phoenix, Arizona, 85021 USA
Tel: 001-602-995-1580
Website: www.arltma.com
Tests: Hair analysis and metabolic typing.

Doctor's Data
Tel: USA: 800-323-2784; elsewhere: 001-630-377-8139
Website: www.doctorsdata.com
Tests: Hair mineral analysis.

Neuroscience
Tel: 00-1 888-342-7272
Website: www.neurorelief.com
Tests: Neurotransmitters

Oncolab
A free testing kit can be ordered from the USA through the website or by calling 00-1-800-922-8378
Website: www.oncolabinc.com
Test: AMAS test.

Trace Element Laboratory
4501 Sunbelt Drive, Addison, Texas, 75001 USA
Tel: 00-1- 972-250-6410
Website: www.traceelements.com
Tests: Hair mineral analysis and metabolic typing.

APPENDIX 7

EQUIPMENT AND SUPPLIERS

UK Juicers has a wide variety of equipment items.
Tel: 01904 757070
Website: www.ukjuicers.com

Theolife specialises in inexpensive masticating enzyme juicers suitable for wheatgrass etc.
Tel: 0845 458 8177
Website: www.theolife.com

The Fresh Network sells equipment and a variety of raw foods, such as raw nut butters.
Tel: 0845 8337017
Website: www.fresh-network.com

[FO] **Blenders – heavy duty.** VitaMix is a high-powered, heavy-duty blender. It will enable you to make many of the foods that are part of the raw food diet. Buy the most powerful blender you can afford; anything less will soon frustrate you.

Dehydrator. Used to dry or 'cook' food below 40°C (105°F) and prevent loss of enzymes and valuable nutrients. Square ones with flat trays, such as the Excalibur, have more uses than circular ones with 'walls' around the trays.

Enemas. Enema kit with long tubing from Manifest Health.
Tel: 01235 838551
Website: www.e-enema.co.uk

Coffee. Un-roasted therapeutic enema coffee, such as Wilson brand, available from Manifest Health.
Tel: 01235 838551
Website: www.manifesthealth.co.uk

Far Infra Red (FIR) saunas. Get FITT sell a 'sleeping-bag' version, which takes up a minimum of space.
Tel: 020 84455412
Website: www.get-fitt.com

Juice extractor. A heavy-duty screw variety is preferable to the rotating centrifugal basket. These can also be used for making nut butters, humus, etc. Examples include Champion 2000, Samson, Matstone, Greenstar elite etc.
Websites: www.ukjuicers.com
www.theolife.com
www.juicemaster.com
www.fresh-network.com

Sprouting equipment. Automatic ones with electrical timer for watering your crop are available, e.g. Freshlife Sprouter. See:
www.savant-health.com/categories/Health-Equipment/Sprouting-/
Simpler equipment is also available from many health-food shops or some kitchen departments.

Water purification. Reverse Osmosis water purifier – this is very much more efficient than a filter, which is only partially and briefly effective. However the purified water should be remineralised to make up for the nutritional minerals that are lost in the process.

East Midlands Water
Tel: 0166 2763334
Website: www.eastmidlandswater.com

The Retreat Company
Tel: 0116 2599211
Website: www.theretreatcompany.com

Fresh Water Company
Tel: 0870 4423633
Website: www.freshwaterfilter.com

Or consider energised filtered water such as Grander Water from www.granderwater.co.uk

The Water Ionizer Company

Website: www.thewaterionizer.co.uk produces equipment that divides tap water into (a) pure, ionised alkaline water for consumption and (b) acid water suitable for household cleaning purposes.

APPENDIX 8

PRODUCTS BY XANDRIA WILLIAMS

BOOKS

Living with Allergies, Allen and Unwin (1986 and 1990)
What's in My Food?, Nature and Health Books (1988)
Choosing Health Intentionally, Simon and Schuster (1990), Letts Publishing (1992)
Choosing Weight Intentionally, Simon and Schuster (1990), Letts Publishing (1992)
How to prevent Osteoporosis, Wellspring Publishers (1991)
Stress – Recognise and Resolve, Letts Publishing (1993)
Love, Health and Happiness, Hodder and Stoughton (1995)
Beating the Blues, Vermillion (1995)
The Four Temperaments, St Martin's Press (1996)
Fatigue: The Secret of Getting Your Energy Back, William Heinemann (1996)
You're Not Alone, Cedar (1997)
Eating Right: Nutrition, Time-Life Books (1997)
Natural Cures for Common Ailments, Time-Life Books (1997)
Liver Detox Plan, Vermillion (1998)
From Stress to Success, 10 steps to a relaxed and happy life, Thorsons (2001)
Building Stronger Bones, Hamlyn (2002)
Overcoming Candida, Element Books (2002)
The Herbal Detox Plan, Ebury (2003)
Ideal Weight, Ideal Shape, Wellbeing Golden Keys (2004)
Vital Signs for Cancer, protect yourself from the onset or recurrence of cancer, Piatkus (2010)

SUPPLEMENTS

Liver Support formulated by Xandria Williams. Available in the UK from 0-800-212-742, or overseas from 44-1663-718850 or from many health-food shops.

AdrenoMax formulated by Xandria Williams is a supplement for adrenal support. It is available from Nutri Imports on 0-800-212-742 (from the UK) or 44-1663-718-850.

REFERENCES

[1] http://clinicalevidence.bmj.com/ceweb/about/knowledge.jsp

[2] Greer, S. et al., Psychological Response to Breast Cancer and 15-year Outcome. Lancet, 1990; 335 (8680): 49-50

[3] LeShan, L., *Cancer as a Turning Point*. Plume/Penguin, 1994

[4] http://www.eurekalert.org/pub_releases/2007-07/mcog-eeb071807.php

[5] McDougall, S.R., Anderson, A.R.A., Chaplain, M.A.J., Mathematical modelling of dynamic adaptive tumour-induced angiogenesis: Clinical implications and therapeutic targeting strategies. Journal of Theoretical Biology 2006; 241(s): 564-89

[6] Greenblatt, M., Shubik, P., Tumor Angiogenesis: Trans filter diffusion studies by the transparent chamber technique. J. Nat'l Cancer Inst. 1968; 41: 111-124

[7] Takaoka, A., Hayakawa, S., Yanai, H., Stoiber, D., Negishi, H., Kikuchi, H., Sasaki, S., Imai, K. et al., *Integration of interferon-alpha/beta signalling to p53 responses in tumour suppression and antiviral defence.* Nature 2003; 424(6948): 516–23

[8] Morgan, G., Ward, R. and Barton, M., *The contribution of cytotoxic chemotherapy to 5-year survival in adult malignancies.* Clin Oncol (R Coll Radiol), 2004; 16 (8): 549-60

[9] Nicola McCarthy, *Cancer stem cells: Can mutated stem cells produce tumours?* Nature Reviews Cancer 2009; 9: (Feb): 74

[10] Hilary Thomas, Helen M. Coley, Overcoming Multidrug Resistance in Cancer: An Update on the Clinical Strategy of Inhibiting P-Glycoprotein. Cancer Control: Journal of the Moffitt Cancer Center 2003; 10(2)

[11] Seeger, P.G., and Wolz, S., *Successful biological control of cancer by combat against the causes.* 1990 Neuwieder Verlagsgesellschaft, Neuwied, Germany and http://www.health-science-spirit.com/cancersolution.htm

[12] Morgan, G., Ward, R. and Barton, M., *The contribution of cytotoxic chemotherapy to 5-year survival in adult malignancies.* Journal of Clinical Oncology. 2004; 16(8): 549–60

[13] Pert, C., *Molecules of Emotion*. Pocket Books, 1997

[14] Bruce Lipton, *Biology of Belief*. Elite Books, 2005

[15] Harvey, E.B., A comparison of the development of nucleate and non-nucleate eggs of Arbacia punctulata. Biol. Bull. 1940; 79: 166-187

[16] Williams, X., *Duplicate D's*. Nature and Health 1980; 1(10): 11

[17] *Dietary Chromium: An Overview* by Barry Mennen, M.D. Executive Director, Chromium Information Bureau, Inc.

http://www.hbci.com/~wenonah/hydro/crbacker.htm

[18] Wang, J., Yuen, V.G., McNeill, J.H., *Effect of vanadium on insulin sensitivity and appetite.* Metabolism 2001; 50: 667-673

[19] Stenersen, Jorgen, Chemical Pesticides. Mode of action and toxicology. CRC Press, 2004 p.63

[20] http://www.thefreelibrary.com/Chromium+and+biotin+for+type+2+diabetes-a019871556 Townsend Letter 2009; May 1: 1246

[21] William C. Copeland, Joseph T. Wachsman, F. M. Johnson, John S. Penta., *Mitochondrial DNA Alterations in Cancer.* Cancer Investigation: 2002; 20(4): 557-569

[22] Jennifer S. Carew, Peng Huang, *Mitochondrial defects in cancer.* Molecular Cancer 2002; 1: 9

[23] Rui-hua Xu, Helene Pelicano, Yan Zhou, Jennifer S. Carew, Li Feng, Kapil N. Bhalla, Michael J. Keating and Peng Huang., Experimental Therapeutics, Molecular Targets, and Chemical Biology: Inhibition of Glycolysis in Cancer Cells: A Novel Strategy to Overcome Drug Resistance Associated with Mitochondrial Respiratory Defect and Hypoxia. Cancer Res., 2005 65: 613-621

[24] Warburg, O., *On the origin of cancer cells.* Science, 1956; 123: 309-14

[25] Warburg, O., *On the origin of cancer cells.* Science, 1956; 123: 309-14

[26] Otto Warburg. *The Prime Cause and Prevention of Cancer.* Lecture to Nobel Laureates, 1966, June 30

[27] http://healingtools.tripod.com/primecause1.html/

[28] José M. Cuezva, Maryla Krajewska, Miguel López de Heredia, Stanislaw Krajewski, Gema Santamaría, Hoguen Kim, Juan M. Zapata, Hiroyuki Marusawa, Margarita Chamorro and John C. Reed, *The bioenergetic signature of cancer, a marker of tumour progression.* Cancer Research 2002; 62: 6674-6681

[29] John, A.P., Dysfunctional mitochondria, not oxygen insufficiency, cause cancer cells to produce inordinate amounts of lactic acid: the impact of this on the treatment of cancer. Med Hypothesis. 2001; 57(4): 429-432

[30] Muniswamy Madesh, Lakshmi Bhaskar and K.A. Balasubramanian, *Enterocyte viability and mitochondrial function after graded intestinal ischemia and reperfusion in rats.* Moll and Cell Biochem. 1997; 167(1-2): 81-87

[31] Rucker, R.R. and Mueller, G.C., *Effect of Oxygen Tension on HeLa Cell Growth.* Cancer Res., 1960; 20: 944

[32] Genova Diagnostics Laboratory report ONE test. www.genovadiagnostics.com

[33] Otto Warburg, *The Prime Cause and Prevention of Cancer.* Lecture to Nobel Laureates, 1966, June 30

34 http://healingtools.tripod.com/primecause1.html/

35 Navindra P. Seeram, Berry Fruits for Cancer Prevention: Current Status and Future Prospects. J. Agric. Food Chem., 2008; 56(3): 630–635

36 Kim, J.W., Dang, C.V., (2006). *Cancer's molecular sweet tooth and the Warburg effect.* Cancer Res. 66 (18): 8927–30

37 Edwardsson, S., Birkhed, D., Mejare, B., Acid production from Lycasin, maltitol, sorbitol and xylitol by oral streptococci and lactobacilli. Acta Odontol Scand, 1977; 35: 257–263

38 Drucker, D., Verran, J., Comparative effects of the substance-sweeteners glucose, sorbitol, sucrose, xylitol and trichlorosucrose on lowering of pH by two oral Streptococcus mutant strains in vitro. Arch Oral Biol 1980; 24: 965–970

39 Hecht, F.M., Busch, M.P., Rawal, B., Webb, M., Rosenberg, E., Swanson, M., Chesney, M., Anderson, J., Levy, J., Kahn, J.O. *Use of laboratory tests and clinical symptoms for identification of primary HIV infection.* AIDS. 2002; 16(8): 1119-29

40 Bodansky, O., *Serum Phosphohexose isomerase in cancer. I. Method of determination and establishment of range of normal values.* Cancer, 1954; 7: 1191

41 Damle, S.R., Talavdekar, R.V., Panse, T.B., *The studies on glycolytic enzymes in relation to cancer. II. Comparative study of phosphohexose-isomerase, aldolase, isocitric dehydrogenase, serum glutamic oxaloacetic and pyruvic transaminase, and alkaline phosphatase in liver.* Indian J Cancer. 1971; 8(1): 21-9

42 Anokhin, V.N., *Use of coefficients of enzymatic activity for differential diagnosis of liver diseases.* Lab Delo. 1976; (7): 401-4

43 Harish Goel, G. S. Kohli and Harbans Lal, *Serum phosphohexose isomerase levels in patients with head and neck cancer.* The Journal of Laryngology & Otology, 1986; 100: 581-586

44 Muir, Grainger G., (1966). *Possible use of phosphohexose isomerase as a preliminary to exfoliative cytology in screening for cervical carcinoma.* J Clin Pathol. 1966; 19(4): 378–383

45 Maity, C., Boo-Chai, Khoo., *Tissue and serum levels of phospho-hexo-isomerase and lactate dehydrogenase in breast cancer patients: Their diagnostic importance.* Plastic & Reconstructive Surgery. 1990; 86(3): 614

46 Matthias Baumann, Karl Brand, Josef Giedl, Paul Hermanek, Stefan Ruf, Johannes Scheele, Suse Hoferichter, Franz P. Gall, *Significance of Serum Phosphohexose Isomerase in Gastrointestinal Cancer at Different Stages.* Oncology, 1988; 45(3): 153-158

47 P. C. Verma, T. Ojha, D. Yadav and D. D. Hemani, *Study of serum phosphohexose isomerase (PHI) levels in the management of head and neck malignancies.* Indian Journal of Otolaryngology and Head & Neck Surgery, 2001; 53(1): 40-46

[48] M. H. Gault, M. W. Cohen, L. M. Kahana, F. T. Leelin, J. F. Meakins, and M. Aronovitch, Lactic-Acid Dehydrogenase, Phosphohexose Isomerase, Alkaline Phosphatase and Glutamic Oxaloacetic Transaminase Serum Enzymes in Patients with Carcinoma of Lung. Can Med Assoc J. 1967; 96(2): 87–94

[49] Kiberstis, P.A., *Medicine Rethinking Cancer Metastasis.* Science Signalling, 2008; 1(39): 341

[50] Klein, C.A., *The Metastasis Cascade.* Science 2008; 321(5897): 1785-1787

[51] Daily Diagnosis, Leading News, American Society for Clinical Pathology. *Novel roles of the autocrine motility factor/phosphoglucose isomerase in tumor malignancy.* Endocrine-Related Cancer. 11 (4) 749 -759;

Daily Diagnosis, Leading News, American Society for Clinical Pathology. August 29, 2008;

E.K. Schandl., *The Cancer Profile and its Clinical Application.* Townsend Letter, 2010 Aug/Sept;

R.A.S. Hemat, 2004, *Orthomolecularism in Principle and Practice.* Authorhouse, 2008

[52] Schandl, E.K., *Clinical laboratory results data bank.* Unpublished, in preparation.

[53] Hideomi Watanabe, Kenji Takehana, Masayo Date, Tetsuya Shinozaki, and Avraham Raz, *Tumor Cell Autocrine Motility Factor Is the Neuroleukin/Phosphohexose Isomerase Polypeptide.* Cancer Res., 1996; 56: 2960

[54] Bardelli, A., Longati, P., Albero, D., Goruppi, S., Schneider, C., Ponzetto, C. & Comoglio, P.M., *HGF receptor associates with the anti-apoptotic protein BAG-1 and prevents cell death.* EMBO Journal, 1996; 15: 6205–6212

[55] Bikfalvi, A., Klein, S., Pintucci, G. & Rifkin, D.B., *Biological roles of fibroblast growth factor-2.* Endocrine Reviews 1997; 18: 26–45

[56] Parrizas, M., Saltiel, A.R. & LeRoith, D., Insulin-like growth factor 1 inhibits apoptosis using the phosphatidylinositol 3-kinase and mitogen-activated protein kinase pathways. Journal of Biological Chemistry 1997; 272: 154–161

[57] Descamps, S., Toillon, R.A., Adriaenssens, E., Pawlowski, V., Cool, S.M., Nurcombe, V., Le Bourhis, X., Boilly, B., Peyrat, J.P. & Hondermarck, H., *Nerve growth factor stimulates proliferation and survival of human breast cancer cells through two distinct signalling pathways.* Journal of Biological Chemistry 2001; 276: 17864–17870

[58] Harrington, E.A., Bennett, M.R., Fanidi, A. & Evan, G.I., *c-Myc-induced apoptosis in fibroblasts is inhibited by specific cytokines.* EMBO Journal 1994; 13: 3286–3295

[59] T. Yanagawa, T. Funasaka, S. Tsutsumi, H. Watanabe and A Raz, *Novel roles of the autocrine motility factor/phosphoglucose isomerase in tumor malignancy.* Endocrine-Related Cancer, 2004; 11(4): 749 -759

[60] Haga, A., Funasaka, T., Niinaka, Y., Raz, A. & Nagase, H., Autocrine motility factor signaling induces tumor apoptotic resistance by regulations Apaf-1 and

Caspase-9 apoptosome expression. International Journal of Cancer, 2003; 107: 707–714

[61] Folkman, J. & Klagsbrun, M., *Angiogenic factors.* Science, 1987; 235: 442–447

[62] Folkman, J., What is the evidence that tumors are angiogenesis dependent? J. Nat.Cancer Inst., 1990; 82: 4–6

[63] Folkman, J. & Shing, Y., *Angiogenesis.* J. Biol. Chem., 1992; 267: 10931–10934

[64] Leung, D.W., Cachianes, G., Kuang, W.J., Goeddel, D.V. & Ferrara, N., *Vascular endothelial growth factor is a secreted angiogenic mitogen.* Science, 1989; 246: 1306–1309

[65] H.M. Pinedo, Dennis J. Slamon, *Translational Research: The Role of VEGF in Tumor Angiogenesis.* The Oncologist, 2000; 5(1): 1-2

[66] T. Yanagawa, T. Funasaka, S. Tsutsumi, H. Watanabe and A. Raz., *Novel roles of the autocrine motility factor/phosphoglucose isomerase in tumor malignancy.* Endocrine-Related Cancer 11 (4) 749 -759

[67] Funasaka, T., Haga, A., Raz, A., Nagase, H., *Tumor autocrine motility factor induces hyperpermeability of endothelial and mesothelial cells leading to accumulation of ascites fluid.* Biochem. Biophys. Res. Commun., 2002; 26; 293(1): 192-200

[68] E.K. Schandl., *The Cancer Profile and its Clinical Application.* Townsend Letter, 2010 Aug/Sept.: 84-86

[69] R.A.S. Hemat, Orthomolecularism in Principle and Practice. Authorhouse, 2004

[70] Landt, S., Jeschke, S., Koeninger, A., Thomas, A., Heusner, T., Korlach, S., Ulm, K., Schmidt, P., Blohmer, J.U., Lichtenegger, W., Sehouli, J., Kuemmel, S., *Tumor-specific correlation of tumor M2 pyruvate kinase in pre-invasive, invasive and recurrent cervical cancer.* Anticancer Res., 2010; 30(2): 375-81

[71] Joachim Schneider, Harald Morr, Hans-Georg Velcovsky, Günter Weisse, and Erich Eigenbrodt, Quantitative Detection of Tumor M2-Pyruvate Kinase in Plasma of Patients with Lung Cancer in Comparison to Other Lung Diseases. Cancer Detection and Prevention 2000; 24(6): 531-535

[72] Hardt, P.D., Ngoumou, B., Rupp, J., Schnell-Kretschmer, H., Klör, H.U., *Tumor M2-PK: A promising tumor marker in the diagnosis of gastrointestinal cancer.* http://www.augen.med.uni-giessen.de/med3/poster/publ_pdf/050.pdf

[73] Pezzilli, R., Migliori, M., Morselli-Labate, A.M., Campana, D., Ventrucci, M., Tomassetti, P., Corinaldesi, R., *Diagnostic value of tumor M2-pyruvate kinase in neuroendocrine tumors. A comparative study with chromogranin.* Anticancer Res. 2003; 23(3C): 2969-72

[74] Goldblatt, H. and Cameron, G., Induced malignancy in cells from rat myocardium subjected to intermittent anaerobiosis during long propagation in vitro. J. of Expt. Med. 1953; 97(4): 525-552

[75] Seeger, P.G. and Wolz, V., *Successful Biological Control of Cancer by Combat against the Causes.* 1990 Neuwieder Verlagsgesellschaft, Neuwied, Germany

[76] Angelo, John., Dysfunctional mitochondria, not oxygen insufficiency, cause cancer cells to produce inordinate amounts of lactic acid. The impact of this on the treatment of cancer. Medical Hypotheses, 2001; 57 (4): 429-431

[77] Josephine S. Modica-Napolitano and Keshav K. Singh., *Mitochondrial dysfunction in cancer.* Mitochondrion. 2004; 4: 755-762

[78] Jennifer S. Carew and Peng Huang., *Mitochondrial defects in cancer.* Molecular Cancer 2002,1: 9

[79] Kulawiec, M., Owens, K.M., Singh, K.K., *Cancer cell mitochondria confer apoptosis resistance and promote metastasis.* Cancer Biol. Ther. 2009; 8(14): 1378-85

[80] Ma, Y., Bai, R.K., Trieu, R., Wong, L.J., *Mitochondrial dysfunction in human breast cancer cells and their transmitochondrial cybrids.* Biochim Biophys Acta. 2010 Jan; 1797(1): 29-37

[81] Jian-Jun Yu, Tao Yan, Ying-Chuan Jiang, *Mitochondrial function score combined with Gleason score for predicting the progression of prostate cancer.* Zhonghua nan ke xue National journal of andrology. 2010; 16(3): 220-222

[82] Ladiges, W., Wanagat, J., Preston, B., Loeb, L., Rabinovitch, P., *A mitochondrial view of aging, reactive oxygen species and metastatic cancer.* Aging Cell. 2010; 9(4): 462-5

[83] Wallace, D.C., A mitochondrial paradigm of metabolic and degenerative diseases, aging, and cancer: a dawn for evolutionary medicine. Annual Rev Genetics 2005; 39: 359-407

[84] Lee, H.C., Chang, C.M., Chi, C.W., *Somatic mutations of mitochondrial DNA in aging and cancer progression.* Ageing Res Rev. 2010 Nov; 9 Suppl 1: S47-58. 8

[85] Nageswara, R., Madamanchi, Marschall, S., Runge., *Mitochondrial Dysfunction in Atherosclerosis.* Circulation Research 2007; 100: 460

[86] Karamanlidis, G., Nascimben, L., Couper, G.S., Shekar, P.S., del Monte, F., Tian, R., *Defective DNA replication impairs mitochondrial biogenesis in human failing hearts.* Circ Res. 2010; 106(9): 1541-8

[87] D.J. Michelson, S. Ashwal., *The pathophysiology of stroke in mitochondrial disorders.* Mitochondrion, 2004; 4: 665-74

[88] Katsutaro Morino, Kitt Falk Petersen, Sylvie Dufour, Douglas Befroy, Jared Frattini, Nadine Shatzkes, Susanne Neschen, Morris F. White, Stefan Bilz, Saki Sono, Marc Pypaert, and Gerald I. Shulman., *Reduced mitochondrial density and increased IRS-1 serine phosphorylation in muscle of insulin-resistant offspring of type 2 diabetic parents.* J Clin Invest. 2005; 115(12): 3587–3593

[89] Schapira, A.H., *Mitochondrial dysfunction in neurodegenerative disorders.* Biochim Biophys Acta. 1998 Aug 10; 1366(1-2): 225-33

[90] Müller, W.E., Eckert, A., Kurz, C., Eckert, G.P., Leuner, K., *Mitochondrial dysfunction: common final pathway in brain aging and Alzheimer's disease--therapeutic aspects*. Mol Neurobiol. 2010 Jun; 41(2-3): 159-71

[91] Lin, T.K., Liou, C.W., Chen, S.D., Chuang, Y.C., Tiao, M.M., Wang, P.W., Chen, J.B., Chuang, J.H., *Mitochondrial dysfunction and biogenesis in the pathogenesis of Parkinson's disease*. Chang Gung Med J. 2009; 32(6): 589-99

[92] M. N. Valcárcel-Ares, C. Vaamonde-García, R. R. Riveiro-Naveira, B. Lema, F. J. Blanco, M. J. López-Armada, *A novel role for mitochondrial dysfunction in the inflammatory response of rheumatoid arthritis*. Ann Rheum Dis. 2010; 69: A56

[93] Mario D. Cordero, Manuel De Miguel, Ana M. Moreno Fernández, Inés M. Carmona López, Juan Garrido Maraver, David Cotán, Lourdes Gómez Izquierdo, Pablo Bonal, Francisco Campa, Pedro Bullon, Plácido Navas and José A Sánchez Alcázar, *Mitochondrial dysfunction and mitophagy activation in blood mononuclear cells of fibromyalgia patients: implications in the pathogenesis of the disease*. Arthritis Research & Therapy 2010, 12: R17

[94] Mabalirajan, U., Dinda, A.K., Kumar, S., Roshan, R., Gupta, P., Sharma, S.K., Ghosh, B., *Mitochondrial structural changes and dysfunction are associated with experimental allergic asthma*. J Immunol. 2008; 181(5): 3540-8

[95] Ergün Sahin, Ronald A. DePinho, Linking functional decline of telomeres, mitochondria and stem cells during ageing. Nature, 2010; 464: 520-528

[96] St. Clair, D.K., Oberley, L.W., Manganese superoxide dismutase expression in human cancer cells. A possible role of mRNA processing. Free Radical Research Communications 1991; 12-13(2): 771-8

[97] Oberley, L.W., Oberley, T.D., Buettner, G.R., Cell differentiation, aging and cancer. The possible roles of superoxide and superoxide dismutases. Med Hypotheses 1980; 6(3): 249-268

[98] Ibid. *Cell division in normal and transformed cells: the possible role of superoxide and hydrogen peroxide.* Med Hypotheses 1981: 7(1): 21-42

[99] Oberley, L.W., Buettner, G.R., Role of superoxide dismutase in cancer: a review. Cancer Res., 1979; 39: 1141-49

[100] Borrello, S., De Leo, M.E., Galeotti, T., *Defective gene expression of MnSOD in cancer cells*. Mol Aspects Med 1993; 14(3): 253-8

[101] Shoffner, J., Lott, Voljavec, A., et al., Spontaneous Kearns-Sayre/chronic external ophthalmoplegia plus syndrome associated with a mitochondrial DNA deletion: a slip-replication model and metabolic therapy. Proc Natl Acad Sci USA, 1989, 86: 7952-56

[102] Kobayashi, M., Morishita, H., Okajima, K., et al., *Successful treatment with succinate supplement in a patient with a deficiency of Complex I (NADH-CoQ reductase)*. Int Cong Inborn Errors Metab, 4th, Sendai, Japan, 1987: 148

[103] Quillin Patrick, *Cancer's sweet tooth.* Nutrition Science News, 2000(4): 1-8

[104] Tannenbaum, A., Silverstone, H., The influence of the degree of caloric restriction on the formation of skin tumors and hepatomas in mice. Cancer Res 1949; 9:724–727

[105] Weindruch, R., Walford, R., Dietary restriction in mice beginning at 1 year of age: effect on life-span and spontaneous cancer incidence. Science 1982; 215: 1415–1418

[106] Bandaru, S., Reddy, Chung-Xiou Wang, and Hiroshi Maruyama., *Effect of Restricted Caloric Intake on Azoxymethane-induced Colon Tumor Incidence in Male F344 Rats.* Cancer Research, 1987; 47: 1226-1228

[107] Hilf, R., *The actions of insulin as a hormonal factor in breast cancer.* In: Pike M.C., Siiteri P.K., Welsh C.W.,eds. Hormones and Breast Cancer, 1981. Cold Spring Harbor Laboratory. pp. 317–337

[108] Zapf, J., Froesch, E.R., Insulin-like growth factors/somatomedins: structure, secretion, biological actions and physiological role. Hormone Research 1986. 24; (24): 121–130

[109] Goustin, A.S., Leof, E.B., Shipley, G.D., Moses, H.L., *Growth Factors and Cancer.* Cancer Research, 1986: 1015–1029

[110] Quinn, K.A., Treston, A.M., Unsworth, E.J. et al., *Insulin-like growth factor expression in human cancer cell lines.* J Biol. Chem. 1998; (271): 11477–83

[111] Pap, V., Pezzino, V., Constantino, A. et al., *Elevated insulin receptor content in human breast cancer.* J Clin. Invest. 1990; 86 (86): 1503–1510

[112] Gross, G.E., Boldt, D.H., Osborne, C.K., *Pertubation by insulin of human breast cancer cell kinetics.* Cancer Research 1984 (44): 3570–3575

[113] Kevin J. Cullen, Douglas Yee, William S. Sly, James Perdue, Brian Hampton, Marc E. Lippman, and Neal Rosen, *Insulin-like Growth Factor Receptor Expression and Function in Human Breast Cancer.* Cancer Res 1990; 50(1): 48

[114] Rasmussen, A.A., Cullen, K.J. (1998), *Paracrine/autocrine regulation of breast cancer by the insulin-like growth factors.* Breast Cancer Res Treat. 1998; 47(3): 219–33

[115] Yee, D., *The insulin-like growth factors and breast cancer - revisited.* Breast Cancer Res Treat. 1998; 47(3): 197–199

[116] Lyons, C.N., Mathieu-Costello, O., Moyes, C.D., *Regulation of skeletal muscle mitochondrial content during aging.* J Gerontol A Biol Sci Med Sci. 2006; 61(1): 3-13

[117] Spindler, S.R., *Caloric restriction: from soup to nuts.* Ageing Res Rev. 2010; 9(3): 324-53

[118] Chen, G., Wang, F., Trachootham, D., Huang, P., *Preferential killing of cancer cells with mitochondrial dysfunction by natural compounds.* Mitochondrion. 2010; 10(6): 614-25

[119] Li, C.J., Zhang, Q.M., Li, M.Z., Zhang, J.Y., Yu, P., Yu, D.M., *Attenuation of myocardial apoptosis by alpha-lipoic acid through suppression of mitochondrial oxidative stress to reduce diabetic cardiomyopathy.* Chin Med J (Engl). 2009; 122(21): 2580-6

[120] Rodriguez, M.C., MacDonald, J.R., Mahoney, D.J., Parise, G., Beal, M.F., Tarnopolsky, M.A., *Beneficial effects of creatine, CoQ10, and lipoic acid in mitochondrial disorders.* Muscle Nerve. 2007; 35(2): 235-42

[121] Hagen, T.M., Moreau, R., Suh, J.H., Visioli, F., *Mitochondrial decay in the aging rat heart: evidence for improvement by dietary supplementation with acetyl-L-carnitine and/or lipoic acid.* Ann N Y Acad Sci. 2002; 959: 491-507

[122] Robert Rucker, Winyoo Chowanadisai, Masahiko Nakano, *Potential Physiological Importance of Pyrroloquinoline Quinone.* Alternative Medicine Review,2009; 14(3): 268

[123] Chowanadisai, W., Bauerly, K.A., Tchaparian, E., Wong, A., Cortopassi, G.A., Rucker, R.B., *Pyrroloquinoline quinone stimulates mitochondrial biogenesis through cAMP response element-binding protein phosphorylation and increased PGC-1alpha expression.* J Biol Chem. 2010; 285(1): 142-52

[124] Fryda, Dr. Waltrout, 1987, *Adrenalin deficiency as the cause of cancer formation, 4th Edition.* Pub. Kunst and Alltag, Munich ISBN 3-88410-079-3

[125] Fryda, Dr. Waltraut, *Diagnosis: Cancer.* ISBN 9781599268972, available from www.Xlibris.com

[126] Xandria Williams, *From Stress to Success.* Thorsons, 2001

[127] Dr. A von Metzler of the Max-Planck institute for brain research in Frankfurt and Dr. Cordula Nitsch of the same institute in Munich, GEP No 181, 12:1988; Naturwissenschaften. No 72, p.542, 1985; Arzt heute, 4. p.2, 1986, and Leben. 3-4 1986

[128] Xandria Williams, *From Stress to Success.* Thorsons, 2001

[129] Lawrence LeShan, *Cancer as a Turing Point.* 1994. Plume/Penguin

[130] Colthurst, J., *Cancer Positive.* Michael O'Mara Books, 2003

[131] Yasuo Ohashi et al., Habitual Intake of Lactic Acid Bacteria and Risk Reduction of Bladder Cancer. Urologia Internatinalis, 2002; 68(4): 273-280

[132] J. Singh, A. Rivenson, M. Tomita, S. Shimamura, N. Ishibashi and B.S. Reddy, Bifidobacterium longum, a lactic acid-producing intestinal bacterium inhibits colon cancer and modulates the intermediate biomarkers of colon carcinogenesis. Carcinogenesis, 1997; 18(4): 833-841

[133] http://www.cancer.gov/Templates/drugdictionary.aspx?CdrID=486744

[134] Abo, T., *Your Immune Revolution.* 2007. Chapter 2, 48-78. Kokoro Publishing

[135] Ronald A. Berk, *The active ingredients in humor: psychophysiological benefits and risks for older adults.* Educational Gerontology, 2001; 27(3 and 4): 323 – 339

[136] Bennett, M.P. and Lengacher, C., *Humor and Laughter May Influence Health: II. Complementary Therapies and Humor in a Clinical Population.* Evidence-based Complementary and Alternative Medicine; 3(2): 187-190

[137] Buxman, K., *Humor as a cost-effective means of stress management.* Managing Employee Benefits. 1998; 6(2): 74-78

[138] Cousins, N., Anatomy of an Illness as perceived by the patient. 1979. Norton and Co.

[139] Webster, J.I., Tonelli, L., Sternberg, E.M., *Neuroendocrine regulation of immunity.* Annu. Rev. Immunol., 2002; 20: 125–163

[140] Charo, I.F., Ransohoff, R.M., *The many roles of chemokines and chemokine receptors in inflammation.* N. Engl. J. Med. 2006: 354: 610–621

[141] Granger, D.N., Role of xanthine oxidase and granulocytes in ischemia-reperfusion injury. Am. J. Physiol. 1988; 255: H1269-H1275

[142] Christopher W. Pugh, Peter J. Ratcliffe, *Regulation of angiogenesis by hypoxia: role of the HIF system.* Nature Medicine, 2003; 9: 677 – 684

[143] Wang, Y., Wan, C., Deng, L., Liu, X., Cao, X., Gilbert, S.R., Bouxsein, M.L., Faugere, M.C., Guldberg, R.E., Gerstenfeld, L.C., Haase, V.H., Johnson, R.S., Schipani, E., Clemens, T.L., *The hypoxia-inducible factor alpha pathway couples angiogenesis to osteogenesis during skeletal development.* J. Clin. Invest., 2007; 117(6): 1616-26

[144] Tiffany N. Seagroves, Heather E. Ryan, Han Lu, Bradly G. Wouters, Merrill Knapp, Pierre Thibault, Keith Laderoute, and Randall S. Johnson, *Transcription Factor HIF-1 Is a Necessary Mediator of the Pasteur Effect in Mammalian Cells.* Molecular and Cellular Biology, 2 001; 21(10): 3436-3444

[145] Beard, J., *The Enzyme Treatment of Cancer.* London: Chatto and Windus, 1911

[146] *Recherches dur le Traitement du Cancer*, etc. Paris. (1829); Editoral Archiv fuer pathologische Anatomie und Physiologie und fuer klinische Medizin 8 (1855) 23

[147] Durante, F., 1874, Nesso fisio-pathologico tra la struttura dei nei materni e la genesi di alcuni tumori maligni. Arch Memor Observ Chir. Pract. 11: 217-26

[148] John Beard, The Enzyme Theory of Cancer and its scientific basis. New Spring Press, 2010

[149] Sell. S., *Stem Cell Handbook.* Totowa, 2003, N.J. Human Press vol .9

[150] www.scienceblog.com/cms/scientists_find_stem_cells_in_human_breast_cancer

[151] Beard, J., *The Action of Trypsin.* Br. Med J., 1906;4: 140-41

[152] Wiggin, F.H., Case of Multiple Fibrosarcoma of the Tongue, With Remarks on the Use of Trypsin and Amylopsin in the Treatment of Malignant Disease. JAMA, 1906; 47: 2003-08

[153] Cutfield, A., *Trypsin Treatment in Malignant Disease.* Br. Med. J., 1907; 5: 525

[154] Little, W.L., A Case Of Malignant Tumor, with Treatment. JAMA, 1908; 50: 1724

155 Gotze, H., Rothman, S.S., Enterohepatic Circulation of Digestive Enzymes as a Conservative Mechanism. Nature 1976; 257: 607-609

156 Krichevsky, A., Birken, S., O'Connor, J., Acevedo, H.F., Bikel, K., Luatbader, J., Hartree, A., Canfield, R,E., Development, characterization and application of monoclanal antibodies to the native and synthetic beta COOH-terminal portion of human chorionic gonadotropin (hCG) that distinguish between the native and desialylated forms of hCG. Endocrinol 1994; 134: 1139-1145

157 Acevedo, H.F., Tong, J.Y., Hartsock, R.J., Human chorionic ganadotropin-beta subunit gene statement in cultured human fetal and cancer cells of different types and angina. Cancer 1995; 76: 1467-1475

158 Schandl, E.K., *The cancer profile and its clinical applications.* Townsend Newsletter. 2010; Aug-Sept.

www.townsendletter.com/AugSept2010/cancerprofile0810.html

159 Regelson, W., *Have we found the "definitive cancer biomarker"? The diagnostic and therapeutic implications of human chorionic gonadotropin-beta statement as a key to malignancy.* Cancer 1995; 76: 1299-1301

160 Navarro, M., 72nd Science Meeting of the Cavite Med. Soc.; 1959; Trece Martires City, Philippines

161 Williams, R.R., McIntire, K.R., Waldmann, T.A., et al., *Tumor-associated antigen levels (CEA, HCG, alpha-feto protein) antedating the diagnosis of cancer in the Framingham study.* J. Natl. Cancer Inst., 1977; 58(6): 1547–1551

162 Emil K. Schandl, *The Cancer Profile and its Clinical Application.* Townsend Letter, 2010, Aug/Sept

163 Acavedo, H.F. et al., *Flow cytometry method for the analysis of membrane-associated HCG, its subunits and fragments on human cancer cells.* Cancer. 1992; 69: 1818–1828

164 Acavedo, H.F. et al., *HCG-β gene expression in cultured human fetal and cancer cells.* Cancer. 1995;,76:,1467–1475

165 Marcillac, I. et al., *Free human chorionic gonadotropin β subunit in gonadal and nongonadal neoplasms.* Cancer Res. 1992; 52: 3901–3907

166 Martinez Flores, A. et al., *Development and validation of an in vitro culture model for the study of the differentiation of human trophoblast.* [In Spanish.] Ginecol. Obstet. Mex., 2006; 74(12): 657–665

167 Bjurlin, M.A. et al., *Histological pure seminoma with an elevated beta-HCG of 4497IU/l.* Urology. 2007; 70(5): 1007.e13–1007.e15

168 P. Biava, *Cancer and the Search for Lost Meaning.* North Atlantic Books. 2009

169 Beavon, I.R., *The E-cadherin-catenin complex in tumour metastasis: structure, function and regulation.* Eur. J. Cancer, 2000; 36 (13): 1607–20

[170] Daniel G. Miller, *Cancer in Hiroshima: 35 years after the bomb.* InterScience, 2006; 12(3): 224-227

[171] Alessandra Cucina, Pier-Mario Biava, Fabrizio D'Anselmi, Pierpaolo Coluccia, Filippo Conti, Roberta di Clemente, Alfredo Miccheli, Luigi Frati, Alberto Gulino, Mariano Bizzarri. *Zebrafish embryo proteins induce apoptosis in human colon cancer cells (Caco2).* Apoptosis (2006) 11:1617–1628

[172] Kelley, W., *Cancer: Curing the Incurable Without Surgery, Chemotherapy, or Radiation.* 2001. New Century Promotions

[173] Morrison-Kelley, C., *Cancer Cure Without Surgery-chemotherapy-radiation.* 2002. http://www.road-to-health.com/am/publish/article_56.shtml

[174] Kelley, W., *One Answer to Cancer with Cancer Cure Suppressed.* 1999. The Road to Total Health Inc.

[175] Kelley, W.D., *New Hope for Cancer Victims: An Ecological Approach to the Successful Treatment of Malignancy.* 1969

[176] Navarro, M., 72nd Science Meeting of the Cavite Med Soc; 1959; Trece Martires City, Philippines

[177] Kelley, W.D., *One Answer To Cancer. Latest update - 33,000 cancer cases over three decades.* 1999. New Century Promotions 3711 Alta Loma Drive Bonita, CA

[178] Kelley, W.D. with Fred Rohe, *Cancer: Curing the Incurable, without surgery, chemotherapy or radiation.* 2005, ISBN 09669422-9-9

[179] Roberts, Melina, A., *A critique of the Kelley Nutritional-Metabolic Cancer Program.* Townsend Letters; June 2003

[180] Saruc, M., Standop, S., Standop, J., Nozawa, F., Itami, A., Pandey, K.K., Batra, S.K., Gonzalez, N.J., Guesry, P., Pour, P.M., *Pancreatic enzyme extract improves survival in murine pancreatic cancer.* Pancreas. 2004; 28.4: 401-12

[181] Nicholas J. Gonzalez, *One Man Alone: An Investigation of Nutrition, Cancer, and William Donald Kelley.* New Spring Press, 1986

[182] N. Gonzales, L. Isaacs, *The Trophoblast and the origins of cancer: One solution to the medical enigma of our times.* New Spring Press. 2009

[183] Shively, F.L., *Multiple Proteolytic Enzyme Therapy Of Cancer.* Dayton, Johnson-Watson, 1969

[184] *The inhibition of lactic acid formation in cancer and muscle.* Biochem. J.,1930; 24(1):141–157

www.pubmedcentral.nih.gov/picrender.fcgi?artid=1254366&blobname=biochemj01 128-0173.tif

[185] Gonzalez, N.J., Isaacs, L.L., *Evaluation of pancreatic proteolytic enzyme treatment of adenocarcinoma of the pancreas, with nutrition and detoxification support.* Nutr. Cancer. 1999; 33(2): 117-24. Comment on: Nutr. Cancer. 1999; 33(2): 115-6

[186] Ulf-Håkan Stenman, *Tumor-associated Trypsin Inhibitor*. Clinical Chemistry, 2002; 48: 1206-1209

[187] Yamamoto, H., Iku, S., Adachi, Y., Imsumran, A., Taniguchi, H., Nosho, K., Min, Y., Horiuchi, S., Yoshida, M., Itoh, F., Imai, K., *Association of trypsin expression with tumour progression and matrilysin expression in human colorectal cancer*. J Pathol. 2003; 199(2): 176-84

[188] Y.C. Lee, H.W. Pan, S.Y. Peng, P.L. Lai, W.S. Kuo, Y.H. Ou, H.C. Hsu, *Overexpression of tumour-associated trypsin inhibitor (TATI) enhances tumour growth and is associated with portal vein invasion, early recurrence and a stage-independent prognostic factor of hepatocellular carcinoma*. European Journal of Cancer, 2007; 43(4): 736-744

[189] P. Venesmaa, P. Lehtovirta, U.H. Stenman, A. Leminen, M. Forss and O. Ylikorkala. *Tumour-associated trypsin inhibitor (TATI): comparison with CA125 as a preoperative prognostic indicator in advanced ovarian cancer*. Br. J. Cancer 1994, 70: 1188-1190

[190] Townsend Letter for Doctors. July 1990

[191] Jackson, P.E., Groopman, J.D., *Aflatoxin and liver cancer*. Baillieres Best Pract Res Clin Gastroenterol. 1999; 13(4): 545-55

[192] Schulsinger, D.A., Root, M.M., and Campbell, T.C., *Effect of dietary protein quality on development of aflatoxin B1-induced hepatic preneoplastic lesions*. J. Natl. Cancer Inst. 1989; 81: 1241-1245

[193] Campbell, T.C. and Campbell, T.M., *The China Study*. Benbella Books, 2006, p.60

[194] http://www.vegparadise.com/news22.html

[195] Renato Baserga, Francesca Peruzzi, Krysztof Reiss, *The IGF-1 receptor in cancer biology*. Int. J. Cancer, 2003; 107(6): 873-877

[196] Susan E. Hankinson and others, *Circulating concentrations of insulin-like growth factor I and risk of breast cancer*. Lancet, 1998; 351(9113): 1393-1396

[197] http://www.vegparadise.com/news22.html

[198] Hawrylewicz, E.J., Huang, H.H., Kissane, J.Q. et al., *Enhancement of the 7,12-dimethylbenzene(a)anthracene (DMBA) mammary tumorigenesis by high dietary protein in rats*. Nutr. Reps. Int., 1982; 26: 793-806

[199] X.M. Zhang, D. Stamp, S. Minkin, A. Medline, D.E. Corpet, W.R. Bruce, M.C. Archer, *Promotion of Aberrant Crypt Foci and Cancer in Rat Colon by Thermolyzed Protein*. J. Ntnl. Cancer Inst., 1992; 84(13): 1026-1030

[200] K.H. Sabeena Farvin, Caroline P. Baron, Nina Skall Nielsen, Jeanette Otte and Charlotte Jacobsen, *Antioxidant activity of yoghurt peptides: Part 2 – Characterisation of peptide fractions*. Food Chemistry, 2010; 123(4): 1090-1097

[201] K.H. Sabeena Farvin, Caroline P. Baron, Nina Skall Nielsen and Charlotte Jacobsen. *Antioxidant activity of yoghurt peptides: Part 1-in vitro assays and evaluation in ω-3 enriched milk*. Food Chemistry 2010; 123(4): 1081-1089

[202] Struewing, J.P., Hartge, P., Sholom Wacholder, D., Baker, S.M., Berlin, M., McAdams, M., Timmerman, M.M., Lawrence, B.S., Brody, C., Tucker, M.A., *The Risk of Cancer Associated with Specific Mutations of BRCA1 and BRCA2 among Ashkenazi Jews.* N.Eng.J.Med. 1997; 336(20): 1401-1408

[203] Mary-Claire King, Joan H. Marks, Jessica B. Mandell, *Breast and Ovarian Cancer Risks Due to Inherited Mutations in BRCA1 and BRCA2.* Science, 2003; 302(5645): 643 – 646

[204] Bunz, F., Dutriaux, A., *Requirement for p53 and p21 to sustain G_2 arrest after DNA damage.* Science 1998, 282: 1497-1501

[205] Elbendary, A.A., Cirisano, A.C., et al., *Relationship between p21 expression and mutation of the p53 suppressor gene in normal and malignant ovarian epithelial cells.* Clin. Can. Res.; 2(9): 1571-1575

[206] Anttila, M.A., Kosma, V-M, Hongxiu, J., Puolakka, J., Juhola, M., Saarikoski, S., and Syrjänen, K., *p21/WAF1 expression as related to p53, cell proliferation and prognosis in epithelial ovarian cancer.* Br J Cancer. 1999; 79(11/12): 1870–1878

[207] Västrik, I., Kaipainen, A., Penttilä, T.L., Lymboussakis, A., Alitalo, R., Parvinen, M., Alitalo, K., *Expression of the mad gene during cell differentiation in vivo and its inhibition of cell growth in vitro.* J Cell Biol., 1995; 128(6): 1197-208

[208] Angst, B., Marcozzi, C., Magee, A., *The cadherin superfamily: diversity in form and function.* J Cell Sci; 114(4): 629–41

[209] Berx, G., Cleton-Jansen, A.M., Nollet, F., de Leeuw, W.J., van de Vijver, M., Cornelisse, C. and van Roy, F., *E-cadherin is a tumour/invasion suppressor gene mutated in human lobular breast cancers.* EMBO J. 1995; 14(24): 6107-6115

[210] Michael Evans and Iain Rodger, *Complete Healing: Regaining Your Health Through Anthroposophical Medicine.* Thorsons, 2002

[211] Victor Bott, *Anthroposophical Medicine, an extension of the art of healing.* Rudolf Steiner Press. 1978

[212] Michael Evans and Iain Rodger, *Complete Healing: Regaining Your Health Through Anthroposophical Medicine.* Thorsons, 2002

[213] Friedrich Husemann and Otto Wokff, *The Anthroposophical approach to medicine.* 3 vols. The Anthroposophical Press, 1982

[214] Kienle, Kiene and Albonico, *Anthroposophic Medicine.* Schattauer, 2006

[215] Klotter, Jule, *Anthroposophical Medicine.* Townsend Letter for Doctors and Patients, 2006; 24(1): 274

[216] Harold S Burr, *Blueprint for Immortality.* 1991

[217] http://www.wrf.org/men-women-medicine/dr-harold-s-burr.php

[218] http://www.wddty.com/human-energy-fields-fritz-albert-popp.html

[219] Lynne McTaggart, *The Field. Element.* 2001

[220] James L. Oschman, *Trauma energetics*. J. Bodywork and Movement Therapies. 2006; 10(1): 21-34

[221] Rudolf Steiner and Ita Wegman, *Extending Practical Medicine: Fundamental Principles Based on the Science of the Spirit*. Rudolf Steiner Press, 1925, Reprinted 2000

[222] von Rohr et al., *Experiences in the realisation of a research project on anthroposophical medicine in patients with advanced cancer*. Schweiz Med Wochenschr 2000; 130: 1173–84

[223] Friedrich Husemann and Otto Wolff, *The Anthroposophical approach to medicine*. Anthroposophic Press, 3: 43-77

[224] Christine Murphy, *Iscador: Mistletoe in Cancer Therapy*. Lantern Books. 2001

[225] Ernst, E., Schmit, K., Steuer-Vogt, M.K., *Mistletoe for cancer? A systematic review of randomised controlled trials*. Int J Cancer 2003; 107: 262-7

[226] Finall, A.J., McIntosh, S.A., and Thompson, W.D., (2006) *Subcutaneous inflammation mimicking metastatic malignancy induced by injection of mistletoe extract*. British Medical Journal, 333(7582): 1293-4

[227] S. Lori Brown, Marcel E. Salive, Jack M. Guralnik, Robert B. Wallace, Adrian M. Ostfeld and Dan Blazer, *Depressive symptoms in the elderly: Association with total white blood cell count*. Progress in Neuro-Psychopharmacology and Biological Psychiatry, 19(5): 849-860

[228] www.bbc.co.uk/health/emotional_health/bereavement/bereavement_physical.shtml

[229] Sidney Zisook, Stephen R. Shuchter, Michael Irwin, Denis F. Darko, Paul Sledge and Kathy Resovsky, *Bereavement, depression, and immune function*. Psychiatry Research; 1994; 52(1): 1-10

[230] www.lukasklinik.ch

[231] Hirneise, L., *Chemotherapy cures cancer and the world is flat*. 2005. Nexus

[232] Damodaran Chendil, Rama S. Ranga, David Meigooni, Sabapathi Sathishkumar and Mansoor M. Ahmed, *Curcumin confers radiosensitizing effect in prostate cancer cell line PC-3 Oncogene*. 2004; 23: 1599–1607

http://www.nature.com/onc/journal/v23/n8/abs/1207284a.html

[233] S. Krishnan, S. Sandur, S. Shentu, B. Aggarwal, *Curcumin Enhances Colorectal Cancer Cell Radiosensitivity by Suppressing the Radiation-Induced Nuclear Factor-kappaB (NF-kB) Pathway*. International Journal of Radiation Oncology Biology Physics, 2006; 66(3): S547-S547

[234] Swati Girdhani, Mansoor M. Ahmed, Kaushala P. Mishra, *Enhancement of Gamma Radiation-induced Cytotoxicity of Breast Cancer Cells by Curcumin*. Mol. Cell. Pharmacol, 2009;1 (4): 208-217

[235] Simone Fulda and Klaus-Michael Debatin (2004), *Sensitization for anticancer drug-induced apoptosis by the chemopreventive agent resveratrol.* Oncogene 2004; 23, 6702–6711

[236] Klein, C.A., *The Metastasis Cascade.* Science 2008; 321(5897): 1785-1787

[237] Daily Diagnosis, Leading News, American Society for Clinical Pathology, *Novel roles of the autocrine motility factor/phosphoglucose isomerase in tumor malignancy.* Endocrine-Related Cancer 11(4): 749 -759

[237] Daily Diagnosis, Leading News, American Society for Clinical Pathology. August 29, 2008

[237] E.K. Schandl, *The Cancer Profile and its Clinical Application.* Townsend Letter, 2010 Aug/Sept

[237] R.A.S. Hemat, 2004, *Orthomolecularism in Principle and Practice.* Authorhouse, 2008

[238] Kiberstis, P.A., *Medicine Rethinking Cancer Metastasis.* Science Signalling, 2008; 1(39): 341

[239] M.W. Kissin, G. Querci Della Rovere, D. Easton, G. Westbury, *Risk of lymphoedema following the treatment of breast cancer.* British Journal of Surgery, 1986; 73(7): 580-584

[240] Mitchell, G.K., *The role of general practice in cancer care.* Austral. Fam. Physician, 2008; 37: 698-702

[241] Passik, S.D., McDonald, M.V., *Psychosocial aspects of upper extremity lymphedema in women treated for breast carcinoma.* Cancer 1998; 83 (12 suppl American): 2817-20

[242] Gayle Giboney Page, Shamgar Ben-Eliyahu, *Increased surgery-induced metastasis and suppressed natural killer cell activity during proestrus/estrus in rats.* Breast Cancer Research and Treatment 1997; 45(2): 159-167

[243] Ben-Eliyahu S., *The promotion of tumor metastasis by surgery and stress: immunological basis and implications for psychoneuroimmunology.* Brain Behav Immun. 2003; 17(1): S27-36

[244] Michael S. O'Reilly, Lars Holmgren, Yuen Shing, Catherine Chen, Rosalind A. Rosenthal, Marsha Moses, William S. Lane, Yihai Cao, E.Helene, *Sage and Judah Folkman. Angiostatin: A novel angiogenesis inhibitor that mediates the suppression of metastases by a lewis lung carcinoma.* Cell, 1994; 79(2): 315-328

[245] Qadri, S.S., Wang, J.H., Coffey, J.C., Alam, M., O'Donnell, A., Aherne, T., Redmond, H.P., *Surgically induced accelerated local and distant tumor growth is significantly attenuated by selective COX-2 inhibition.* Ann Thorac Surg. 2005; 79(3): 990-5

[246] Nakamura, M., Inufusa, H., Adachi, T., Aga, M., Kurimoto, M., Nakatani, Y., Wakano, T., Nakajima, A., Hida, J.I., Miyake, M., Shindo, K., Yasutomi, M., *Involvement of galectin-3 expression in colorectal cancer progression and metastasis.* Int J Oncol. 1999; 15(1): 143-8

[247] J.F. Dowdall, FRCSI, D.C., Winter, M.D., E. Andrews, FRCSI, W.E. Laug, M.D., J.H. Wang, Ph.D., H.P. Redmond, M.D., *Soluble Interleukin 6 Receptor (sIL-6R) Mediates Colonic Tumor Cell Adherence to the Vascular Endothelium: A Mechanism for Metastatic Initiation?* J. Surg. Res. 2002; 107(1): 1-6

[248] P. Sooriakumaran, *Surgery-induced angiogenesis.* Internat. J.Surg.; 2005 3 (4): 289-290

[249] Retsky, M., Demicheli, R. Hrushesky, H., Baum, M. and Gukas, I., Review: *Surgery Triggers Outgrowth of Latent Distant Disease in Breast Cancer: An Inconvenient Truth?* Cancers 2010: 2(2): 305-337

[250] Retsky, M., Demicheli, R., and Hrushesky, W.G.M., *Does surgery induce angiogenesis in breast cancer? Indirect evidence from relapse pattern and mammography paradox.* Int.J.Surg., 2005; 3(3): 179-187

[251] Devitt, J.E., *The influence of conservative and radical surgery on the survival of patients with breast cancer.* Canad. Med. Ass. J., 1962; 57: 906: 911

[252] Curran, D., van Dongen, J.P., Aaronson, N.K., Kiebert, G., Ffentiman, J.S., Mignolet, F., Bartelink, H., *Quality of life of early-stage breast cancer patients treated with radical mastectomy or breast-conserving procedures: Results of EORTC trial 10801.* Eur. J. Cancer., 1998; 34(3): 307-314

[253] Isabel Monteiro-Grillo, Pedro Marques-Vidal and Marília Jorge, *Psychosocial effect of mastectomy versus conservative surgery in patients with early breast cancer.* Clinical and Translational Oncology, 2005; 7(11): 499-503

[254] Morris, A.D., Morris, R.D., Wilson, J.F., White, J., Steinberg, S., Okunieff, P., Arriagada, R., Lê, M.G., Blichert-Toft, M., van Dongen, J.A., *Breast-conserving therapy vs mastectomy in early-stage breast cancer: a meta-analysis of 10-year survival.* Cancer J Sci Am. 1997; 3(1): 6-12

[255] Onik, G., Vaughan, D., Lotenfoe, R., Dineen, M., Brady, J., *Male lumpectomy: focal therapy for prostate cancer using cryoablation.* Urology. 2007 Dec; 70(6 Suppl): 16-21

[256] Moss, R., *Questioning Chemotherapy.* 2000, Equinox Press

[257] Loeb, S., *Chemotherapy handbook.* Springhouse, PA: 1994. Springhouse Corp.

[258] Stephen K. Carter, *The carcinogenic potential of cytotoxic chemotherapy and its implications for therapeutic decision-making.* Cancer Chemotherapy and Pharmacology 1984; 12 (2): 67-69

[259] Schmall, D., Habs, M., Lorenz, M., Wagner, I., *Occurrence of second tumors in man after anticancer drug treatment.* Cancer Treat Rev 1982; 9: 167–195

[260] Sieber, S.M., *The action of antitumor agents: A double edged sword.* Med Pediatric Oncol 1977; 3: 123–131

[261] Boice, J.D., Greene, M.H., Killen, J.Y., *Leukemia and preleukemia after adjuvant treatment of gastrointestinal cancer with Methyl-CCNU.* N Engl J Med 1983; 309: 1079–1084

[262] Boivin, J-F., Hutchison, G.B., *Leukemia and other cancers after radiotherapy and chemotherapy for Hodgkin's disease.* J Natl Cancer Inst 1981; 67: 751–761

[263] Reimer, R.R., Hoover, R., Fraumeni, J.F. Jr,, Young, R.C., *Acute leukemia after alkylating-agent therapy of ovarian cancer.* N Engl J Med 1977; 297: 177–181

[264] Valagussa, P., Santoro, A., Kenda, R., *Second malignancies in Hodgkin's disease: a complication of certain forms of treatment.* Br Med J 1980; 280: 216–219

[265] Morgan, G., Ward, R., Barton, M., *The contribution of cytotoxic chemotherapy to 5-year survival in adult malignancies.* Clin Oncol (R Coll Radiol). 2004; 16(8): 549-60

[266] Fields, K.K., Elfenbein, G.J., Lazarus, H.M., Cooper, B.W., Perkins, J.B., Creger, R.J., Ballester, O.F., Hiemenz, J.H., Janssen, W.E. and Zorsky, P.E., *Maximum-tolerated doses of ifosfamide, carboplatin, and etoposide given over 6 days followed by autologous stem-cell rescue: toxicity profile.* Journal of Clinical Oncology, 1995; 13: 323-332

[267] Testa, N.G., Hendry, J.H., Molineux, G., *Long-term bone marrow damage in experimental systems and in patients after radiation or chemotherapy.* Anticancer Res. 1985; 5(1): 101-10

[268] Mitchell, G.K., *The role of general practice in cancer care.* Austral. Fam. Physician, 2008; 37: 698-702

[269] DeVita, V.T., Jr., et al. [eds]., *Cancer: principals and practice of oncology.* 1993, Philadelphia: J.B. Lippincott

[270] Loeb, S., *Chemotherapy handbook.* 1994, Springhouse, PA: Springhouse Corp.

[271] Wittes, R.E.[ed.]., *Manual of oncologic therapeutics 1991/1992.* Philadelphia: J.B. Lippincott

[272] Physicians' Desk Reference. 1995

[273] Rubin, P. and Casarett, G. W., *Clinical Radiation Pathology.* 1968, W. B. Saunders

[274] Joanna Banerjee, Eija Pääkkö, Marika Harila, Riitta Herva, Juho Tuominen, Antero Koivula, Marjatta Lanning and Arja Harila-Saari, *Radiation-induced meningiomas: A shadow in the success story of childhood leukaemia.* Neuro-Oncology 2009; 11(5): 543-549

[275] Smith, P.G., *Leukemia and other cancers following radiation treatment of pelvic disease.* Cancer. 1977; 39(4): 1901-5

276 Christoph Richter, Jeen-Woo Park, and Bruce N. Ames, *Normal oxidative damage to mitochondrial and nuclear DNA is extensive.* Proc. Nati. Acad. Sci. USA, 1988; 85: 6465-6467

277 Tinsley, P.W., and Maerker, G., *Effect of low-dose γ-radiation on individual phospholipids in aqueous suspension.* J. Am. Oil Chem. Soc. 1993; 70(2): 187-191

278 Marathe, D., Mishra, K.P., *Radiation-induced changes in permeability in unilamellar phospholipid liposomes.* Radiat Res 2002; 158(5): 666

279 Yurkova, I., Shadyro, O., Kisel, M., Brede, O. and Arnhold, J., *Radiation-induced free-radical transformation of phospholipids: MALDI-TOF MS study.* Chemistry and Physics of Lipids, 2004; 132(2): 235-246

280 J. Kevin Leach, Glenn Van Tuyle, Peck-Sun Lin, Rupert Schmidt-Ullrich and Ross B. Mikkelsen, *Ionizing Radiation-induced, Mitochondria-dependent Generation of Reactive Oxygen/Nitrogen.* Cancer Research 2001; 61: 3894-3901

281 Lothar Hirneise, *Chemotherapy cures cancer and the world is flat.* Nexus. 2005; 176-184 [refs in German edition]

282 Hille, A., Herrmann, M.K., Kertesz, T. et al., *Sodium butyrate enemas in the treatment of acute radiation-induced proctitis in patients with prostate cancer and the impact on late proctitis. A prospective evaluation.* Strahlenther Onkol 2008; 184(12): 686–92

283 Ossama Al-Mefty, Jane E. Kersh, Anupam Routh, and Robert R. Smith, *The long-term side effects of radiation therapy for benign brain tumors in adults.* J. Neurosurgery. 1990; 3(4): 502-512

284 John B. Little, *Radiation carcinogenesis.* Carcinogenesis, 2000; 21(3): 397-404

285 Read, A.P., Strachan, T., *"Chapter 18: Cancer Genetics".* Human molecular genetics 2. New York: Wiley. (1999). ISBN 0-471-33061-2

286 R. L. Ullrich, *Radiation-induced instability and its relation to radiation carcinogenesis.* Int.J.Rad.Biol. 1998; 74(6): 747-754

287 Kohn, H.I., Fry, R.J.M., *Radiation carcinogenesis.* N.Engl. J. Med. 1984; 310: 504-511

288 Carmel Mothersill, Colin Seymour, *Radiation-induced bystander effects, carcinogenesis and models.* Oncogene (2003) 22, 7028–7033

289 Alfred I. Neugut, Todd Murray, Jason Santos, Howard Amols, Mary K. Hayes, John T. Flannery, Eliezer Robinson, *Increased risk of lung cancer after breast cancer radiation therapy in cigarette smokers.* Cancer, 2006; 73(6): 1615-1620

290 Habibul Ahsan, Alfred I. Neugut, *Radiation Therapy for Breast Cancer and Increased Risk for Esophageal Carcinoma.* Annals.Int.Med. 1998; 128(2): 114-117

291 Mitchell, G.K., *The role of general practice in cancer care.* Austral. Fam. Physician, 2008; 37: 698-702

292 Chajes, V., Thiebaut, A.C.M., Rovital, M., Gauthier, E., et al., *Association between serum trans-monunsaturated fatty acids and breast cancer risk.* Cancer Epidem. Biomarkers and Prevention, 2007; 16(7): 1312-1320

293 Tareke, E., Rydberg, P., Jarkssib, P., Eriksson, S., Tornqvist, M., *Acryklamide: a cooking carcinogen.* Chem.Tes. in Toxicology, 2000, June; 13(6): 517-22

294 Tareke et.al., *Analysis of acrylamide, a carcinogen formed in heated foodstuffs.* J. of Ag Food. Chem., 2002; 50(17): 4998-5006

295 World Cancer Research Fund, *Food, Nutrition and the Prevention of Cancer: A Global Perspective.* Washington, DC: American Institute for Cancer Research 1997

296 Boffetta, P., et al, Fruit and vegetable intake and overall cancer risk in the European Prospective Investigation Into Cancer and Nutrition. J Natl Cancer Inst. 2010; 102: 1-9

297 Canene-Adams, K., Lindshield, B.L., Wang, S., Jeffery, E.H., Clinton, S.K., & Erdman, J.W. Jr., *Combinations of tomato and broccoli enhance antitumor activity in Dunning R3327-H prostate adenocarcinomas.* Cancer Research, 2007; 67(2), 836–843

298 Kimber, L. Stanhope, Jean Marc Schwarz, Nancy L. Keim, Steven C. Griffen, Andrew A. Bremer, James L. Graham, Bonnie Hatcher, Chad L. Cox, Artem Dyachenko, Wei Zhang, John P. McGahan, Anthony Seibert, Ronald M. Krauss, Sally Chiu, Ernst J. Schaefer, Masumi Ai, Seiko Otokozawa, Katsuyuki Nakajima, Takamitsu Nakano, Carine Beysen, Marc K. Hellerstein, Lars Berglund and Peter J. Havel, *Consuming fructose-sweetened, not glucose-sweetened, beverages increases visceral adiposity and lipids and decreases insulin sensitivity in overweight/obese humans.* J Clin Invest. 2009; 119(5): 1322–1334

299 Wang, X.Q., Terry, P.D., Yan, H., *Review of salt consumption and stomach cancer risk: epidemiological and biological evidence.* World J Gastroenterol. 2009; 15(18): 2204-13

300 Jansson, B., *Potassium, sodium, and cancer: a review.* J Environ Pathol Toxicol Oncol. 1996; 15(2-4): 65-73

301 Shoba, G., Joy, D., Joseph, T., Majeed, M., Rajendran, R., Srinivas, P.S., *Influence of piperine on the pharmacokinetics of curcumin in animals and human volunteers.* Planta Med. 1998; 64(4): 353-6

302 *Antiproliferative and apoptotic effects of selective phenolic acids on T47D human breast cancer cells: potential mechanisms of action.* Breast Cancer Res. 2004; 6(2): R63-74

303 Lee, Y.S., *Role of NADPH oxidase-mediated generation of reactive oxygen species in the mechanism of apoptosis induced by phenolic acids in HepG2 human hepatoma cells.* Arch Pharm Res. 2005; 28(10): 1183-9

304 Tomisato Miura, Mitsuru Chiba, Kosuke Kasai, Hiroyuki Nozaka, Toshiya Nakamura, Toshihiko Shoji, Tomomasa Kanda, Yasuyuki Ohtake and Tatsusuke

Sato, *Apple procyanidins induce tumor cell apoptosis through mitochondrial pathway activation of caspase-3 Carcinogenesis.* 2008; 29(3): 585-593

[305] Zhao, J., Sharma, Y., Agarwal, R., *Mol Significant inhibition by the flavonoid antioxidant silymarin against 12-O-tetradecanoylphorbol 13-acetate-caused modulation of antioxidant and inflammatory enzymes, and cyclooxygenase 2 and interleukin-1alpha expression in SENCAR mouse epidermis: implications in the prevention of stage I tumor promotion.* Carcinog. 1999; 26: 321-333

[306] Jiang, C., Agarwal, R., Lu, J., *Anti-angigenic potential of a cancer chemopreventive flavonoid antioxidant, silymarin: inhibition of key attributes of vascular endothelial cells and angiogenic cytokine secretion by cancer epithelial cells.* Biochem Biophys Res Commun. 2000; 276: 371-378

[307] Miccadei, S., Di Venere, D., Cardinali, A., Romano, F., Durazzo, A., Foddai, M.S., Fraioli, R., Mobarhan, S., Maiani, G., *Antioxidative and apoptotic properties of polyphenolic extracts from edible part of artichoke (Cynara scolymus L.) on cultured rat hepatocytes and on human hepatoma cells.* Nutr Cancer. 2008; 60(2): 276-83

[308] Wei Wang, Terrell R. Bostic and Liwei Gu, *Antioxidant capacities, procyanidins and pigments in avocados of different strains and cultivars.* Food Chemistry, 2010; 122(4): 1193-1198

[309] Ding, H., Chin, Y.W., Kinghorn, A.D., & D'Ambrosio, S.M., *Chemo preventive characteristics of avocado fruit.* Seminars in Cancer Biology, 2007; 17(5): 386–394

[310] Christiana Winkler, Barbara Wirleitner, Katharina Schroecksnadel, Harald Schennach and Dietmar Fuchs, *In vitro Effects of Beet Root Juice on Stimulated and Unstimulated Peripheral Blood Mononuclear Cells.* Fuchs American Journal of Biochemistry and Biotechnology 2005; 1(4): 180-185

[311] Kapadia, G.J., Tokuda, H., Konoshima, T. and Nishino, H., *Chemoprevention of lung and skin cancer by Beta vulgaris (beet) root extract.* Cancer Lett., 1996; 100: 211-214

[312] Crowell, P.L., et al., *Human metabolism of the experimental cancer therapeutic agent d-limonene.* Cancer Chemother Pharmacol 1994; 35: 31-7

[313] Hou, Z., Lambert, J.D., Chin, K.V., & Yang, C.S., *Effects of tea polyphenols on signal transduction pathways related to cancer chemoprevention.* Mutation Research/DNA Repair. 2005, 555: 3–19

[314] Milner, J.A., Garlic: *Its anticarcinogenic and antitumorigenic properties.* Nutrition Reviews, 1996; 54: S82–S86

[315] Milner, J.A., *A historical perspective on garlic and cancer.* Journal of Nutrition, 2001; 131: 1027S–1031S

[316] *Protective effects of ellagic acid and other plant phenols on benzo[a]pyrene-induced neoplasia in mice.* Carcinogenesis. 1983; 4(12): 1651-3

[317] Mori, H., Kawabata, K., Yoshimi, N., Tanaka, T., Murakami, T., Okada, T., Murai, H., *Chemopreventive effects of ferulic acid on oral, and rice germ on large bowel carcinogenesis.* Anticancer Res. 1999; 19(5A): 3775-8

[318] Delmas, D., Lancon, A., Colin, D., Jannin, B., & Latruffe, N., *Resveratrol as a chemo preventive agent: A promising molecule for fighting cancer.* Current Drug Targets, 2006; 7: 423–442

[319] Signorelli, P. & Ghidoni, R., *Resveratrol as an anticancer nutrient: Molecular basis, open questions and promises.* Journal of Nutritional Biochemistry, 2005; 16: 449–466

[320] Pezzuto, J.M., *Resveratrol as a cancer chemo preventive agent.* In B.B. Aggarwal & S. Shishodia (Eds.), *Resveratrol in health and disease.* 2006: 233–383, New York, Marcel Dekker

[321] Kuo, P.C., Liu, H.F., Chao, J.I., *Survivin and p53 modulate quercetin-induced cell growth inhibition and apoptosis in human lung carcinoma cells.* J Biol Chem. 2004; 279(53): 55875-85

[322] Shishodia, S., Majumdar, S., Banerjee, S., Aggarwal, B.B., *Ursolic acid inhibits nuclear factor-kappaB activation induced by carcinogenic agents through suppression of IkappaBalpha kinase and p65 phosphorylation: correlation with down-regulation of cyclooxygenase 2, matrix metalloproteinase 9, and cyclin D1.* Cancer Res. 2003; 63; 15: 4375–83

[323] Pathak, A.K., Bhutani, M., Nair, A.S., et al., *Ursolic acid inhibits STAT3 activation pathway leading to suppression of proliferation and chemosensitization of human multiple myeloma cells.* Mol. Cancer Res. 2007; 5(9): 943–55

[324] Ma, C.M., Cai, S.Q., Cui, J.R., Wang, R.Q., Tu, P.F., Hattori, M., Daneshtalab, M., *The cytotoxic activity of ursolic acid derivatives.* Eur. J. Med. Chem. 2005; 40: 582–589

[325] Bhuvaneswari, V. & Nagini, S., *Lycopene: A review of its potential as an anticancer agent.* Current Medicinal Chemistry, Anticancer Agent. 2005; 5: 627–635

[326] Ralph Muecke, Lutz Schomburg, Jens Buentzel, Klaus Kisters, Oliver Micke, *Selenium or No Selenium – That Is the Question in Tumour Patients: A New Controversy.* Integrative Cancer Therapies. 2010; 9: 136-141

[327] Whanger, P.D., *Selenium and its relationship to cancer: An update dagger.* British. Journal of Nutrition, 2004; 91: 11–28

[328] Gleissman, H., Segerström, L., Hamberg, M., Ponthan, F., Lindskog, M., Johnsen, J.I., Kogner, P., *Omega-3 fatty acid supplementation delays the progression of neuroblastoma in vivo.* Int J Cancer. 2010 May 24

[329] Manna, S., Chakraborty, T., Ghosh, B., Chatterjee, M., Panda, A., Srivastava, S., Rana, A., *Dietary fish oil associated with increased apoptosis and modulated expression of Bax and Bcl-2 during 7,12-dimethylbenz(alpha)anthracene-induced mammary carcinogenesis in rats.* Prostaglandins Leukot Essent Fatty Acids 2008; 79: 5-14

330 Yuri, T., Danbara, N., Tsujita-Kyutoku, M., Fukunaga, K., Takada, H., Inoue, Y., Hada, T., Tsubura, A., *Dietary docosahexaenoic acid suppresses N-methyl-N-nitrosourea-induced mammary carcinogenesis in rats more effectively than eicosapentaenoic acid.* Nutr Cancer, 2003; 45: 211-7

331 Noguchi, M., Minami, M., Yagasaki, R., Kinoshita, K., Earashi, M., Kitagawa, H., Taniya, T., Miyazaki, I., *Chemoprevention of DMBA-induced mammary carcinogenesis in rats by lowdose EPA and DHA.* Br J Cancer.1997; 75: 348-53

332 Toriyama-Baba, H., Iigo, M., Asamoto, M., Iwahori, Y., Park, C.B., Han, B.S., Takasuka, N., Kakizoe, T., Ishikawa, C., Yazawa, K., Araki, E., Tsuda, H., *Organotropic chemopreventive effects of n-3 unsaturated fatty acids in a rat multi-organ carcinogenesis model.* Jpn J Cancer Res 2001; 92: 1175-83

333 Mami Takahashi, Toshinari Minamoto, Naoyuki Yamashita, Kazunaga Yazawa, Takashi Sugimura and Hiroyasu Esumi, *Reduction in Formation and Growth of 1,2-Dimethylhydrazine-induced Aberrant Crypt Foci in Rat Colon by Docosahexanoic Acid.* Cancer Res., 1993, June; 53: 2786

334 Iigo, M., Nakagawa, T., Ishikawa, C., Iwahori, Y., Asamoto, M., Yazawa, K., Araki, E., Tsuda, H., *Inhibitory effects of docosahexaenoic acid on colon carcinoma 26 metastasis to the lung.* Br J Cancer, 1997; 75: 650-5

335 Kelavkar, U.P., Hutzley, J., Dhir, R., Kim, P., Allen, K.G., McHugh, K., *Prostate tumor growth and recurrence can be modulated by the omega-6:omega-3 ratio in diet: athymic mouse xenograft model simulating radical prostatectomy.* Neoplasia 2006; 8: 112-24

336 Toriyama-Baba, H., Iigo, M., Asamoto, M., Iwahori, Y., Park, C.B., Han, B.S., Takasuka, N., Kakizoe, T., Ishikawa, C., Yazawa, K., Araki, E., Tsuda, H., *Organotropic chemopreventive effects of n-3 unsaturated fatty acids in a rat multi-organ carcinogenesis model.* Jpn J Cancer Res 2001; 92: 1175-83

337 T. Akihisa, H. Tokuda, M. Ogata, M. Ukiya, M. Iizuka et al., *Cancer chemopreventive effects of polyunsaturated fatty acids.* Cancer Letters. 2004; 205(1): 9-13

338 Ramos, E.J., Middleton, F.A., Laviano, A., Sato, T., Romanova, I., Das, U.N., Chen, C., Qi, Y., Meguid, M.M., *Effects of omega-3 fatty acid supplementation on tumor-bearing rats.* J Am Coll Surg. 2004; 199: 716-23

339 Wolk, A., Larsson, S.C., Johansson, J.E., Ekman, P., *Long-term fatty fish consumption and renal cell carcinoma incidence in women.* JAMA 2006; 296: 1371-6

340 Fradet, V., Cheng, I., Casey, G., Witte, J.S., *Dietary Omega-3 Fatty Acids, Cyclooxygenase-2 Genetic Variation, and Aggressive Prostate Cancer Risk.* Clin Cancer Res 2009; 15: 2559

341 Wolk, A., Larsson, S.C., Johansson, J.E., Ekman, P., *Long-term fatty fish consumption and renal cell carcinoma incidence in women.* JAMA 2006; 296: 1371-6

[342] Chinthalapally V. Rao, Barbara Simi, Tin-Tin Wynn, Kathy Garr, and Bandaru S. Reddy, *Modulating Effect of Amount and Types of Dietary Fat on Colonic Mucosal Phospholipase A_2, Phosphatidylinositol-specific Phospholipase C Activities, and Cyclooxygenase Metabolite Formation during Different Stages of Colon Tumour Promotion in Male F344 Rats.* Cancer Res., 1996; 56: 532

[343] Gleissman, H., Segerström, L., Hamberg, M., Ponthan, F., Lindskog, M., Johnsen, J.I., Kogner, P., *Omega-3 fatty acid supplementation delays the progression of neuroblastoma in vivo.* Int J Cancer. 2010, May 24

[344] Vanderveen, J.E., *Regulation of flaxseed as a food ingredient in the United States.* In: *Flaxseed in Human Nutrition.* eds Cunnane, S.C. and Thompson, L.U., AOCS Press, Champaign, IL, 1995: 363-366

[345] Yuri, T., Danbara, N., Tsujita-Kyutoku, M., Fukunaga, K., Takada, H., Inoue, Y., Hada, T., Tsubura, A., *Dietary docosahexaenoic acid suppresses N-methyl-N-nitrosourea-induced mammary carcinogenesis in rats more effectively than eicosapentaenoic acid.* Nutr Cancer 2003; 45: 211-7

[346] Boyd, D.B., *Insulin and cancer.* Integrative Cancer Strategies 2003; 2(4): 315-329

[347] Kaaks, R., *Nutrition, insulin, IGF-1 metabolism and cancer risk: A summary of epidemiological evidence.* Novartis Foundation Symposium, 2004; 262: 247–260

[348] Rosana Chirinos, Jorge Galarza, Indira Betalleluz-Pallardel, Romina Pedreschi and David Campos, *Antioxidant compounds and antioxidant capacity of Peruvian camu camu (Myrciaria dubia (H.B.K.) McVaugh) fruit at different maturity stages.* Food Chemistry; 2010, June 15; 120(4): 1019-1024

[349] Ginter, E., et al., *Natural hypocholesterolemic agent: pectin plus ascorbic acid.* International Journal of Viticulture and Natural Resource, 1979; 49: 406-408

[350] Guess, B.W., Scholz, M.C., Strum, S.B., Lam, R.Y., Johnson, H.J., Jennrich, R.I., *Modified citrus pectin (MCP) increases the prostate-specific antigen doubling time in men with prostate cancer: a phase II pilot study.* Prostate Cancer Prostatic Dis. 2003; 6: 301-304

[351] Nangia-Makker, P., Hogan, V., Honjo, Y., et al., *Inhibition of human cancer cell growth and metastasis in nude mice by oral intake of modified citrus pectin.* J Natl Cancer Inst. 2002; 94: 1854-1862

[352] Pienta, K.J., Naik, H., Akhtar, A., et al., *Inhibition of spontaneous metastasis in a rat prostate cancer model by oral administration of modified citrus pectin.* J Natl Cancer Inst. 1995; 87: 348-353

[353] X Williams. *Liver Detox Plan.* 1998, Vermillion

[354] Cesar de Oliveira, Richard Watt, Mark Hamer, *Toothbrushing, inflammation, and risk of cardiovascular disease: results from Scottish Health Survey.* BMJ 2010; 340: 2451

[355] Bokemeyer, C., Aapro, M.S., Courdi, A., Foubert, J., Link, H., Osterborg, A., Repetto, I., Soubeyran, P., *EORTC guidelines for the use of erythropoietic proteins in anaemic patients with cancer.* Europ. J. Cancer, 2007; 43(2): 258-270

356 Weinberg, E.D., *The role of iron in cancer*. Eur J Cancer Prev. 1996; 5(1): 19-36

357 www.findarticles.com/p/articles/mi_m1200/is_n9_v145/ai_14878110/?tag=content; col1

358 Ebisuzaki, K., *Aspirin and methylsulfonylmethane (MSM): a search for common mechanisms, with implications for cancer prevention.* Anticancer Res. 2003; 23(1A): 453-8

359 Scott M. Auerbach, Kathleen A. Carrado, Prabir K. Dutta, eds., *Handbook of zeolite science and technology.* CRC Press, 2003

360 Ivkovic, S., Deutsch, U., Silberbach, A., Walraph, E., Mannel, M., *Dietary supplementation with the tribomechanically activated zeolite clinoptilolite in immunodeficiency: Effects on the immune system.* Advances in Therapy, 2004; 21(2): 135

361 Kathryn H. Schmitz, Jeremy Holtzman, Kerry S. Courneya, Louise C. Masse, Sue Duval and Robert Kane., *Controlled Physical Activity Trials in Cancer Survivors: A Systematic Review and Meta-analysis.* Cancer Epidemiol Biomarkers Prev 2005; 14(7): 1588-1595

362 Friedenreich, C.M., *Physical activity and cancer prevention: from observational to intervention research.* Cancer Epidemiol Biomarkers Prev. 2001; 10:287-301

363 Dimeo, F., Rumberger, B.G., Keul, J., *Aerobic exercise as therapy for cancer fatigue.* Med Sci Sports Exerc. 1998 Apr; 30(4): 475-8

364 Hayes, S.C., Rowbottom, D., Davies, P.S., Parker, T.W., Bashford, J., *Immunological changes after cancer treatment and participation in an exercise programme.* Med Sci Sports Exerc 2003; 35: 2–9

365 Na, Y.M., Kim, M.Y., Kim, Y.K., Ha, Y.R., Yoon, D.S., *Exercise therapy effect on natural killer cell cytotoxic activity in stomach cancer patients after curative surgery.* Arch Phys Med Rehabil 2000; 81: 777– 9

366 Williams, X., *From Stress to Success.* 2001. Thorsons

367 LeShan, L., *Cancer as a Turning Point.* 1994. Plume/Penguin

368 LeShan, L., *Cancer as a Turning Point.* 1994. Plume/Penguin

369 Williams. X., *From Stress to Success.* 2001. Thorsons

370 Williams, X., *Liver Detox Plan.* 1998 Vermilion

371 http://www.ars.usda.gov/SP2UserFiles/Place/12354500/Data/ORAC/ORAC07.pdf

372 Johnson, Paul D., in *Artemis*, P. Simopoulos, C. Gopalan. *Plants in Human Health and Nutrition Policy.* 2003; 91: 63–74

373 www.healthaliciousness.com/nutritionfacts/sbsl.php?one=9002&two=9206&three= 9017. Nutrition Facts Comparison Tool

374 Kuskoski, E.M., Asuero, A.G., Morales, M.T., Fett, R. (2006), *Wild fruits and pulps of frozen fruits: antioxidant activity, polyphenols and anthocyanins.* Cienc Rural 2006; 6(4)

[375] Tarwadi, K., Agte, V., *Antioxidant and micronutrient potential of common fruits available in the Indian subcontinent.* Int J Food Sci Nutr 2007; 58(5): 341–9

[376] Ghosal, S., Triethi, V.K., and Chauhan, S., *Active xconstituents of Emblica officinalis: Part 1.-The chemistry and antioxidative effects of two new hydrolysable tannins, Emblicanin A and B.* Indian Journal of Chemistry 1996; 35B: 941-948

[377] Habib-ur-Rehman, Yasin, K.A., Choudhary, M.A., et al., *Studies on the chemical constituents of Phyllanthus emblica.* Nat. Prod. Res. 2007; 2 (9): 775–81

[378] Saeed, S., Tariq, P., *Antibacterial activities of Emblica officinalis and Coriandrum sativum against Gram negative urinary pathogens.* Pak J Pharm Sci, 2007; 20 (1): 32–5

[379] Penolazzi, L. et al., *Induction of apoptosis of human primary osteoclasts treated with extracts from the medicinal plant Emblica officinalis.* BMC Compl Altern Med 2008; 8: 59

[380] Ganju, L., Karan, D., Chanda, S., Srivastava, K.K., Sawhney, R.C., Selvamurthy, W., *Immunomodulatory effects of agents of plant origin.* Biomed Pharmacother. 2005; 57(7): 296–300

[381] Yokozawa, T., Kim, H.Y., Kim, H.J., et al., *Amla (Emblica officinalis Gaertn.) attenuates age-related renal dysfunction by oxidative stress.* J Agric Food Chem. 2007; 55(19): 7744–52

[382] Rao, T.P., Sakaguchi, N., Juneja, L.R., Wada, E., Yokozawa, T., Amla (Emblica officinalis Gaertn.) extracts reduce oxidative stress in streptozotocin-induced diabetic rats. J Med Food, 2005; 8 (3): 362–8

[383] Jacob, A., Pandey, M., Kapoor, S., Saroja, R., *Effect of the Indian gooseberry (amla) on serum cholesterol levels in men aged 35-55 years.* Eur J Clin Nutr, 1988; 42(11): 939–44

[384] Qureshi, S.A., Asad, W., Sultana, V., *The Effect of Phyllantus emblica Linn on Type - II Diabetes, Triglycerides and Liver - Specific Enzyme.* Pakistan Journal of Nutrition. 2009; 8(2): 125–128

[385] Rosana Chirinos, Jorge Galarza, Indira Betalleluz-Pallardel, Romina Pedreschi and David Campos, *Antioxidant compounds and antioxidant capacity of Peruvian camu camu (Myrciaria dubia (H.B.K.) McVaugh) fruit at different maturity stages.* In Food Chemistry, 2010; 120(4): 1019-1024

[386] In-depth nutrition information on raw blueberries Nutritiondata.com

[387] Russell, W.R., Labat, A., Scobbie, L., Duncan, S.H., *Availability of blueberry phenolics for microbial metabolism in the colon and the potential inflammatory implications.* Mol Nutr Food Res. 2007; 51(6): 726–31

[388] Seeram, N.P., Adams, L.S., Zhang, Y., et al., *Blackberry, black raspberry, blueberry, cranberry, red raspberry, and strawberry extracts inhibit growth and stimulate apoptosis of human cancer cells in vitro.* J Agric Food Chem. 2006; 54 (25): 9329–39

[389] Neto, C.C., *Cranberry and blueberry: evidence for protective effects against cancer and vascular disease.* Mol Nutr Food Res. 2007; 51 (6): 652–64

[390] Seeram, N.P., Adams, L.S., Zhang, Y., et al. (December 2006), *Blackberry, black raspberry, blueberry, cranberry, red raspberry, and strawberry extracts inhibit growth and stimulate apoptosis of human cancer cells in vitro.* J Agric Food Chem. 2006; 54 (25): 9329–39

[391] Yi, W., Fischer, J., Krewer, G., Akoh, C.C., *Phenolic compounds from blueberries can inhibit colon cancer cell proliferation and induce apoptosis.* J Agric Food Chem. 2005; 53(18): 7320–9

[392] Schmidt, B.M., Erdman, J.W., Lila, M.A., *Differential effects of blueberry proanthocyanidins on androgen sensitive and insensitive human prostate cancer cell lines.* Cancer Lett. 2006; 231(2): 240–6

[393] http://whfoods.org/genpage.php?tname=nutrientprofile&dbid=23

[394] Cerdá, B., Tomás-Barberán, F.A., Espín, J.C., *Metabolism of antioxidant and chemopreventive ellagitannins from strawberries, raspberries, walnuts, and oak-aged wine in humans: identification of biomarkers and individual variability.* J Agric Food Chem. 2005; 53(2): 227-35

[395] Gary D. Stoner, Hasan Mukhtar, *Polyphenols as cancer preventive agents.* J. Cell Biochem. 2004, 59 (S22): 169-180

[396] Bhagavathi A. Narayanana, Otto Geoffroya, Mark C. Willingham, Gian G. Reb, Daniel W. Nixona, *p53/p21(WAF1/CIP1) expression and its possible role in G1 arrest and apoptosis in ellagic acid treated cancer cells.* Cancer Letters, 1999; 136 (2): 215-221

[397] Duthie, S.J., Jenkinson, A.M., Crozier, A., et al., *The effects of cranberry juice consumption on antioxidant status and biomarkers relating to heart disease and cancer in healthy human volunteers.* Eur J Nutr 2006; 45 (2): 113–22

[398] Seeram, N.P., Adams, L.S., Zhang, Y., et al., *Blackberry, black raspberry, blueberry, cranberry, red raspberry, and strawberry extracts inhibit growth and stimulate apoptosis of human cancer cells in vitro.* J Agric Food Chem 2006; 54(25): 9329–39

[399] Ferguson, P.J., Kurowska, E.M., Freeman, D.J., Chambers, A.F., Koropatnick, J., *In vivo inhibition of growth of human tumor lines by flavonoid fractions from cranberry extract.* Nutr Cancer, 2006; 56 (1): 86–94

[400] Lou, H.C., *Correction of increased plasma pyruvate and lactate levels using large doses of thiamine in patients with Kearns-Sayre Syndrome.* Arch Neurol, 1981, 38, 469

[401] Arts, W., Scholte, H., Bogaard, J. et al., *NADH-CoQ reductase deficient myopathy: Successful treatment with riboflavin.* Lancet, 1983, 2: 581-82

[402] Driver, C. and Georgiou, A., *How to re-energize old mitochondria without shooting yourself in the foot.* Biogerontology, 2002, 3: 103-106

[403] Martin, D., Towey, M., Horrobin, D. and Lynch, M., *A diet enriched in alpha lipoic acid reverses the age-related compromise in antioxidant defenses in rat cortical tissue.* Nutr Neurosci, 2000, 3: 3, 193-206

[404] Cohen, B. and Gold, D., *Mitochondrial cytopathy in adults: What we know so far.* Cleveland Clinic J Medicine, 2001, 68(7): 625-642

[405] James South, *Idebenone: The Ultimate Anti-Aging Supplement?* Vitamin Research News, April 2001

[406] Opalka, J., Gellerich, F., Zierz, S., *Age and sex dependency of carnitine concentrations in human serum and skeletal muscle.* Clinical Chemistry, 2001,47: 12, 2150-2153

[407] Chakraborti, S., Batabyal, S., Ghosh, S., Chakraborti, T., *Protective role of N-acetylcysteine against the age-related decline in oxidative phosphorylation in pulmonary smooth muscle mitochondria.* Med Sci Res, 1999, 27: (1), 39-40

[408] Cossarizza, A., Franceschi, C., Monti, D., et al., *Protective effect of N-Acetylcysteine in tumor necrosis factor-alpha-induced apoptiosis in U937 cells: The role of mitochondria.* Experimental Cell Research, 1995, 220: 232-240

[409] Sugrue, M. and Tatton, W., *Mitochondrial membrane potential in aging cells.* Biol Signals Recept, 2001, 10(3-4): 176-188

[410] Mittendorfer, B. and Klein, S., *Effect of aging on glucose and lipid metabolism during endurance exercise.* Int J Sport Nutr Ex Metab, 2001, 11 (Suppl), S86-S91

[411] Lu, J., Chen, C., Xu, H. et al., *Effects of prolonged physical training on antioxidation in aged mice myocardial mitochondria.* Tianjin Tiyu Xueyuan Xuebao, 1999, 14 (2), 23-25

INDEX

Page number in **bold** refer to chapter or section headings.

M

S

salt	257
sauerkraut	178, 281
screening	54
selenium	181, 262
serine	172
serotonin	121
side effects	56
slippery elm powder	268
Slow Oxidiser	247
small intestine	73
SNS (sympathetic nervous system)	113, 125
sodium bicarbonate	294
soul or astral field	188, 190
spices	259
spirit	188, 191
spirulina	266
starches	73, 74
stearic acid	172
Steiner, Rudolph	187
stem cells	45, 102, 134, 135, 142, 143, 151, 153, 196
steroids	81
stool	72
stool analysis	274
stress	51, 63, 115, 121, **124**, 125, 127, 152, 272, 275
strokes	102
succinic acid	83
succinyl CoA	83
sucrose (sugar)	73, 74, 87, 93
sugars	72
sulphur-rich amino acids	173
sunflower oil	264
superoxide dismutase	105
superoxide radicals	105
surgery	42, 56, 120, 127, 148, **206**
sweets	74
Sympathetic Dominant	247

T

U

Z